Forgiveness

Forgiveness

Theory, Research, and Practice

Edited by

Michael E. McCullough
Kenneth I. Pargament
Carl E. Thoresen

THE GUILFORD PRESS
New York London

© 2000 The Guilford Press
A Division of Guilford Publications, Inc.
72 Spring Street, New York, NY 10012
www.guilford.com

Printed in the United States of America

This book is printed on acid-free paper.

Last digit is print number: 9 8 7 6 5 4 3 2 1

Library of Congress Cataloging-in-Publication Data

Forgiveness : theory, research, and practice / edited by Michael
E. McCullough, Kenneth I. Pargament, Carl E. Thoresen.
    p.   cm.
  Includes bibliographical references and index.
  ISBN 1-57230-510-X
  1. Forgiveness. I. McCullough, Michael E. II. Pargament,
Kenneth I. (Kenneth Ira), 1950–   III. Thoresen, Carl E.

BF637.F67 F67 1999
155.9′2–dc21

                      99-047188
                         CIP

To Billie, with a heart full of love
—M. E. M.

*To my wife, Aileen, and two sons, Jonathan and Benjamin,
with gratitude for their gifts of love.*
—K. I. P.

*To Kay Armstrong Thoresen, who for over 40 years has,
fortunately for me, proved to be highly skilled
in the art and science of forgiveness.
Also to Eknath Easwaran, whose profound wisdom
has exemplified how love, compassion, and forgiveness
together yield life's most longed for destination.*
—C. E. T.

About the Editors

Michael E. McCullough, PhD, is Director of Research at the National Institute for Healthcare Research in Rockville, Maryland. Dr. McCullough investigates forgiveness, the association of religion and spirituality with physical and mental health, and the influence of religion and spirituality on counseling, psychotherapy, and care at the end of life. He is senior author of *To Forgive Is Human* (InterVarsity Press), with Steven J. Sandage and Everett L. Worthington, Jr., and coauthor of *Religion and Health: A Century of Research Reviewed* (Oxford University Press), with Harold G. Koenig and David B. Larson. Dr. McCullough is also the moderator of *ForgivenessResearch*, an e-mail discussion group for a network of researchers who are involved in research on forgiveness. His current work is funded by the John Templeton Foundation, the Nathan Cummings Foundation, and the Fetzer Institute.

Kenneth I. Pargament, PhD, is Professor of Psychology at Bowling Green State University and Director of Clinical Training of the clinical psychology PhD program. He has published extensively in the psychology of religion, stress, and coping, and is the author of *The Psychology of Religion and Coping: Theory, Research, Practice* (The Guilford Press). A fellow of the American Psychological Association and the American Psychological Society, he is past president of Division 36 (Psychology of Religion) of the American Psychological Association and received its William James Award for excellence in research in the psychology of religion. Dr. Pargament also conducts workshops for clergy and mental health professionals and psychotherapy with clergy and congregation members, and consults with churches and synagogues.

Carl E. Thoresen, PhD, is Professor of Education, Psychology, and Psychiatry/Behavioral Sciences at Stanford University. His research interests involve assessment and management of the Type A behavior pattern, greater methodological diversity in behavioral health/medicine research, and the role of spiritual and religious factors in health, broadly defined. Currently he is studying, in a large clinical trial of coronary patients, what effects, if any, spirituality has on morbidity and mortality. He is also examining the effects of forgiveness training with adults as well as adult volunteering ("selfless service") on health and well-being. He is the author of 7 books and over 150 articles and book chapters, including a forthcoming chapter on spirituality and health in the American Psychological Association's *Handbook of Health Psychology*. He recently edited a special issue of the *Journal of Health Psychology* on spirituality and health.

Contributors

M. Amir Ali, PhD, Institute of Islamic Information and Education, Chicago, Illinois

Donald H. Baucom, PhD, Psychology Department, University of North Carolina at Chapel Hill, Chapel Hill, North Carolina

Roy F. Baumeister, PhD, Department of Psychology, Case Western Reserve University, Cleveland, Ohio

Guy L. Beck, PhD, Department of Religious Studies, College of Charleston, Charleston, South Carolina

Jack W. Berry, PhD, Virginia Commonwealth University, Richmond, Virginia

Prabha S. Chandra, MD, Department of Psychiatry, National Institute of Mental Health and Neurosciences, Bangalore, India

Eugene G. d'Aquili, MD, PhD (deceased), Department of Psychiatry, Hospital of the University of Pennsylvania, Philadelphia, Pennsylvania

Verushka deMarici, PhD, Department of Psychiatry, Hospital of the University of Pennsylvania, Philadelphia, Pennsylvania

Elliot N. Dorff, PhD, Department of Philosophy, University of Judaism, Bel Air, California

Robert A. Emmons, PhD, Department of Psychology, University of California–Davis, Davis, California

Julie Juola Exline, PhD, Department of Psychology, Case Western Reserve University, Cleveland, Ohio

Michèle Girard, PhD, Laboratoire Cognition et Décision de l'École Pratique des Hautes Études, Université François-Rabelais, Tours, France

Kristina Coop Gordon, PhD, Psychology Department, University of Tennessee, Knoxville, Tennessee

Leslie S. Greenberg, PhD, Department of Psychology, York University, Toronto, Ontario, Canada

Charles Hallisey, PhD, Department of Sanskrit and Indian Studies, Harvard University, Cambridge, Massachusetts

Alex H. S. Harris, doctoral candidate, School of Education, Stanford University, Stanford, California

William T. Hoyt, PhD, Department of Counseling Psychology, University of Wisconsin–Madison, Madison, Wisconsin

Frederic Luskin, PhD, Stanford Center for Research on Disease Prevention, School of Medicine, Stanford University, Stanford, California

Wanda M. Malcolm, PhD, NW GTA Hospital Corporation, Brampton Memorial Campus, Brampton, Ontario, Canada; Tyndale College and Seminary, Toronto, Ontario, Canada

Michael E. McCullough, PhD, National Institute of Healthcare Research, Rockville, Maryland

Étienne Mullet, PhD, Laboratoire Cognition et Décision de l'École Pratique des Hautes Études, Université François-Rabelais, Tours, France

Vasudha Narayanan, PhD, Department of Religion, University of Florida, Gainesville, Florida

Andrew B. Newberg, MD, Division of Nuclear Medicine and Department of Psychiatry, Hospital of the University of Pennsylvania, Philadelphia, Pennsylvania

Stephanie K. Newberg, MEd, MSW, private practice, Philadelphia, Pennsylvania

Kenneth I. Pargament, PhD, Department of Psychology, Bowling Green State University, Bowling Green, Ohio

John Patton, PhD, Columbia Theological Seminary, Decatur, Georgia

K. Chris Rachal, MA, Department of Counseling Psychology and Guidance Services, Ball State University, Muncie, Indiana

Mark S. Rye, PhD, Department of Psychology, University of Dayton, Dayton, Ohio

Steven J. Sandage, PhD, Bethel Theological Seminary, St. Paul, Minnesota

Douglas K. Snyder, PhD, Department of Psychology, Texas A & M University, College Station, Texas

Lydia R. Temoshok, PhD, Department of Psychiatry, University of Maryland School of Medicine, Baltimore, Maryland; Behavioral Medicine Program, Institute of Human Virology, Division of Clinical Research, Baltimore, Maryland

Carl E. Thoresen, PhD, School of Education, Stanford University, Stanford, California

James G. Williams, PhD, Department of Religious Studies, Syracuse University, Syracuse, New York

Everett L. Worthington, Jr., PhD, Department of Psychology, Virginia Commonwealth University, Richmond, Virginia

Preface

We bid farewell to the most consequential century in human history. With the ability to harness nuclear power, paired with our appetites for petroleum-based fuels, and the grim, inescapable fact that the world's supplies of food and fresh water are simply unable to keep up with the current population growth, humans have now become a bona fide force of nature, capable of altering (permanently) the complexion and even vital status of the planet. If we do not develop ways to control our passions and the fruits of our ingenuity, we may succeed in writing ourselves out of history.

We also bid farewell to the bloodiest century in human history. More human beings died in ethnic conflicts, civil strife, dictatorial power grabs, and world wars during the 20th century than in all other centuries combined. Anyone who approaches the subject matter of this book with skepticism can surely be forgiven; we are, after all, living in the aftermath of the most unforgiving of centuries.

Even so, the 21st century still remains very much a blank slate, ours to make of it what we will. If humanity can make use of scientific ingenuity (and force of will) to curtail its reliance on dirty fuels, slow population growth, and reduce the size of its ecological footprint, perhaps there is hope for a sustainable future both for humankind and for the planet. Similarly, if we can make use of scientific advances (and force of will) to reduce ethnic strife, political violence, and world conflict, perhaps the 21st century will find its way out of the 20th century's crimson shadow.

In achieving these latter goals, perhaps forgiveness will play a role.

This volume, as its name suggests, explores the possibilities for creating a scientific understanding of forgiveness, its precursors, its consequences, and its potential applications for reducing human misery. We believe that scientific research, conducted with rigor and skepticism, might play a role in improving our understanding of how forgiveness operates in persons of all ages, from the youngest of children to the oldest of the old; in dyads, marriages, families, communities, and nations.

We are also cautiously optimistic that this scientific understanding might be used to improve the lot of humanity. For example, perhaps educational institutions for the young could successfully teach the skills of forgiveness as one way to reduce conflict and hostility, as well as to promote understanding and respect. Perhaps older adults could be helped to experience forgiveness as one way to diminish unresolved hurt and pain that burdens many in the last years of life. Successful approaches would surely benefit from the kind of scientific advances this volume advocates.

*   *   *

The idea for this book arose from discussions with Seymour Weingarten and Rochelle Serwator at The Guilford Press, who had been in dialogue with the first editor (M. E. M.) since 1995 regarding the possibilities for a work on the topic. In 1996 and 1997, the first editor solicited the collaboration of the other editors (K. I. P. and C. E. T.), who were also interested in forgiveness from their own academic perspectives.

The first thing to decide was what an edited volume on the social science of forgiveness should address. From our initial discussions, we concluded that a sustainable future for the scientific study of forgiveness would require active dialogue with other vibrant areas of basic and applied psychology. Thus, we began to identify researchers and scholars who, by virtue of their immersion in their own specialties and their own interests in forgiveness, could explore the interface of forgiveness research with the subject matter, goals, and methods of their own disciplines. Stated simply, we asked the contributors of this volume to help readers become acquainted with the existing theory, research, and practice on forgiveness, and then to help them set their sights on the frontiers of forgiveness. If the volume succeeds in this single goal, then the time and effort that have gone into preparing it have been well spent.

The perceptive reader of the present volume will be struck by its almost exclusively psychological perspective. In part, the focus on psychological understandings of forgiveness reflects the academic backgrounds of the editors and contributors, but it also accurately reflects the fact that scientific scholarship on forgiveness has, to date, been dominated by psychological inquiries. We hope other scientific disciplines will join the dialogue with louder voices in years to come.

During the editing of this book, we have become indebted to many. We must thank especially our home institutions—the National Institute for Healthcare Research, Bowling Green State University, and Stanford University. Norman Anderson, Warren Brown, Betty Gridley, Ed Haertel, Bill Hoyt, David Kenny, Joshua Smyth, and several other colleagues provided helpful feedback on portions of the book. We extend thanks to them. In addition, we owe a debt of gratitude to the John Templeton Foundation, which, through various forms of assistance, has helped us to bring this volume to light. We also thank Seymour Weingarten, Rochelle Serwator, and Carolyn Graham at The Guilford Press for encouragement and assistance throughout every stage of preparing this volume.

Finally, we are sincerely grateful to our authors, who contributed time, energy, and thought to making this collection a reality. We thank you.

MICHAEL E. MCCULLOUGH
KENNETH I. PARGAMENT
CARL E. THORESEN

Contents

III. APPLICATIONS IN COUNSELING, PSYCHOTHERAPY, AND HEALTH

IV. CONCLUSION

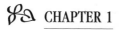

CHAPTER 1

The Psychology of Forgiveness

History, Conceptual Issues, and Overview

Michael E. McCullough, Kenneth I. Pargament, and Carl E. Thoresen

We are awash in public apologies and expressions of forgiveness. In the news magazines, we read stories of men's organizations that have offered apologies to "Women" on behalf of "Men" for failing to live up to their responsibilities as husbands and fathers. In the newspaper, we read that a community in Kentucky offers forgiveness to a young man who has shot and killed several of his classmates. The host of a daytime television show gives contestants the opportunity to offer public apologies to relationship partners whom they have betrayed or offended in some way, and urges the recipients of these apologies to forgive. And of course, we know from all media that President Clinton has apologized to his family, Monica Lewinsky, and the entire nation for his lack of honesty in the aftermath of being caught in an extramarital affair. Clearly, apologies and expressions of forgiveness are in vogue. Right or wrong, genuine or contrived, they seem to have an irresistible human interest and political cache.

Does the current deluge of apologies and expressions of forgiveness indicate that the citizens of the world really are becoming more forgiving? Are women (and men) becoming any more adept at forgiving their fathers and husbands (or mothers and wives)? Are historically disadvantaged racial groups learning to forgive groups that have historically oppressed them? Are people any more adept today at forgiving their close relationship partners? Are we more willing to forgive an apologetic and apparently contrite President, despite character defects?

These issues raise other questions in the minds of laypersons: Are our own, private transactions of apology and forgiveness taking us anywhere? Are relationships being restored? Are racial groups learning to trust one another more effectively? Is violence being reduced? Are families happier? Are marriages more stable? Are people coping with their lives better? In short, does forgiveness deliver what it promises? People apologize—both publicly and privately—because apologies are supposed to *do* something. People hope that these expressions of forgiveness are effective in making the world (or at least the part of the world in which each of us lives) a slightly better place to be.

Social scientists are asking the same questions in slightly more subtle ways: What psychological factors are involved in forgiveness? What are its personality and biological substrates? How does the capacity to forgive develop across the life span? Is it largely guided by individual factors, situational factors, or the interaction of personality and situation? Does forgiveness have consequences that are relevant for mental health, physical health, and social relationships? Can forgiveness be effectively encouraged in counseling and psychotherapy? If so, to what ends? Is forgiveness an unmitigated psychological and social good, or does it involves costs to the forgiver, the person forgiven, or society?

Scientific research on forgiveness has never been more relevant. Perhaps this is why many psychologists have had an increased scientific interest in the concept of forgiveness during the last decade. The scientific foundation that has begun to be poured in recent years could lead to wonderful scientific advancements in the years to come, helping us to understand more about the basic nature of forgiveness, how it develops, and its consequences for human health, well-being, and relationships. This volume is designed to review these developing foundations and help the forgiveness researchers of the present and future to steer a scientifically productive course.

In this introductory chapter, we take on three tasks. First, we present a brief history of scientific inquiry into the psychology of forgiveness. Second, we briefly discuss the definitional status of the forgiveness construct, and offer a metadefinition that is intended to highlight the commonalities among the various approaches that researchers are using to define and operationalize forgiveness. Third, we comment on the major threats to the development of a self-sustaining psychology of forgiveness and introduce the collection of chapters that appear in the remainder of this volume.

THE PSYCHOLOGY OF FORGIVENESS: A BRIEF HISTORY

The concept of forgiveness received no systematic attention from scientific psychologists for most of the discipline's short history. Given Freud's prolific scholarly output and his ability to shed light on nearly everything psychological, it is altogether striking that he wrote nothing about forgiveness. The same could be said of innovators such as William James, G. Stanley Hall, E. L. Thorndike, Lewis Terman, and Gordon Allport. Nothing seemed entirely off limits to these innovators, so why nothing about forgiveness? In the fields of mental health, we also find little attention to the phenomenon of human forgiveness from leaders such as Carl Jung, Karen Horney, Alfred Adler, or Viktor Frankl. On one hand, we might simply conclude that these scholars had other projects to attend to and thus were not able to focus attention on many important human phenomena (including forgiveness).

On the other hand, substantive reasons might exist for the relative neglect of forgiveness in the early decades of scientific psychology. One might point to the fact that forgiveness seems to have been neglected throughout all of academia, not just the social sciences (Enright & North, 1998). One might also point to traditional links between forgiveness and religious belief, and to the social sciences' aversion to religious matters (e.g., Gorsuch, 1988). One might point to the difficulties that might be associated with gathering reliable data about forgiveness, particularly during the era when scientific psychology insisted on the analysis of observable behaviors. Finally, one might point to the fact that the 20th century has been the bloodiest and probably the most unforgiving century in human history, perhaps leading people to conclude that forgiveness constituted little more than a nice sentiment. All of these factors might have played a role in discouraging systematic inquiry into the psychology of forgiveness. In any case, the concept of forgiveness would have to wait many decades for sustained, systematic attention.

It would be pointless to dwell on the neglect of forgiveness by the major leaders and innovators in psychology, but it would be naïve to assume that the social scientists who have been investigating forgiveness during the last 15 years invented the concept *ex nihilo*. There is a history of forgiveness in the psychological sciences, albeit a short and skimpy one. The history of forgiveness in psychology and the social sciences can be divided into two periods. The first of these periods, roughly spanning the five decades between 1932 and 1980, consisted of many theoretical papers and modest empirical work designed to shed light on aspects of forgiveness. A second period, roughly spanning the two decades from 1980 to the present, reflects more intensive and serious consideration of the concept of forgiveness.

Early Forgiveness Inquiries: 1932–1980

As far back as the 1930s, psychologists and mental health professionals in the United States and Europe did from time to time discuss the human phenomenon of forgiveness. For example, Piaget (1932) and Behn (1932) all discussed how the capacity to forgive grew out of the development of moral judgment. Litwinski (1945) also made an early attempt to describe the affective structure of the capacity for interpersonal forgiving.

Forgiveness in Pastoral Care

Also, pastoral counselors and mental health experts with religious interests made early attempts to articulate the role that forgiveness might play in helping people to achieve mental health (e.g., Beaven, 1951; Bonell, 1950; Johnson, 1947; Rusk, 1950). Andras Angyal (1952) was one of the champions of the view that helping psychotherapy clients to experience forgiveness from God was an important antidote to the pathological guilt that was thought to underlie much psychopathology. Effective psychotherapy would, in Angyal's view, create an environment in which clients experience opportunities (1) to feel forgiven for their ethical or moral failures and (2) to forgive others.

Other scholars from the field of pastoral care also addressed the potential salutary benefits of forgiveness. One of the most noteworthy is Emerson (1964). In his largely theoretical book, Emerson also reported the results of a study using a Q-sort method that was designed to examine the associations between forgiveness and psychological well-being. Despite its lack of sophistication and a failure to use modern inferential statistics, this study was probably the first scientific inquiry into the association of forgiveness with mental health and well-being.

Forgiveness in Heider

In a chapter on benefit and harm in *The Psychology of Interpersonal Relations*, Heider (1958) outlined a variety of attributional principles that underlie the quest for revenge after one has incurred an interpersonal transgression. In this context, Heider described forgiveness as foregoing vengeful behavior, which he posited to be an implicit expression of the victim's self-worth or an attempt to be faithful to an ethical standard. However, Heider did not elaborate on these concepts very much, and the concept of forgiveness received no explicit theoretical attention. Although Heider's work was absolutely seminal to the field of social psychology, the short shrift given to forgiveness was clearly not sufficient to stimulate scientific imagination.

Forgiveness and Human Values

One of the more systematic forays into the psychology of forgiveness arose out of the work of Milton Rokeach, whose investigations into the nature of human values (e.g., Rokeach, 1973) were guided by several versions of the Rokeach Value Survey (e.g., Rokeach, 1967). The Rokeach Value Survey consists of two sets of human values. The "instrumental" set refers to preferred modes of conduct. The "terminal" set refers to preferred end states for life. Participants complete the form by ranking each of the 18 values within the instrumental values and the terminal values. The value of being "forgiving" is one of the 18 instrumental values. Given the huge number of studies that have employed Rokeach's tools for studying human values, it is surprising that more is not made of this work in modern discussions of forgiveness, since it probably reveals much about (1) differences in how various groups of people value forgiveness, and (2) how the value of being forgiving fits into wider systems of human values.

Forgiveness and the Prisoner's Dilemma

Forgiveness was made the topic of a limited amount of theoretical and empirical attention through the work of Tedeschi and others (e.g., Gahagan & Tedeschi, 1968; Horai, Lindskold, Gahagan, & Tedeschi, 1969) who conceptualized forgiveness as a cooperative response following a competitive response in the Prisoner's Dilemma Game. In this mixed-motives game, two players are repeatedly faced with the dilemma of choosing either a competitive or a cooperative strategy. The object is to win as many points as possible. If both partners cooperate, they might each win, for example, 3 points. If one defects while the other cooperates, the defector might win 5 points while the cooperator receives 0 points. If both defect, then each might win 1 point. Thus, there are certain advantages to cooperating (depending on one's partner's willingness to cooperate) and to competing (depending on one's partner's disposition to compete). When a partner cooperates even after the opponent has made a competitive move, this has been called a "forgiving" response, and it has been shown to lead to beneficial outcomes in certain game-playing environments (e.g., Axelrod, 1980a, 1980b). Despite this innovative approach to conceptualizing forgiveness (and the number of studies that have used variants of the Prisoner's Dilemma Game protocol), it has not yet been used to produce fundamental insights about the nature of forgiveness.

Clearly, the professional literature through 1980 reveals that thinking about forgiveness is not something that just "happened" in the final decades of the 20th century. Many scholars have considered forgiveness over the years, and it would be a mistake not to examine their work closely. Nevertheless, the attention paid to forgiveness in the years 1932–

1980 was piecemeal. Researchers did not begin to devote serious, sustained energy to the concept of forgiveness until the last 20 years of the 20th century.

Increased Interest in the Psychology of Forgiveness: 1980–Present

By the 1980s, the number of papers and book-length treatments of forgiveness began to increase substantially. By the end of 1998, in developmental psychology, counseling/clinical psychology, and social psychology, important papers had appeared that dealt explicitly with the phenomenon of forgiveness. The appearance of these theoretical and empirical treatments seemed to suggest that forgiveness was a concept whose popularity was on the rise.

Forgiveness and Moral Development

Enright, Santos, and Al-Mabuk (1989) linked the development of reasoning about forgiveness explicitly to Kohlberg's theorizing about the development of reasoning about justice. Enright and his colleagues adduced data to demonstrate that the capacity to reason in a complex way about forgiveness was associated with more complex reasoning about justice, and also found evidence that reasoning about forgiveness became more complex with age. Enright and his colleagues (e.g., Enright & the Human Development Study Group, 1994), and other developmentalists such as Girard and Mullet (1997) and Spidell and Liberman (1981) have examined theoretically and empirically how the capacity to forgive (and the inclination to seek forgiveness) unfolds across the life span.

Forgiveness in Counseling and Clinical Psychology

One difference between the theoretical and conceptual treatments of forgiveness that appeared in the 1980s and those from earlier years was the heavy speculative focus on the potential links of forgiveness to mental health and mental health treatment in this second historical period. Indeed, most conceptual papers that discussed forgiveness during the 1980s were written by clinicians and/or published in journals typically read by clinicians (McCullough & Worthington, 1994). Influential papers by Fitzgibbons (1986), Hope (1987), and Jampolsky (1980), and trade books by Smedes (1984), and Linn and Linn (1978) pointed to the potentially salutary effects of forgiveness on mental health. Also, research by DiBlasio (1993; DiBlasio & Proctor, 1993) highlighted that many practitioners were open to the use of forgiveness in clinical settings.

By the mid-1990s, bona fide empirical research on the uses of strategies for encouraging forgiveness in counseling and psychotherapy began to appear in scientific journals (e.g., Hebl & Enright, 1993; McCullough & Worthington, 1995). Papers in the leading journal in clinical psychology (e.g., Coyle & Enright, 1997; Freedman & Enright, 1996) demonstrated the potential relevance of forgiveness to clinical work with a variety of populations.

Forgiveness in Personality and Social Psychology

In the 1980s and 1990s, a variety of researchers explored the social-psychological principles underlying forgiveness. Most notable among these were papers by Boon and Sulsky (1997), Darby and Schlenker (1982), and Weiner, Graham, Peter, and Zmuidinas (1991). These studies found that people's willingness to forgive an offender can be explained by variables of a social-cognitive nature, such as the offender's perceived responsibility, intentionality, and motives (Darby & Schlenker, 1982), and the severity of the offense (Boon & Sulsky, 1997). New theory and research designed to integrate multiple theoretical perspectives on forgiveness also began to appear in personality and social psychology journals during these latter years (e.g., McCullough & Worthington, 1999; McCullough, Worthington, & Rachal, 1997; McCullough et al., 1998).

The most consequential event for the scientific study of forgiveness to date might have been a request by the John Templeton Foundation for proposals for scientific research on forgiveness. Following a 1-day research workshop (the proceedings of which are published in Worthington, 1998b), over 100 research teams submitted proposals as part of the Foundation's initiative to fund innovative scientific research on forgiveness. Ultimately, nearly 30 research laboratories were granted funding to conduct 3-year research programs on forgiveness. Still others may receive funding in the future as a part of this effort. It is too early to assess what this financial backing will ultimately accomplish for the field of forgiveness, but it seems clear that, as a result, psychology will possess much more scientific information about forgiveness in the next decade than it currently possesses.

THE DEFINITION PROBLEM

Clearly, scientific research on forgiveness is on the rise. However, at the time of this writing, individual researchers' conceptualizations of forgiveness are quite diverse. In particular, no consensual definition of forgiveness exists (Worthington, 1998a). Indeed, some interpret the lack of consensus in definition to be one of the most pernicious problems in the field today (Elder, 1998; Enright & Coyle, 1998; Enright, Freedman, &

Rique, 1998; Enright, Gassin, & Wu, 1992). It appears that most theorists and researchers now agree with Enright and Coyle (1998) that forgiveness should be differentiated from "pardoning" (which is a legal term), "condoning" (which implies a justification of the offense), "excusing" (which implies that the offender had a good reason for committing the offense), "forgetting" (which implies that the memory of the offense has simply decayed or slipped out of conscious awareness), and "denying" (which implies simply an unwillingness to perceive the harmful injuries that one has incurred). Most also seem to agree that forgiveness is distinct from "reconciliation" (which implies the restoration of a relationship). The fact that no scholars have offered serious disputations of these distinctions in recent years suggests that real conceptual progress has been made in understanding forgiveness.

Remaining Definitional Differences

However, other definitional issues remain. Agreeing on what forgiveness is *not* does not necessarily mean that researchers agree on what forgiveness *is*. For example, Enright and his colleagues (e.g., Enright & Coyle, 1998; Enright et al., 1998) define forgiveness as "a willingness to abandon one's right to resentment, negative judgment, and indifferent behavior toward one who unjustly hurt us, while fostering the undeserved qualities of compassion, generosity, and even love toward him or her" (Enright et al., 1998, pp. 46–47). McCullough and colleagues (McCullough et al., 1997, 1998) define the essence of forgiveness as prosocial changes in one's motivations toward an offending relationship partner (although these motivational changes would most likely result in many of the cognitive and behavioral changes that Enright and colleagues conceptualize as part of forgiveness *per se*). Working from the perspective of marital and family therapy, Hargrave and Sells (1997) define forgiveness as (1) allowing one's victimizer to rebuild trust in the relationship through acting in a trustworthy fashion, and (2) promoting an open discussion of the relational violation, so that the offended partner and the offender can agree to work toward an improved relationship.

Still other researchers and theorists offer other definitions. The many definitions of forgiveness that have been proposed share some similarities but are different in some substantial ways. For example, some researchers who have offered definitions of forgiveness emphasize that it can best be conceptualized as a stage-like unfolding of a sequence of events over time. Others remain agnostic on issues of whether forgiveness has, by definition, a stage-like or developmental character. Similarly, some have emphasized that effort and intentionality are intrinsic elements of an adequate definition (i.e., forgiveness requires conscious effort) even though others are agnostic regarding the essentiality of awareness or volition to forgiveness.

In spite of the many differences among the definitions of forgiveness that various researchers are currently using, a consensual definition might be more feasible than one might initially imagine. All of the existing definitions seem to be built on one core feature: When people forgive, their responses toward (or, in other words, what they think of, feel about, want to do to, or actually do to) people who have offended or injured them become more positive and less negative. Although a specific interpersonal offense (or series of offenses) caused by a specific person (or groups of persons) once elicited negative thoughts, feelings, motivations, or behaviors directed toward the offender, those responses have become more prosocial over time. Therefore, we propose to define forgiveness as *intraindividual, prosocial change toward a perceived transgressor that is situated within a specific interpersonal context.*

When someone forgives a person who has committed a transgression against him or her, it is the forgiver (specifically, in his or her thoughts, feelings, motivations, or behaviors) who changes. In this sense, forgiveness is a *psychological* construct. However, forgiveness has a dual character; it is interpersonal as well as intrapersonal. Forgiveness occurs in response to an interpersonal violation, and the individual who forgives necessarily forgives in relation to someone else. Thus, even while being a psychological phenomenon, forgiveness is interpersonal in the same sense that many other psychological constructs are interpersonal in nature (e.g., trust, prejudice, empathy): Each construct has other people as its point of reference. Although someone might be said to possess trust, prejudice, or empathy, each of these constructs attempts to describe dimensions of persons that are inescapably social in nature. Both the intrapersonal and social aspects of forgiveness are "real"; thus, to intrapersonally and interpersonally conceptualize forgiveness is an eminently reasonable thing to do. Perhaps it is most comprehensive to think of forgiveness as a *psychosocial* construct.

If considered acceptable to the academic community, such a consensual definition of forgiveness would not only enable researchers to be sure that they are discussing the same phenomenon (forgiveness) when using the same language ("forgiveness") but it would also allow other conceptual features that might otherwise be associated definitionally with forgiveness (e.g., stage-like, developmental course; intentionality; primacy of motivational or affective systems; etc.) to be freed from the moorings of definition and transformed instead into researchable hypotheses about the nature of forgiveness. If all researchers can agree that forgiveness is (at the very least) "intraindividual, prosocial change toward a transgressor that is situated within an interpersonal context," then they can proceed to examine empirically whether such change (i.e., forgiveness) is necessarily developmental in nature, whether intentionality is indispensable, and so on, thereby giving these ancillary hypotheses about forgiveness the empirical examinations that they merit. The reader is invited to test this minimalist conceptualization of forgiveness against his or her own definition, and also those definitions provided by contributors to the present volume. Obviously, our goal here is conceptual progress, so we welcome reactions and responses to this proposal.

THE PRESENT VOLUME

Amid the enthusiasm in the concept of forgiveness that appears to be building among many researchers and practitioners in scientific and professional psychology, many problems must be addressed and adequately solved before this initial enthusiasm can be applied to create a solid, coherent base of scientific knowledge regarding forgiveness. Unless these problems are addressed with scientific rigor, the emerging interest in the science and practice of forgiveness is likely to be marginalized from mainstream psychological research and practice.

A first set of problems is largely conceptual and methodological. We have already discussed the definitional problem, but other problems exist as well. For example, the field still lacks a thorough understanding of the influences of religion, culture, and life situation on people's understandings and experiences of forgiveness. Without addressing religious, cultural, and situational variations, scientific notions of forgiveness are likely to be disconnected from lived human experience. Also, initial attempts at developing measures of forgiveness are well under way, but it is not yet clear how forgiveness should be operationalized to maximize scientific progress. A variety of thorny methodological problems exist in operationalizing forgiveness, and these problems must be addressed to create dependable measures of forgiveness constructs.

A second set of problems is largely substantive. Few researchers from mainstream areas of psychological research have offered critical appraisals of the concept of forgiveness and outlined prospects for integrating the concept of forgiveness into our existing knowledge about the basic neurobiological, developmental, social, and personality processes that govern human behavior and mental processes. Moreover, it is not clear what steps should be taken to systematically explore the neurobiological, developmental, social, and personality substrates of forgiveness.

A third set of problems is predominantly related to research on the practical application of forgiveness in counseling, psychotherapy, and prevention. To date, only a few researchers in counseling, psychotherapy, or prevention have explored the possibilities for integrating the concept of forgiveness into the practice of professional psychology and related mental health fields. Additionally, few theorists or researchers have even explored the possibility that forgiveness might, in some instances, lead to clinical harm rather than benefit for the recipients of psychological services. Finally, few researchers have outlined research protocols by which the efficacy of techniques to encourage forgiveness in applied settings might be systematically developed and evaluated.

If these three sets of problems are not addressed as a preparation for creating a "psychology of forgiveness," it is likely that the concept of forgiveness will not be fully integrated into the theory, research, and practice of psychologists. Instead, researchers interested in the concept of forgiveness might find themselves talking only to each other rather than helping to integrate the grammar of forgiveness into mainstream understandings of human psychology and psychological change. Conversely, if such initial field-building steps are taken, the concept of forgiveness could have a rich future in the fields of scientific and professional psychology.

In the present volume, we have drawn together over a dozen chapters that (1) review existing psychological thought and research on forgiveness and (2) outline the conceptual, methodological, and substantive issues that should be addressed to build a strong body of research and practice on forgiveness in the years to come. While the book is optimistic about the possibilities for a psychology of forgiveness, it is also written critically, with a focus on the shortcomings and pitfalls that must be addressed to build a healthy, well-integrated psychology of forgiveness.

Part I of the book tackles conceptual and measurement issues in the psychology of forgiveness. Chapter 2, written by Mark S. Rye, Kenneth I. Pargament, and six religion scholars, compares the views regarding forgiveness embodied in five world religions. This comparative study was designed to illuminate the commonalities and differences in how forgiveness is understood within these great religious traditions. Chapter 3, written by Lydia R. Temoshok and Prabha S. Chandra, examines the contours of forgiveness from within a specific cultural and situational context: that of people living with HIV/AIDS in India. This is a different portrayal of forgiveness than what American theorists and researchers are accustomed to considering, and it is presented here to illustrate exactly how culturally and situationally specific our notions of forgiveness actually can be. Chapter 4, written by Michael E. McCullough, William T. Hoyt, and K. Chris Rachal presents a taxonomy for organizing the possibilities for measuring forgiveness empirically, and then presents a generalizability framework for evaluating the psychometric adequacy of existing measures and those to be developed in the future.

Part II consists of four chapters designed to review and integrate data, and present new theorizing on the psychology of forgiveness from within four domains of basic psychological research. In Chapter 5, Andrew B. Newberg, the late Eugene G. d'Aquili, Stephanie K. Newberg, and Verushka deMarici present new theorizing about the neuroevolutionary basis for the capacity to forgive. In Chapter 6, Étienne Mullet and Michèle Girard review an impressive set of studies examining how the cognitive capacity to forgive develops across the life span, and how people integrate social information in making decisions about whether to forgive an interpersonal transgressor. In Chapter 7, Julie Juola Exline and Roy F. Baumeister discuss how the costs and benefits of forgiveness might be productively and systematically investigated within the field of social psychology. In Chapter 8, Robert A. Emmons presents a framework for how forgiveness might be best studied within the field of personality psychology.

Part III is focused on a critical appraisal of how forgiveness is (and should be) studied and applied in the context of counseling and psychotherapy. In Chapter 9, Wanda M. Malcolm and Leslie S. Greenberg discuss the existing research on the applications of forgiveness to individual psychotherapy, and demonstrate how task analytic methods can be used to determine whether forgiveness itself is a curative factor in forgiveness-based psychotherapies. Chapter 10, by Kristina Coop Gordon, Donald H. Baucom, and Douglas K. Snyder, integrates a variety of approaches to forgiveness in marital therapy and proposes a systematic agenda for studying (and applying) forgiveness-based intervention strategies in that therapeutic context. In Chapter 11, Everett L. Worthington, Jr., Steven J. Sandage, and Jack W. Berry use meta-analytic methods to draw some innovative conclusions about the efficacy of group approaches to encouraging forgiveness. They also present a broad set of guidelines for the application of forgiveness-based strategies in group counseling, psychoeducation, and psychotherapy. In Chapter 12, Carl E. Thoresen, Alex H. S. Harris, and Frederic Luskin describe the need and possibilities for studying forgiveness in the context of health psychology and behavioral medicine—fields interested in basic research and practical interventions for improving physical health. In Chapter 13, John Patton discusses his own therapeutic approach to "using" forgiveness (a phrase that he himself would eschew) in the context of pastoral care and counseling.

Finally, we conclude with a summary of the entire collection. In Chapter 14, we address the major themes that have arisen from the book and what we believe to be the major "frontiers of forgiveness" that should be the priorities for future research and theorizing.

SUMMARY

Like psychology itself, the psychology of forgiveness has a short history. Researchers and theorists have considered this construct many times during psychology's short history, but only recently has forgiveness become a focal topic for scientific research; thus, only in the last few decades has it been possible to write a "history" of forgiveness in scientific psychology. The chapters that constitute the remainder of this volume are presented not to examine the history of forgiveness, but to explore the frontiers of forgiveness. They articulate the cutting edge of theory and research on forgiveness, pointing out the perils and promise of studying and applying forgiveness in theory, research, and practice. The last 20 years were important for the burgeoning psychology of forgiveness, and the next few decades should present interesting, exciting possibilities for scientific discovery. Read on for a tour of the interesting developments to date and for a glimpse of the great things that are still to come.

REFERENCES

Angyal, A. (1952). The convergence of psychotherapy and religion. *Journal of Pastoral Care, 5*(4), 4–14.

Axelrod, R. (1980a). Effective choice in the Prisoner's Dilemma. *Journal of Conflict Resolution, 24,* 3–25.

Axelrod, R. (1980b). More effective choice in the Prisoner's Dilemma. *Journal of Conflict Resolution, 24,* 379–403.

Beaven, R. H. (1951). Christian faith and the psychological study of man. *Journal of Pastoral Care, 5*(Spring), 53–60.

Behn, S. (1932). Concerning forgiveness and excuse. *Archiv fuer die Gesamte Psychologie, 86,* 55–62.

Bonell, J. S. (1950). Healing for mind and body. *Pastoral Psychology, 1,* 30–33.

Boon, S. D., & Sulsky, L. M. (1997). Attributions of blame and forgiveness in romantic relationships: A policy-capturing study. *Journal of Social Behavior and Personality, 12,* 19–44.

Coyle, C. T., & Enright, R. D. (1997). Forgiveness intervention with post-abortion men. *Journal of Consulting and Clinical Psychology, 65,* 1042–1045.

Darby, B. W., & Schlenker, B. R. (1982). Children's reactions to apologies. *Journal of Personality and Social Psychology, 43,* 742–753.

DiBlasio, F. A. (1993). The role of social workers' religious beliefs in helping family members forgive. *Families in Society, 74,* 163–170.

DiBlasio, F. A., & Proctor, J. H. (1993). Therapists and the clinical use of forgiveness. *American Journal of Family Therapy, 21,* 175–184.

Elder, J. W. (1998). Expanding our options: The challenge of forgiveness. In R. D. Enright & J. North (Eds.), *Exploring forgiveness* (pp. 150–161). Madison: University of Wisconsin Press.

Emerson, J. G., Jr. (1964). *The dynamics of forgiveness.* Philadelphia: Westminster Press.

Enright, R. D., & Coyle, C. T. (1998). Researching the process model of forgiveness within psychological interventions. In E. L. Worthington (Ed.), *Dimensions of forgiveness* (pp. 139–161). Radnor, PA: Templeton Foundation Press.

Enright, R. D., Freedman, S., & Rique, J. (1998). The psychology of interpersonal forgiveness. In R. D. Enright & J. North (Eds.), *Exploring forgiveness* (pp. 46–62). Madison: University of Wisconsin Press.

Enright, R. D., Gassin, E. A., & Wu, C. (1992). Forgiveness: A developmental view. *Journal of Moral Education, 21,* 99–114.

Enright, R. D., & Human Development Study Group. (1994). Piaget on the moral development of forgiveness: Identity or reciprocity? *Human Development, 37,* 63–80.

Enright, R. D., & North, J. (1998). Introducing forgiveness. In R. D. Enright & J. North (Eds.), *Exploring forgiveness* (pp. 3–8). Madison: University of Wisconsin Press.

Enright, R. D., Santos, M. J. D., & Al-Mabuk, R. (1989). The adolescent as forgiver. *Journal of Adolescence, 12,* 99–110.

Fitzgibbons, R. P. (1986). The cognitive and emotive uses of forgiveness in the treatment of anger. *Psychotherapy, 23,* 629–633.

Freedman, S., & Enright, R. D. (1996). Forgiveness as an intervention goal with incest survivors. *Journal of Consulting and Clinical Psychology, 64,* 983–992.

Gahagan, J. P., & Tedeschi, J. T. (1968). Strategy and the credibility of promises in the Prisoner's Dilemma game. *Journal of Conflict Resolution, 12,* 224–234.

Girard, M., & Mullet, É. (1997). Propensity to forgive in adolescents, young adults, older adults, and elderly people. *Journal of Adult Development, 4,* 209–220.

Gorsuch, R. L. (1988). Psychology of religion. *Annual Review of Psychology, 39,* 201–221.

Hargrave, T. D., & Sells, J. N. (1997). The development of a forgiveness scale. *Journal of Marital and Family Therapy, 23,* 41–62.

Hebl, J. H., & Enright, R. D. (1993). Forgiveness as a psychotherapeutic intervention with elderly females. *Psychotherapy, 30,* 658–667.

Heider, F. (1958). *The psychology of interpersonal relations.* New York: Wiley.

Hope, D. (1987). The healing paradox of forgiveness. *Psychotherapy, 24,* 240–244.

Horai, J., Lindskold, S., Gahagan, J., & Tedeschi, J. (1969). The effects of conflict intensity and promisor credibility on a target's behavior. *Psychonomic Science, 14,* 73–74.

Jampolsky, G. G. (1980). The future is now. *Journal of Clinical Child Psychology, 9,* 192–184.

Johnson, P. E. (1947). Religious psychology and health. *Mental Hygiene, 31,* 556–566.

Linn, D., & Linn, M. (1978). *Healing life's hurts: Healing memories through the five stages of forgiveness.* New York: Paulist Press.

Litwinski, L. (1945). Hatred and forgetting. *Journal of General Psychology, 33,* 85–109.

McCullough, M. E., Rachal, K. C., Sandage, S. J., Worthington, E. L., Brown, S. W., & Hight, T. L. (1998). Interpersonal forgiving in close relationships: II. Theoretical elaboration and measurement. *Journal of Personality and Social Psychology, 75,* 1586–1603.

McCullough, M. E., & Worthington, E. L., Jr. (1994). Models of interpersonal forgiveness and their applications to counseling: Review and critique. *Counseling and Values, 39,* 2–14.

McCullough, M. E., & Worthington, E. L., Jr. (1995). Promoting forgiveness: A comparison of two brief psychoeducational interventions with a waiting-list control. *Counseling and Values, 40,* 55–68.

McCullough, M. E., & Worthington, E. L., Jr. (1999). Religion and the forgiving personality. *Journal of Personality.*

McCullough, M. E., Worthington, E. L., Jr., & Rachal, K. C. (1997). Interpersonal forgiving in close relationships. *Journal of Personality and Social Psychology, 73,* 321–336.

Piaget, J. (1932). *Le jugement moral chez l'enfant.* Paris: Alcan.

Rokeach, M. (1967). *Value survey.* Sunnyvale, CA: Halgren Test.

Rokeach, M. (1973). *The nature of human values.* New York: Free Press.

Rusk, H. A. (1950). Dynamic therapeutics in chronic disease. *Digest of Neurology and Psychiatry, 18,* 152.

Smedes, L. B. (1984). *Forgive and forget: Healing the hurts we don't deserve.* New York: Harper & Row.

Spidell, S., & Liberman, D. (1981). Moral development and the forgiveness of sins. *Journal of Psychology and Theology, 9,* 159–163.

Weiner, B., Graham, S., Peter, O., & Zmuidinas, M. (1991). Public confession and forgiveness. *Journal of Personality, 59,* 281–312.

Worthington, E. L., Jr. (Ed.). (1998a). *Dimensions of forgiveness.* Radnor, PA: Templeton Foundation Press.

Worthington, E. L., Jr. (1998b). Empirical research in forgiveness: Looking backward, looking forward. In E. L. Worthington (Ed.), *Dimensions of forgiveness* (pp. 321–339). Radnor, PA: Templeton Foundation Press.

PART I

Conceptual and Measurement Issues

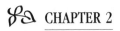 CHAPTER 2

Religious Perspectives on Forgiveness

Mark S. Rye, Kenneth I. Pargament, M. Amir Ali,
Guy L. Beck, Elliot N. Dorff, Charles Hallisey,
Vasudha Narayanan, and James G. Williams

Forgiveness has been encouraged for thousands of years by major world religions. Adherents of these religions have claimed that forgiveness yields numerous emotional and spiritual benefits, and can dramatically transform one's life. In spite of such claims, social scientists have only recently (i.e., within the last 15 years) begun to develop theoretical models and conduct empirical studies on forgiveness. Given that the scientific study of forgiveness is relatively new, it seems prudent for scientists to learn about long-standing religious conceptualizations of forgiveness. Examination of religious perspectives on forgiveness can benefit social scientists in several ways.

First, religious perspectives on forgiveness can shed light on how religion influences the psychological processes involved in forgiveness. Pargament and Rye (1998) have proposed several ways in which religion can contribute to forgiveness. To begin, forgiveness can be sanctified, or imbued, with divine-like qualities. Thus, in theistic religions, forgiveness becomes a means for imitating God, carrying out God's plan, or enhancing one's relationship with the divine. In addition, religion provides numerous role models of individuals who have forgiven despite profound injustices. Religion also offers worldviews that help victims to reframe their attitudes toward their offenders. Furthermore, religious faith can help individuals cope with the uncertainty surrounding the choice to forgive. The resources of divine and/or congregational support may be especially helpful to people working through the forgiveness process. In a study conducted by Rye and Pargament (1998), participants in group forgiveness interventions reported frequent use of religiously based forgiveness strategies, even if these strategies were not encouraged in the intervention. In fact, the most common forgiveness strategy reported was to ask God for help and/or support when trying to forgive. This finding attests to the pervasiveness of people's reliance upon religion when trying to forgive.

Several other researchers have examined the connection between religion and forgiveness (for review, see McCullough & Worthington, in press). These studies suggest that people who are more religious value forgiveness more than do people who are less religious (Gorsuch & Hao, 1993; Poloma & Gallup, 1991; Rokeach, 1973; Shoemaker & Bolt, 1977). Although individuals who are more religious tend to place greater value on forgiveness, it is unclear whether they actually forgive more often than people who are less religious (McCullough & Worthington, in press). Examination of how forgiveness is understood within the major world religions can enhance researchers' efforts to resolve these issues.

Second, examination of religious perspectives on forgiveness can help social scientists to appreciate the richness and diversity of conceptualizations that exist rather than mistakenly characterizing forgiveness as a monolithic construct. Most of the literature describing religious perspectives on forgiveness has focused on Christianity (e.g., Educational Psychology Study Group, 1990; Enright & Zell, 1989; Gassin & Enright, 1995; Jones-Haldeman, 1992; Pingleton, 1989) and Judaism (e.g., Dorff, 1998; Newman, 1987). Only a few authors have examined how other religions view forgiveness (see Enright, Eastin, Golden, Sarinopoulos, & Freedman, 1992; McCullough & Worthington, in press). Furthermore, there is a dearth of articles that compare perspectives on forgiveness across religions.

Third, clinicians risk responding insensitively if they fail to recognize the value religious individuals place on forgiveness and the differences in perspectives that exist across religious traditions. Understanding diverse religious perspectives on forgiveness is particularly helpful when working with clients who may be unaware, inadequately informed, or misinformed about the value and practice of forgiveness from the perspective of their religious community. In such cases, therapists, with appropriate training, consultation, and/or referral, may be able to help clients learn more about the resources of their traditions.

This chapter was written in an attempt to familiarize researchers and practitioners with perspectives on forgiveness espoused by various religions. In contrast, Chapter 13, written by John Patton, focuses on the application of the Christian perspective on forgiveness to pastoral care. Although any number of religions could have been included in this chapter, we (Rye & Pargament) limited our discussion to those major religions with which we felt our readers would be most familiar. We asked scholars in Judaism, Christianity, Islam, Buddhism, and Hinduism to respond to five questions on forgiveness. Scholars were selected who have written extensively about their respective religions and expressed interest in the topic of forgiveness. Two Hindu scholars were recruited because they each had knowledge related to different questions covered in this chapter.

Generating questions that were applicable to all of these religions proved to be a challenging task. Our own Western, Judeo–Christian backgrounds undoubtedly influenced the selection and wording of questions. As Charles Hallisey pointed out, differences in worldviews and language make it difficult to compare Eastern and Western moral concepts directly. However, our scholars made efforts to "bridge the gap" when necessary and to explain why particular questions posed problems.

Obviously, an exhaustive presentation of each religion's perspective on forgiveness was not possible here. Our goal for this chapter was to provide a brief overview of how various religions view forgiveness. Keep in mind that there is considerable diversity within each religious tradition and with respect to how individual scholars interpret religious traditions. By no means are these responses intended to provide the "last word" from each tradition. Thus, we caution the reader against overgeneralizations about particular religious perspectives on forgiveness. Furthermore, in some cultures, elements of different religions and philosophical systems are often combined (Smith, 1994), making it less likely that one's response to being wronged will be guided by a single value system. With these qualifications in mind, we hope that the responses provided by religious scholars will serve to enlighten and, as importantly, to prompt further questions among researchers and practitioners interested in forgiveness.

We asked the religious scholars to respond to the following five questions:

1. How is forgiveness defined according to your tradition?
2. What is the theological basis for forgiveness according to your tradition? Please include examples of major references pertaining to forgiveness in sacred texts.
3. How important or central is forgiveness to your tradition?
4. According to your tradition, should forgiveness be contingent upon repentance by the offender? If so, why? If not, why? Are there other conditions placed on forgiveness?

5. Does forgiveness necessitate reconciliation? In other words, is it possible to forgive while deciding not to reconcile with the offender?

How is forgiveness defined according to your tradition?

Judaism (Dorff)

Some general, philosophical distinctions will be helpful before articulating the stance of the Jewish tradition. We use the terms "pardon" or "excuse" when the violation still stands but no punishment (or no further punishment) is to be imposed. Thus, we say "Excuse me" when we accidentally bump into someone but expect no punishment, and governors pardon prisoners when the violation will still appear in police records but the violator will be freed of further punishment. "Forgiveness" involves one step more: The original violation is itself removed. Thus a creditor who "forgives" a loan thereby expunges the entire debt. Injured parties who forgive may still remember the transgression and even take some precautions to make sure that they will not suffer that way again. If they forgive the perpetrator, though, they accept him or her as possible candidates for an ongoing relationship. Finally, in "reconciliation," the transgressor becomes part of the friendship, family, or community again, despite the bad feelings that have been generated by what he or she did. People may reconcile without forgiving or forgive without reconciling.

The most common Hebrew words for "forgiveness" in classical Jewish texts are *mehillah* and *selihah*. Although they are often used interchangeably in both classical and modern Hebrew, strictly speaking, *mehillah* denotes the wiping away of a transgression—that is, forgiveness, as defined earlier—while *selihah*, especially in its biblical usage, denotes reconciliation.

Christianity (Williams)

The most common words denoting forgiveness in the New Testament are (1) *eleao* (and cognate nouns)—show mercy (78 times), and (2) *aphiemi*—release, discharge, put away (64 times). Another word used infrequently but in a striking way is *splanchnizomai*. Usually understood as "feeling sorry for" or "having compassion on" someone, it is derived from a word for "intestines." It literally means to pour out one's insides, one's intestines.

Forgiveness is generally understood as an act of pardon or release from an injury, offense, or debt. On the part of the forgiving subject, it entails having compassion, releasing someone from any act or attitude that would impede the relationship of those involved. On the part of the forgiven subject, it usually entails showing signs of repentance for the wrong done and acts of contrition and love, in keeping with the graciousness shown by the forgiver.

Islam (Ali)

I would like to deal with the terminology used in this question. The term, "tradition" perhaps applies best to those religions that do not have God-revealed books in their original languages and in which the religion is the outgrowth of teachings and writings of religious leaders who have come and gone over the centuries and new traditions have developed. In the case of Islam, the original revelation, the Qur'an, exists in its original language and the second source, Hadith, remains intact. Islamic teachings, methods of ritual worship, and elements of legal system remain the same as given by Allah through His Messenger, Muhammad (peace and salutations of Allah be upon him, henceforth denoted by [S]).

The concept of forgiveness in the Qur'an is expressed in three terms: (1) *'afw,* used 35 times; (2) *safhu,* used 8 times; and (3) *ghafara,* used 234 times. *'Afw* means to pardon, to excuse for a fault, an offense, or a discourtesy, waiver of punishment, and amnesty. Examples of usage in the Qur'an are verses 42:40, 2:187 and 5:95. *Safhu* means to turn away from a sin or a misdeed, ignore, etc. Examples of usage in the Qur'an are verses 2:109, 15:85, and 43:89. Ghafara or maghfira means to cover, to forgive, and to remit. Examples of usage in the Qur'an are verses 2:263, 42:37, and 43:43. For more details see Lane's *Lexicon*[1] and Hans Wehr's dictionary,[2] among others.

The God, Allah,[3] is the ultimate power Who can forgive. One of Allah's 99 attributes is Al-Ghafoor, the Forgiving One. Forgiveness means closing an account of offense against God or any of His creation. However, forgiveness must meet the criteria of sincerity. God, the All-Knowing, has the knowledge of everything, including whatever a person thinks but does not express in words or deeds. An offense may be against (1) a person; (2) a group of persons or society; (3) other creation of God such as animals, plants, land, atmosphere, bodies of water and the life therein; and (4) God, Allah. Muslims understand that an offense against the creation of God is an offense against God.

Buddhism (Hallisey)

Someone interested in Buddhism encounters two problems in attempting to find a "Buddhist" definition of forgiveness. First, Buddhism is a global religion that has historically used a wide variety of languages and this linguistic diversity represents a conceptual diversity as well. There is no unified foundation against which a single "Buddhist" concept of forgiveness might be sought. The problem of translation that one inevitably faces when exploring the diverse resources of the Buddhist traditions is only magnified when one attempts to find analogs or equivalents for Western moral categories, such as forgiveness. In fact, it is usually the case that exact translations are not found, but the differences in meaning that are discovered lead to a better understanding of the original concept.

It strikes me that, generally, the notion of forgiveness comprises two factors: first, the removal of an expectation of retribution, and second, the renouncing of anger or resentment toward someone who has offended you. Both factors represent changes of attitude, and both are highly valued in Buddhist cultures, but they are generally kept distinct as quite different virtues. In the *English–Sinhalese Dictionary* by G. P. Malalasekcra,[4] to take the Sinhala language used by Buddhists in Sri Lanka as just one example, the translations for "forgive" and "forgiveness" are *sama venava* and *anukampa dakvenava* for the former, and *ksamava* and *dayava* for the latter. More literal translations of each of these terms reveal that together they may approximate the notion of forgiveness, but individually, they do not. *Sama venava* and its cognate, *ksamava*, can both be translated as forbearance, a concept that is more inclusive than forgiveness. The Buddhist notion of forbearance embraces both enduring an action done against one and the renouncing of anger or resentment toward someone who has offended you; usually, forgiveness is understood to include only the overcoming of resentment. *Anukampa* and *dayava* can be translated as compassion or pity, virtues that move one not to react against someone who deserves punishment because of their own actions. In forgiveness, the rejection of retribution stems from overcoming resentment toward an offender. Compassion and pity as Buddhist virtues, however, effect a change in attitude by which the offender is no longer thought of as such. Instead, through compassion and pity, one ideally comes to empathize with the suffering of the offender, and one then takes steps to ease that suffering, even though both the empathy and the action taken to relieve suffering is undeserved. In this vein, one image of compassion is the empathy that one feels for the criminal on his way to his execution, and it is also said that "the truly compassionate take pity even on their would-be murderers."[5] Compassion, in particular, can have the effect of reforming an offender who is shamed by the contrast between his own behavior and the behavior of the wronged person, but this is not a necessary element in compassion.

Hinduism (Beck)

Ksama or *ksamata* is the word most commonly used to signify forgiveness. This is usually combined with words for mercy such as *kripa, prasada, daya,* or compassion, *karuna*. These words either occur in Sanskrit texts (prayers or *stotras*) or in vernacular settings in which many of the original Sanskrit words are used, sometimes in slightly modified form.

What is the theological basis for forgiveness according to your tradition? Please include examples of major references pertaining to forgiveness in sacred texts.

Judaism (Dorff)

The ultimate theological basis for forgiveness is that God Himself is forgiving, and so we, in imitation of God, must be so as well. Thus, the Rabbis note that the Torah demands that we "walk in all His ways" (Deuteronomy 11:22). What does that require? They answer:

> These are the ways of the Holy One: "The Lord is merciful and compassionate, patient, abounding in kindness and faithfulness, assuring love for a thousand generations, forgiving iniquity, transgression and sin, and granting pardon . . . " (Exodus 34:6) . . . Just as God is merciful, you too must be merciful; . . . just as God is compassionate, you too must be compassionate. "The Lord is righteous in all His ways and loving in all His deeds" (Psalms 145:17). As the Holy One is righteous, you too must be righteous. As the Holy One is loving, you too must be loving. (*Sifre, Ekev* 49 on Deuteronomy 11:22)

The Rabbis did not leave this to the realm of pious principles; they translated this into concrete law. Thus, according to the Mishnah, the first compilation of Jewish oral tradition (c. 200 C.E.), if someone assaults another, the assailant must pay the victim for the following: damages, pain, healing, loss of time, and insult. After describing how each of these is to be assessed, the Mishnah states:

> Even though the assailant pays the victim, God does not forgive him until he asks the victim's forgiveness, as it is said, "Therefore, restore the man's wife and he will pray on your behalf" (Genesis 20:7). And how do we know that if the victim does not pardon him, he [the victim] is considered cruel? Because it says, "Abraham then prayed to God, and God healed Avimelekh" (Genesis 20:17). (Mishnah, Bava Kamma 8:7)

Indeed, injured parties who refuse to forgive those who wronged them despite being asked for forgiveness three times in the presence of others, are themselves deemed sinners (Babylonian Talmud, *Bava Kamma* 92a: Mishneh Torah, *Laws of Forgiveness* 2:10). God wants us not only to fulfill the demands of justice, but also to repair our relationships.

Jews need to forgive not only to imitate God, but also because God's law requires forgiveness. "You shall not take vengeance or bear a grudge against your neighbor. Love your neighbor as yourself" (Leviticus 19:18), the Torah demands. Thus, according to the Rabbis, "All who act mercifully [forgivingly] toward their fellow creatures will be treated mercifully by Heaven, and all who do not act mercifully toward their fellow creatures will not be treated mercifully by Heaven" (Babylonian Talmud, *Shabbat* 151b).

One should note several other central passages in Jewish literature regarding forgiveness. In biblical times, God's forgiveness of us was secured through the offering of animal sacrifices in the Temple (Leviticus 4–6). In addition, the rituals of the Day of Atonement required fasting, cessation from work, and a special rite of purging of sins (Leviticus 16, 23:27–32).

When the Temple was destroyed, prayer took the place of animal sacrifices. Thus in the daily liturgy recited three times each day (the *Amidah*), the Jew asks God for forgiveness: "Forgive us, our Father, for we have sinned; pardon us, for we have transgressed." In addition, the Ten Days of Repentance between the Jewish New Year (*Rosh Ha-Shanah*) and the Day of Atonement (*Yom Kippur*), usually falling in September, focus on this theme.

Christianity (Williams)

The God of love, who restores the image of God in man through Christ (Colossians 1:15), enables and inspires human beings to forgive. This power or spirit of forgiveness is mediated through Christ, the church, and potentially anyone who truly acts as a neighbor (Luke 10:25–37).

The most important reference is Jesus's petition for his crucifiers from the cross, "Father, forgive [from *aphiemi*] them, for they know not what they do" (Luke 23:34). Other important references include the following:

> *Matthew 6:12*   In the Lord's Prayer: Forgive us our debts, as we forgive our debtors.
> *Luke 11:4*   In the Lord's Prayer: Forgive us our sins, for we ourselves forgive everyone who is indebted to us.
> *Mark 11:25*   Although the Gospel of Mark does not have the Lord's Prayer or Our Father, this verse is parallel to the Our Father in Matthew and Luke: When you are praying, forgive whoever has wronged you.
> *Matthew 18:21–22*   Peter asks whether one should forgive his brother seven times and Jesus replies no, 77 times (or 70 times seven).
> *Matthew 18:27, 32*   In parable of the unmerciful servant, the mas-

ter forgives the servant an enormous monetary debt, but then the servant is unwilling to forgive someone else a relatively small amount.

The references to these passages all use some form of *aphiemi*. There are also numerous passages in the New Testament that extol God's compassion, or human acts of mercy or compassion; these often express or imply forgiveness. Among the most important are the following:

> *Luke 10:33* In the parable of the good Samaritan, the Samaritan had compassion (*esplagchnisthe*) on the man beaten and robbed and left half dead.
> *Luke 10:37* After telling the parable of the Samaritan, Jesus asks the lawyer who proved to be a neighbor to the man left beside the road. The lawyer replies, "The one who showed mercy (*poiesas to eleos*) on him." Since the Samaritans and the Jews were extremely hostile to each other, and the half-dead man was a Jew, this act implies forgiveness of the hostility and its justifications.
> *Luke 15:20* In the parable of the prodigal son, the father welcomes back the younger son who has gone off and wasted his inheritance: "His father saw him, and had compassion (*esplagchnisthe*), and ran and embraced him . . . "
> *Titus 3:5* God saved us not because of our righteous deeds but "by virtue of his compassion" (*eleos*).

Islam (Ali)

The theological basis of forgiveness is in the Qur'an and Hadith. Qur'an is the word of God revealed to Prophet Muhammad[S] and is in Arabic. Translation of the Qur'an is not Qur'an, because God did not reveal it in any other language but Arabic. A translation may contain the message of the Qur'an, but it is the word of the translator, not the word of God. Qur'an, in many places, needs explanation, which is done by the Prophet Muhammad[S] and recorded in Hadith collections. Hadith contains reports of Prophet Muhammad's sayings, deeds, and approvals, and is the second source of Islamic knowledge and legal system. A selection of teachings about forgiveness from the Qur'an and Hadith are given below.

Allah forgives:

And vie with one another to attain to your Sustainer's forgiveness and to a paradise as vast as the heavens and the earth, which has been readied for the God-conscious who spend [in His way] in time of plenty and in time of hardship, and hold in check their anger, and pardon their fellow men because God loves the doers of good; and who, when they have committed a shameful deed or have [otherwise] sinned against themselves, remember

God and pray that their sins be forgiven—for who but God could forgive sins? And do not knowingly persist in doing whatever [wrong] they may have done. These it is who shall have as their reward forgiveness from their Sustainer, and gardens through which running waters flow, therein to abide; and how excellent a reward for those who labor! (the Qur'an[6] 3:133–136)

Leadership must be forgiving:

And it was by God's grace that thou [O Muhammad] didst deal gently with thy followers: for if thou hadst been harsh and hard of heart, they would indeed have broken away from thee. Pardon them, then, and pray that they be forgiven. And take counsel with them in all matters of public concern; then, when thou hadst decided upon a course of action, place thy trust in God; for, verily God loves those who place their trust in Him. (the Qur'an 3:159)

General teachings of forgiveness:

Keep to forgiveness, and enjoin kindness, and turn away from the ignorant. And if it should happen that a prompting from Satan stirs thee up [to anger], seek refuge with Allah: behold, He is All-Hearing, All-Knowing. (the Qur'an 7:199–200)

But withal, if one is patient in adversity and forgives—this, behold, is indeed something to set one's heart upon. (the Qur'an 42:43)

Family situations:

O You who believe! Behold among your spouses and your children are enemies unto you: so beware of them! But if you pardon [their faults], and forbear, and forgive—then, behold, Allah is Forgiving, Merciful. (the Qur'an 64:14)

Teachings of the Prophet Muhammad[(S)]:

Abu Kabsha 'Ameri reported that the Messenger of Allah said: . . . and no man pardons an oppression seeking thereby the pleasure of Allah but Allah will increase his honor therewith on the Day of Resurrection . . . [7]

Oqbah Ibn 'Amer reported that the Messenger of Allah said: You shall keep relationship with one who cut it off from you, you shall give one who disappointed you, and you shall pardon one who oppressed you.[8]

Abu Hurayra reported that the Messenger of Allah said: The strong one is not he who knocks out his adversary; the strong one is he who keeps control over his temper.[9]

Prophet Muhammad set an excellent example of a forgiving person in his personal matters. He lived in Makkah (erroneously spelled as Mecca) for 13 years after his appointment as the Messenger and Prophet of Allah for mankind. During this period, he was persecuted, his followers were persecuted and some were killed, and, finally, his enemies wanted to kill him. During the first 8 years in his adopted town, Madinah (misspelled as Medina), his enemies chased him, brought armies against him, and he narrowly escaped. During twenty-some battles over 8 years, he lost many of his close associates and relatives by the hands of Makkans and their allies. After the conquest of Makkah, he declared general amnesty for those who did not take up arms against him during his entry in Makkah. Haykal wrote:

> All these thousands of men, of Muslims in battle array, stood on the ready waiting for that one word to wipe out the whole Makkah and its people within minutes. Muhammad, however, was no less than Muhammad! He was no less than the Prophet of God! No alienation, antagonism, or hostility could find any permanent abode in his heart. His heart was absolutely free of injustice, of malice, of tyranny or false pride. In the most decisive moment, God gave him power over his enemy. But Muhammad chose to forgive, thereby giving to all mankind and all the generations the most perfect example of goodness, of truthfulness, of nobility and magnanimity.[10]

Buddhism (Hallisey)

It is always a problem to speak of "theology" in a Buddhist context since, in quite foundational ways, Buddhism is a nontheistic religion. Buddhists have almost never been interested in a creator who made the world with any kind of moral design. They have seen the world as fundamentally just, and this justice is maintained by karma, in which good actions are rewarded with good fruits and bad with bad fruits. Thus the idea of a "theological" basis, in a Buddhist context, can be taken first in this sense of a metaphysical and valuational account of the world governed by karma.

The two virtues of forbearance and pity are both grounded in Buddhist ideas about the world as a realm of suffering. The Buddha's First Noble Truth is that "all this is suffering," a statement that acknowledges that the reality of suffering pervades all experience in the world. Buddhism, as a religion, is dedicated to ending suffering in all its forms. The chief function of compassion is to ease pain and suffering in others, while the chief function of forbearance is to desist from causing more suffering, both for oneself and others, by reacting to offenses in comparable ways. That resentment, the opposite of forgiveness, is never satisfied, but always has double effect, for oneself and for others, can be seen in a verse from the *Dhammapada*, an anthology of sayings attributed to the Buddha himself:

> In those who harbor such thoughts: "He reviled me, he beat me, he overpowered me, he robbed me," anger is never stilled. . . . Hatred never

ceases by hatred in this world. Through loving kindness it comes to an
end. This is an ancient Law.[11]

Resentment directly causes suffering to a person because of the mental torment that it engenders, but more directly, resentment can motivate
a person to action that by karma, the law of moral cause and effect, will
cause suffering in the future to the person wronged. To hate another for
his or her actions is to create conditions for the experience of being hated
by others in the future. It is thus always in a person's self-interest to overcome resentment through compassion and forbearance.

Compassion and forbearance are also considered "perfections" (*para-
mitas*), moral qualities which have been cultivated to a maximal degree by
Buddhas, the "awakened ones" who represent the apex and goal of the
Buddhist religious life. The acquisition of these perfections transforms
the process of liberation and enlightenment from one that only benefits
an individual to one that is, in the words of one Buddhist text, "for the
welfare and benefit of the whole world." In this regard, we can see a second theological basis for compassion and forbearance in Buddhism. They
are qualities that one cultivates, in imitation of the career of previous
Buddhas, for the sake of others as much as oneself. But even here, forbearance and compassion are more prerogatives than duties, because no
one is required to attempt to become a Buddha.

When approached with the yardstick of the relatively simple canons
of sacred texts in Islam, Judaism, and Christianity, Buddhists may appear
to accept an extraordinarily wide number of texts as containing authorita-
tive statements. All Buddhists do not accept the same texts, however, and
there is no single canon on which all Buddhist religious systems build. In
fact, there are very few individual texts that can be found in every Buddhist tradition, not even those statements a modern historian would take
as the record of the teaching of Gautama Buddha, the founder of Buddhism. Moreover, the size of individual canons accepted by particular
traditions—whether these are defined on sectarian grounds (e.g., Zen Buddhism) or cultural grounds (e.g., Tibetan Buddhism)—can be huge in their
own right, and we might think of them more as a library than as a "canon"
or "scripture."

It is thus impossible to give a list of major references pertaining to
forbearance and compassion in Buddhist texts. This is not to say that
there has been less than agreement that these two qualities are desirable
parts of a flourishing human life. A selection about forbearance from
Arya Sura's *Jatakamala*, a medieval Indian narrative collection, can give a
taste of how these two virtues were portrayed:

The true ornament in this present life, of one who is wellborn, handsome,
in the prime of life, exceptionally powerful or wealthy, is a regard for vir-

tue. Trees are adorned with blossom, low-hanging rain clouds with streaks of lightning, lakes with lotuses and their drunken bees, and human beings with perfections that have been brought to perfection. Whether it be health, age, wealth, beauty or birth . . . [these are] by no means due to a person's natural disposition, nor to outside influences, but rather to show how he has behaved in the past. Once one has realized that this is the immutable law of existence and that life is transient and prone to decay, one should desist from evil and feel disposed to do good. This is the path to fame and happiness. On the other hand, a corrupt heart acts like a fire, burning up both one's own and other people's good completely. If, therefore, one is afraid of evil, one should take pains to avoid such corruption, by cultivating its opposite. Just as a fire, however fierce, is quenched when it meets a large river brimful of water, so a raging heart grows calm if one inclines to forbearance, that mainstay in this life and the next. Practice forbearance and you will avoid evil by cutting it off at the root. The result will be that you arouse no ill feeling because of your friendly disposition. You will be loved and honored for it and thereby win happiness.[12]

Hinduism (Narayanan)

The number of different traditions and viewpoints found within Hinduism make it difficult to define "the theological basis" for forgiveness. However, there are some commonalties across Hindu traditions. To begin, concepts such as forgiveness, duty, righteousness, forbearance, compassion, and patience are discussed in the epics and the dharma sastras (treatises on righteousness). For those who wish to follow the path of dharma (righteousness), it is essential to practice all of these. Also, karma (law of cause and effect), which pervades Hindu thought, is relevant here. Through karma, individuals face the consequences of their actions in subsequent reincarnations. Therefore, one can presume that lack of forgiveness, negative feelings, and unresolved, seething anger can only spill over into future births. Finally, there are numerous examples of divine forgiveness in Hindu sacred texts. In the Sri Vaishnava tradition (a fairly large "denomination"), Lord Vishnu has all the qualities of grace, mercy, and so on, but it is his wife, the Goddess Lakshmi/Sri, who is said to epitomize the quality of forgiveness and grace. Iconographically, she is depicted on the heart (chest) of Vishnu. It should be noted that there are nontheistic Hindu traditions that, by definition, do not focus on the issue of divine forgiveness.

Hinduism (Beck)

Evidence for the divine bestowal of forgiveness (*ksamata*) on repentant human beings is found much earlier in Hinduism than in the biblical record, as far back as the Vedic period (ca. 5000–1000 B.C.E.) in India. In the Rig-Veda, there are prayers of forgiveness directed toward Lord Varuna, a mighty regent sitting on his throne in the highest heaven. As the Guardian of Rita (cosmic order), Varuna could free humans from the bondage of the sins of lying and drunkenness that were a disturbance to this order. He was very gracious to those who repented, and for them, he removed all sins accruing from several generations. Varuna also had hundreds of remedies for the humbled sinner and could take away or prolong life. The righteous hoped to see him in the next world, reigning in bliss.

A famous prayer to Varuna for forgiveness from one of the earliest portions of the *Rig-Veda* (7.89) is as follows:

> Let me not yet, King Varuna, enter into the House of Clay: Have mercy, spare me, Mighty Lord. When Thunderer! I move along tremulous like a wind-blown skin, Have Mercy, spare me, Mighty Lord. O Bright and Powerful God, through want of strength I erred and went astray: Have mercy, spare me, Mighty Lord. Thirst found thy worshipper though he stood in the midst of water-floods: Have mercy, spare me, Mighty Lord. O Varuna, whatever the offence may be which we as men commit against the heavenly host, When through our want of thought we violate thy laws, punish us not, O God, for that iniquity.[13]

The Dharma-Sastras, lawbooks governing the four castes and stages of life written during the classical period of Hinduism, dealt with sins (*papa*) and atonements (*prayascitta*). The *Manu-Samhita* (ca. 500 B.C.E.–200 C.E.), said to be composed by the ancient lawgiver Manu, describes expiations leading to forgiveness from both the gods and society that included acts of charity and purification, vows of fasting and abstinence, and performance of rituals and recitations, with subsequent societal acceptance of such acts. References to Varuna in this book reaffirm a continuity with the Vedic forgiveness.

How important or central is forgiveness to your tradition?

Judaism (Dorff)

Since the Day of Atonement is the holiest day of the Jewish liturgical year, forgiveness is clearly a central theme in Judaism. Since God's forgiveness of us on that day can only occur if we have been forgiven by those we have offended, it is not only God's forgiveness that occupies this central place in Judaism, but also human forgiveness. Indeed, according to the Rabbis, ever since Abraham forgave Avimelekh, forgiveness has been a distinguishing mark of Abraham's descendants—a special gift of God bestowed upon them (Genesis 20:17; Babylonian Talmud, *Bezah* 32b; *Yevamot* 79a; Numbers *Rabbah* 8:4).

Christianity (Williams)

Forgiveness is at the religious, theological, and ethical core of the Christian tradition. It represents the possibility and reality of change and transformation of the individual in relation to others and others in relation to the individual.

Islam (Ali)

Those who desire to be forgiven for their offenses must learn to forgive others. Especially, if they seek forgiveness from God, they should learn to forgive others for their offenses. If they desire that God overlook their weaknesses, they should learn to overlook weaknesses of others. Forgiveness is important for two reasons:

1. Very importantly, for the afterlife or the life hereafter. One forgives to seek forgiveness. Seeking forgiveness is a sign of humility, and forgiving others is a sign of magnanimity.
2. Seeking forgiveness and forgiving others brings happiness in the worldly life. In addition, forgiving improves relations with people by bringing good reputation and respect.

In the ancient world, tribes and families carried on blood feuds for generations because they could not forgive. Islam taught a middle path between turning the other cheek and never ending blood feud, that is, revenge to the extent harm done is allowed but forgiveness is preferred. Allah said in the Qur'an:

> The recompense for an injury is an injury equal thereto (in degree): but if a person forgives and makes reconciliation, his reward is due from Allah: for (Allah) loves not those who do wrong. (42:40, A. Yusuf Ali)

> But [remember that an attempt at] requiting evil may, too, become an evil: hence whoever pardons [his foe] and makes peace, his reward rests with God—for, verily, He does not love evildoers. (42:40, Muhammad Asad)

Both translations of the same verse are correct. One gives more literal meaning (Yusuf Ali) and the other gives more interpretive meaning (Muhammad Asad). To take revenge of an offense is allowed only to the extent of damage done but not to be exceeded. However, there is a great probability of exceeding the damage; thereby, the victim becomes an offender. Forgiveness is a protection and brings great reward from Allah.

Buddhism (Hallisey)

As is probably already clear, the complex category of forgiveness per se is not a central category in the Buddhist tradition, but the two categories of forbearance and compassion are both central and important, especially because of their association with the nature and actions of a Buddha. Indeed, compassion might be said to be at the foundation of all Buddhist practice.

Hinduism (Narayanan)

As mentioned earlier, those who wish to follow the path of dharma must practice forgiveness, compassion, forbearance, and so on. Therefore, forgiveness is considered to be important in the Hindu tradition.

According to your tradition, should forgiveness be contingent upon repentance by the offender? If so, why? If not, why? Are there other conditions placed on forgiveness?

Judaism (Dorff)

A victim is obligated to forgive only when the transgressor goes through the process of *teshuvah*, return. If the transgressor fails to go through the process of return, the victim may still choose to forgive as an act of charity. Sometimes that is ill-advised, as it may discourage the perpetrator from ever engaging in the process of return and may even make him or her think that one may commit that same offense many times over without cost. When the offense is less serious, forgiveness may be granted by the victim just so that he or she can get on with life—or because restoring the relationship is more important to him or her than getting the perpetrator to own up to the offense. In general, though, the Jewish tradition does not look favorably on "free" forgiveness; it insists that transgressors earn forgiveness by going through the process of return. That is ultimately best for the perpetrator, and it protects other potential victims from abuse. The process of return, as described in Chapter 2 of Maimonides's *Laws of Forgiveness,* involves the following steps:

1. Acknowledgment that one has done something wrong.
2. Public confession of one's wrongdoing to both God and the community.
3. Public expression of remorse.
4. Public announcement of the offender's resolve not to sin this way again. These four steps may take place amid crying and entreaties for forgiveness and, in the most serious of cases, may even include changing one's name.
5. Compensation of the victim for the injury inflicted, accompanied by acts of charity to others.
6. Sincere request of forgiveness by the victim—with the help of the victim's friends and up to three times, if necessary (and even more if the victim is one's teacher).
7. Avoidance of the conditions that caused the offense, perhaps even to the point of moving to a new locale.
8. Acting differently when confronted with the same situation again.

Christianity (Williams)

According to the model of Christ on the cross (Luke 23:34), forgiveness, or at least the petition for God the Father to forgive, does not depend first of all on repentance by the offender. However, in various concrete situations, there arises the problem that Dietrich Bonhoeffer spoke of as "cheap grace,"[14] which here means "cheap forgiveness." It should not be offered mechanically, or from the motive of becoming a martyr and thus better than some opponent, and so on.

Islam (Ali)

This question implies cases of clear-cut offense by one side against the other, but real-life situations are not always as clear. Two parties may disagree, sincerely, about the offended and the offender. In such cases, arbitration and conflict resolution may be required. Allah teaches Muslims in the Qur'an:

> Hence if two groups of believers fall to fighting, make peace between them: but then, if one of the two [groups] goes on acting wrongfully towards the other, fight against the one that acts wrongfully until it reverts to God's command; and if they revert, make peace between them with justice, and deal equitably [with them]: for verily, God loves those who act equitably! (49:9)

If there is repentance, it will bring a better bond between the two parties. However, forgiveness does not require repentance by the offender.
When asking Allah for forgiveness, repentance is required.

Buddhism (Hallisey)

The selection from Arya Sura's *Jatakamala,* quoted earlier, indicates that
forbearance does not depend on any repentance or remorse on the part
of the offender. This is even more the case when one forbears in the moment of being wronged, as when one endures violence without resistance.
Above all, forbearance allows one to exercise compassion. This is also illustrated by Arya Sura, when he tells the story of an ascetic who is tortured by an enraged king to test his dedication to forbearance; the story is
hyperbolic, to be sure, but it does allow us to see clearly that forbearance
and compassion can be practiced independently of any action or change
of heart on the part of an offender:

> Even with his right hand cut off, [the future Buddha], keeping true to his
> vow of forbearance, felt less pain than sorrow as he envisaged the frightful
> and inexorable suffering in store for the pampered king who had cut it
> off. . . . He felt sorry for the king, as for a sick man deserted by his doctors,
> and kept silent. . . . The king then duly proceeded to lop off his other
> hand, both his arms, his ears and nose, and his feet. But as the sharp sword
> fell upon his body, that perfect saint felt neither grief nor anger: he knew
> full well that the mechanism of the body must have an end, and he was well
> used to exercising forbearance toward people. Even as he silently looked
> on while his body was hacked to pieces, his spirit remained unbroken in its
> constant forbearance. And because of his kindly disposition, he felt no
> sorrow. But to see the king fallen from the path of virtue caused him an-
> guish. Compassionate souls, who have great powers of judgment, are not
> so much troubled by the hardship they themselves experience as that
> which befalls others.[15]

Hinduism (Narayanan)

The Goddess Sri (more popularly known as Lakshmi) is said to forgive
even when there is no repentance on the part of the soul that perpetuates
the atrocity. Obviously, this is more than normative and is divine. Her acts
of forgiveness are sometimes contrasted rhetorically with the Lord
Vishnu, who forgives only when there is repentance. Additional information on this topic can be found in the following essays: "The Goddess Sri:
Blossoming Lotus and Breast Jewel of Vishnu"[16] and "Sri: Giver of Fortune, Bestower of Grace."[17]

There are two paradigmatic cases of forgiveness in the epic Ramayana. Lakshmi/Sri, in her incarnation as Sita (the wife of Rama in the epic Ramayana) is said to have forgiven (1) a crow, even as it was harming her, and (2) the demon-women of Lanka, even as they were harassing her. These instances serve as "proof" for the later devotees to speak about divine grace. In theological terms, therefore, forgiveness is granted both with and without repentance, by the Lord and the Goddess.

In human relations, one can be more realistic, and there are other stories to illustrate these issues. In his earthly incarnation as Rama, Vishnu forgives Sugriva after he has shown repentance. Sugriva offers to help Rama and later forgets about it. Rama waits for a long time, is angered by the delay, then sends his brother Lakshmana to remind Sugriva about his forgotten promise. Sugriva apologizes and is warmly forgiven by Rama. There is complete reconciliation. However, in the epic Mahabharata, when the Kaurava princes dishonor the queen Draupadi in a royal court and exult about it, she does not forgive them. Nor is there expectancy that she would forgive them when there is no repentance on their side.

Does forgiveness necessitate reconciliation? In other words, is it possible to forgive while deciding not to reconcile with the offender?

Judaism (Dorff)

Forgiveness does not necessitate reconciliation, nor does reconciliation require forgiveness. That is, I may forgive an offender but decide that I do not want to associate any longer with him or her. We always, after all, have the right to choose our friends. When the offender is a family member, this right is more restricted, for the nature of families requires that we do our best to get along with them, even if we do not like particular members of the family very much. Similarly, longtime friendships do impose a moral obligation on us to do our best to get past an offense and restore the relationship. Family members and good friends deserve that effort by virtue of their support over the years and their assumption of the duty of future support. Nevertheless, even in those circumstances, some offenses may cause us to refuse to reconcile with a person even though we do consciously and sincerely forgive her or him. Forgiveness, after all, does not require forgetting the offense, and some memories are too painful to permit further close relationships. Forgiveness does require minimal civility, though, even toward those who have done egregious things to us.

Conversely, I may choose to reconcile with a person even though I do not forgive him or her. My failure to forgive would be a fault on my part if the offender went through the process of return described earlier. If the

offender did not do that, however, I would be under no obligation to forgive. Even so, I may decide that my love for the person and my hope for
future relationships with him or her prompt me to reconcile, despite the
unforgivable thing she or he has done.

One painful example of this last circumstance is the relationship of
contemporary Jews with contemporary Germans. Since the vast majority
of Jews and Germans living today were not even alive during the Holocaust, most Germans do not have the moral standing to ask for forgiveness; after all, they did not do anything wrong. They may nevertheless feel
guilt for the acts of their parents and grandparents. Similarly, most contemporary Jews do not have the moral standing to forgive the Germans;
they were not the ones who directly suffered from the acts of the Nazis. In
many cases, though, family members died horrible deaths at the Nazis'
hands, and so Jews may still feel a certain disdain and fear of the Germans. While forgiveness between contemporary Germans and Jews is
therefore not logically possible, reconciliation is both possible and necessary. Germans and Jews can decide to remember the past but to build new
relationships on a much more positive footing in the present and the future. Reconciliation would be reasonable if contemporary Germans did
all in their power to compensate victims of the Holocaust, prevent a repe-
tition of those horrors, and establish new grounds for positive relationships. That is exactly what post-Holocaust German governments have
done through their program of reparations, their diplomatic support of
the State of Israel, and their welcoming of Soviet Jews into their midst.
Reconciliation is difficult without forgiveness—and many Jews still feel ret-
icent to go to Germany or even to buy German products—but it is possible
and sometimes, as in this case, desirable.

Christianity (Williams)

There are no preconditions for forgiveness. However, forgiveness is a pre-
condition of reconciliation. Christians should never close themselves off
from the possibility of reconciliation, even though they should be realistic
in recognizing that sometimes reconciliation may not occur.

Islam (Ali)

Reconciliation is desirable but not essential to forgiveness. If the victim feels
that the offender has serious character flaws and it is not in his or her best interest, he or she does not have to reconcile. Sometimes it is best for one's
own sanity not to carry on normal relationships with certain kinds of characters, but one should not totally dissociate from Muslim brethren.

Buddhism (Hallisey)

Answering this question depends on what one considers reconciliation to be. Obviously, as my previous answer suggests, mutual reconciliation is not a necessity for the working of compassion. But if one views reconciliation as an expression of the worth and needs of the offender, then this is the distinctive character of compassion. As the *Jatakamala* says, "It is other people's suffering which makes good people suffer: it is that which they cannot endure, not their own suffering."[18] In short, the Buddhist traditions are in general agreement that one must be rather strict in controlling one's own emotions and actions, but at the same time quite tolerant and understanding of the actions of others, especially those which hurt us.

Hinduism (Narayanan)

As mentioned earlier, Hinduism is composed of numerous traditions, many of which would interpret this question differently. Thus, it is impossible to present a "rule of thumb" regarding forgiveness and reconciliation that is practiced and accepted by all of the different traditions. Examples of stories in Hinduism that pertain to forgiveness and reconciliation are generally theological in nature.

DISCUSSION

We (Rye & Pargament) wish to make a few comments regarding similarities and differences in perspectives on forgiveness across religions. Our comments should be viewed with caution since (1) we are social scientists, not scholars in comparative religion; and (2) the format of this chapter did not allow for extensive commentary by religious scholars. However, it is our hope that this discussion will serve as a starting point for an interfaith dialogue about the nature of forgiveness.

Forgiveness is consistent with the worldviews of all the religions represented in this chapter. It is explicitly addressed in Judaism, Christianity, Islam, and Hinduism. In Buddhism, forgiveness is subsumed by the concepts of forbearance and compassion. Furthermore, forgiveness is important to each of these religions. Our Christian and Jewish scholars indicated that forgiveness is central to their traditions. Similarly, forbearance and compassion are central to Buddhism. In Islam, receiving forgiveness from Allah is a foundational theological concern. Interpersonal forgiveness is valued by Islam primarily because Allah values forgiveness. In addition, Islam values interpersonal forgiveness because it can repair relationships and facilitate peace. However, the decision to forgive one's offender is a prerogative of the victim rather than a binding religious duty. In Hinduism, forgiveness appears to be equally as important to dharma as compassion, duty, patience, and other ethical concepts.

Not surprisingly, religions with similar origins provide similar justifications for forgiveness. In the Abrahamic religions (i.e., Judaism, Christianity, Islam), humans are expected to imitate God, who is forgiving by nature. Additionally, people receive forgiveness from God as a function of their willingness to forgive each other. Indeed, forgiveness leads to rewards in the present lifetime and/or after death. In contrast, forgiveness in Buddhism is necessary in order to end suffering of self and others, and to achieve enlightenment. In Hinduism, forgiveness is necessary if one chooses to follow the path of righteousness. According to both Buddhism and Hinduism, unresolved issues such as anger will reappear in subsequent reincarnations through karma.

Christianity, Islam, and Buddhism appear to encourage forgiveness irrespective of whether the offender expresses contrition. Judaism, on the other hand, maintains clearly defined rules for when a victim should forgive. As outlined in Maimonides's *Laws of Forgiveness*, a victim is obligated to forgive only after the offender has expressed contrition and gone through the process of return. Although a victim may choose to forgive even if the offender has failed to go through the process of return, this is discouraged—particularly if the offense was severe. Some sacred Hindu stories depict divine forgiveness without contrition, and other stories indicate that contrition is an important prerequisite for receiving forgiveness from God. Humans are held to different standards than gods, and it appears that humans are not required to forgive when the offender fails to show contrition.

The sacred texts of some religions depict individuals who have forgiven despite experiencing profound injustices. In these religions, it appears that forgiveness is not dependent upon the severity of the offense. Examples include Christ's forgiveness of his executioners, Muhammad's forgiveness of those who persecuted him, and the Buddhist proverb about the ascetic tortured by an enraged king. Hinduism's stance on this matter is unclear. Beck noted that according to *Manu-Samhita* 11.55, some sins were considered unforgivable if intentional (i.e., killing of a Brahmin priest, drinking liquor, stealing, sexual intercourse with the wife of one's spiritual mentor, and associating with someone who has committed any of these sins). However, it remains uncertain how these beliefs are regarded in contemporary Hinduism. Jews who were victims of the Nazi Holocaust during World War II have had to struggle with this issue in a profound way, as captured in Simon Wiesenthal's book (1976) entitled *The Sunflower*. Jews continue to debate whether forgiveness is possible or desirable following such horrific injustice.

Finally, there were differing opinions among the scholars as to whether forgiveness necessitates reconciliation. Our Jewish and Islamic scholars indicated that reconciliation was not a requirement of forgiveness. Our Buddhist scholar indicated that compassion and reconciliation are closely related, although he noted that one can be compassionate in the absence of reconciliation. Our Christian scholar indicated that forgiveness must always allow for the possibility of reconciliation. However, he acknowledged that reconciliation may not always occur. It should be noted that other Christian authors make clearer distinctions between forgiveness and reconciliation (e.g., Smedes, 1996). Narayanan pointed out that there was no "rule of thumb" on this matter that could be applied to the diverse Hindu traditions.

In conclusion, we hope that researchers and clinicians interested in forgiveness begin to consider the rich conceptualizations of forgiveness as provided by religious traditions. We believe there is wisdom in the perspectives of religious traditions, which were considering important questions long before psychology existed as a formal science. As Huston Smith (1994) pointed out, the willingness to listen is the first step toward understanding religious traditions. Religious understandings of concepts such as forgiveness might provide social scientists with invaluable insights into the nature of human experience. At the very least, they deserve further exploration.

NOTES

1. Edward William Lane, *Arabic–English Lexicon* (Lahore, Pakistan: Islamic Book Center, 1982). Originally published by William and Norgate, London, England, 1863.
2. J. M. Cowan, ed., *The Hans Wehr Dictionary of Modern Written Arabic*, 3rd ed. (Ithaca: Spoken Language Services, Inc., 1976).
3. Allah, al-lah, is the name of Supreme Being in Arabic language; in English, the God or in Hebrew, Eloh or Elohim. Allah is the Creator, the Evolver, the Shaper of everything in the universe. In this article, the names Allah and God have been used as synonyms.
4. G. P. Malalasekcra, *English–Sinhalese Dictionary* (Colombo: Gunasena, 1982).
5. Peter Khoroche, trans., *When the Buddha was a Monkey: Arya Sura's Jatakamala* (Chicago: University of Chicago Press, 1989), 177.
6. This chapter uses the following Qur'an translation: Muhammad Asad, trans., *The Message of the Qur'an* (Gibralter: Dar Al-Andalus, 1980). Other Qur'an translations consulted were by Abdullah Yusuf Ali, trans., *The Holy Qur'an, Text, Translation and Commentary* (Brentwood, MD: Amana Corporation, 1989) and Muhammad Marmaduke Pickthal, trans., The Glorious Qur'an. Text and Explanatory Translation, various publishers.
7. Fazle Karim, trans., *Mishkat al-Masabih* under the title *Al-Hadis*, Vol. 1, No. 339 (Lahore, Pakistan: The Book House, 1938), 548.
8. Fazle Karim, trans., *Al-Hadis*, No. 192w, p. 548.
9. Imam Al-Nawawi, *Riyadh-Us-Saleheen*, S. M. Madni-Abbasi, trans., Vol. 1, No. 45 (Karachi, Pakistan: International Islamic Publishers [Pvt.] Ltd., 1990), 43.
10. Muhammad Husayn Haykal, *The Life of Muhammad*, Isma'il Ragi A. al-Faruqi, trans. (North American Trust Publications, 1976), 408.
11. A. P. Buddhadatta, trans., *Dhammapadam: An Anthology of Sayings of the Buddha* (Colombo: Apothecaries, n.d.), 2.
12. Peter Khoroche, trans., *When the Buddha was a Monkey: Arya Sura's Jatakamala*, 197.

13. Ralph T. H. Griffith, trans. *The Hymns of the Rig-Veda* (Delhi: Motilal Banarsidass, 1973 Reprint), 378.
14. Dietrich Bonhoeffer, *The Cost of Discipleship,* R. H. Fuller, trans. (New York: Macmillan, 1963).
15. Peter Khoroche, When the Buddha was a Monkey: Arya Sura's Jatakamala, 202–203.
16. Vasudha Narayanan, "The Goddess Sri: Blossoming Lotus and Breast Jewel of Vishnu," in *The Divine Consort: Radha and The Goddesses of India,* eds. John S. Hawley and Donna Wulff (Berkeley Religious Studies Series, 1982).
17. Vasudha Narayanan, "Sri: Giver of Fortune, Bestower of Grace," in *Devi: Goddesses of India,* eds. John S. Hawley and Donna Wulff (University of California Press, 1996).
18. Peter Khoroche, *When the Buddha was a Monkey: Arya Sura's Jatakamala,* 178.

REFERENCES

Dorff, E. N. (1998). The elements of forgiveness: A Jewish approach. In E. L. Worthington, Jr. (Ed.), *Dimensions of forgiveness* (pp. 29–55). Radnor, PA: John Templeton Press.

Educational Psychology Study Group. (1990). Must a Christian require repentance before forgiving? *Journal of Psychology and Christianity, 9,* 16–19.

Enright, R. D., Eastin, D. L., Golden, S., Sarinopoulos, I., & Freedman, S. (1992). Interpersonal forgiveness within the helping professions: An attempt to resolve differences of opinion. *Counseling and Values, 36,* 84–103.

Enright, R. D., & Zell, R. L. (1989). Problems encountered when we forgive one another. *Journal of Psychology and Christianity, 8,* 52–60.

Gassin, E. A., & Enright, R. D. (1995). The will to meaning in the process of forgiveness. *Journal of Psychology and Christianity, 14,* 38–49.

Gorsuch, R. L., & Hao, J. Y. (1993). Forgiveness: An exploratory factor analysis and its relationship to religious variables. *Review of Religious Research, 34,* 333–347.

Jones-Haldeman, M. (1992). Implications from selected literary devices for a new testament theology of grace and forgiveness. *Journal of Psychology and Christianity, 11,* 136–146.

McCullough, M. E., & Worthington, E. L., Jr. (in press). Religion and the forgiving personality. *Journal of Personality.*

Newman, L. E. (1987). The quality of mercy: On the duty to forgive in the Judaic tradition. *Journal of Religious Ethics, 15,* 155–172.

Paloma, M. M., & Gallup, G. H., Jr. (1991). *Varieties of prayer: A survey report.* Philadelphia: Trinity Press International.

Pargament, K. I., & Rye, M. S. (1998). Forgiveness as a method of religious coping. In E. L. Worthington, Jr. (Ed.), *Dimensions of forgiveness* (pp. 59–78). Radnor, PA: John Templeton Press.

Pingleton, J. P. (1989). The role and function of forgiveness in the psychotherapeutic process. *Journal of Psychology and Theology, 17,* 27–35.

Rokeach, M. (1973). *The nature of human values.* New York: Free Press.

Rye, M. S., & Pargament, K. I. (1998). *Forgiveness and romantic relationships in college: Can it heal the wounded heart?* Manuscript submitted for publication.

Shoemaker, A., & Bolt, M. (1977). The Rokeach Value Survey and perceived Christian values. *Journal of Psychology and Theology, 5,* 139–142.

Smedes, L. B. (1996). *The art of forgiving.* Nashville, TN: Moorings.

Smith, H. (1994). *The illustrated world's religions: A guide to our wisdom traditions.* New York: HarperCollins.

Wiesenthal, S. (1976). *The sunflower.* New York: Schocken Books.

The Meaning of Forgiveness in a Specific Situational and Cultural Context

Persons Living with HIV/AIDS in India

Lydia R. Temoshok and Prabha S. Chandra

It is clear that the interpersonal as well as the intrapsychic dynamics of forgiveness will vary according to one's culture, as well as one's life situation (age, gender, socioeconomic status, health status, marital and family status, etc.). The main goal of this chapter is to explore the meaning of forgiveness in a specific cultural context—India, and in a specific health status situation—being infected with human immunodeficiency virus (HIV), the virus that causes acquired immune deficiency syndrome (AIDS). A secondary purpose is to describe the conceptual foundations for developing an assessment methodology that would be appropriate, applicable, and valid for health status situations and cross-cultural contexts.

The HIV/AIDS epidemic constitutes an unprecedented biopsychosocial phenomenon impacting not only health but also all aspects of life for persons living with HIV/AIDS (PLWHA), including marriage and intimate relations, childbearing and parenthood, work and social functioning, as well as psychological and spiritual well-being (Temoshok, 1990, 1998). As a health status situation, HIV/AIDS provides perhaps the quintessential paradigm for studying the impact of forgiveness on quality of life. It may be said that perceptions of HIV/AIDS are much like perceptions of cancer in the United States 50 years ago: a usually fatal, essentially incurable disease associated with stigma and a sense of hopelessness (although advances in treatment options with combination therapies have improved the capacity to treat a significant proportion of HIV-infected individuals, but primarily in developed versus developing nations). Unlike cancer, however, HIV is an infectious disease, transmissible by two of the most intrinsic human forces—sexuality and procreation. The intense fear and stigma surrounding transmission in these most intimate of human connections have cast the multidimensional concept of forgiveness in a central role for those living with HIV/AIDS and their loved ones. How do HIV-infected (HIV+) women and men come to terms with the natural desires to give life and to see life continue through their children, and the realistic fear that their children may be born infected with HIV, or if spared that fate, may become orphans at a young age (Goldschmidt, Temoshok, & Brown, 1993)? How do HIV-infected individuals come to terms with—and forgive—those who infected them, and with God or other spiritual beings who allowed this tragedy to occur?

HIV/AIDS IN INDIA

The Epidemiological Context

The dimensions of the HIV epidemic defy the imagination: By the beginning of 1998, over 30 million people worldwide were infected with HIV, the virus that causes AIDS, and according to estimates by the United Nations Program on HIV/AIDS (UNAIDS) and the World Health Organization (WHO) (UNAIDS & WHO, 1998), 11.7 million people had already lost their lives to the disease. HIV infections are concentrated in the developing world, mostly in countries least able to afford care for infected people. Most recently, infection rates are rising rapidly in Eastern Europe, southern Africa, and in much of Asia, including India, the focus of this chapter.

Although surveillance is patchy, it is estimated that about 4 million people in India are living with HIV, making India the country with the largest number of HIV-infected people in the world (UNAIDS & WHO, 1998). In September 1998, WHO Director General Gro Brundtland said that as many as 7 million Indians may be HIV-infected (Agence France-Presse, 1998). Recent testing of pregnant women in Pondicherry shows infection rates of around 4%.

The Most Vulnerable Populations

HIV in India has been attributable mainly to heterosexual transmission, although in some states, particularly the northeastern state of Manipur, the epidemic took off quickly among male drug injectors. Among the most affected segments of the population are sex workers and truck drivers (UNAIDS & WHO, 1998).

Truck Drivers

Among truck drivers in the southern sate of Madras, HIV prevalence quadrupled from 1.5% in 1995 to 6.2% just 1 year later (UNAIDS & WHO, 1998). Nationally, the current infection rate for truck drivers is 10 per 1,000, many times higher than the infection rate of 0.5 cases per 1,000 in the general population (Rao, Pilli, Rao, & Chalam, 1999).

With one of the largest road networks in the world and an estimated 5 million long-distance truck drivers, it is not surprising that the spread of HIV in India has generally followed the truck routes. Truck drivers, who are away from their families for long durations, often turn to commercial sex workers along the highways for sexual recreation. A 1994 survey of 5,709 long-distance truck drivers found that 87% of the men had multiple partners but only 11% used condoms during encounters with commercial sex workers (Rao et al., 1999). Among unmarried men ages 21–30 years, 78% reported having had between 31 and 60 sexual partners during the prior 12 months. It is thought that truck drivers acquire the infection from sex workers in urban settings where HIV prevalence is highest, and subsequently spread the disease along their truck routes to uninfected sex workers, as well as to their current and/or future wives and partners when they return home, usually to more rural villages (Mann & Tarantola, 1996). In nearly all marital situations involving HIV, it is the man who infects his wife or partner after he acquires the infection through sex workers (Chandra, 1996).

Sex Workers

Throughout the world, women who are sex workers are at high risk of becoming infected with HIV and other sexually transmitted diseases, and of suffering a lower quality of life than infected women who are not sex workers (d'Cruze-Grote, 1996). HIV seroprevalence from 1986 to 1994 among women sex workers in Asia was highest in Madurai, India (54.7%), and above 30% in several other regions in India (Mann & Tarantola, 1996).

The sex industry in India, along with other Asian countries, displays often appalling conditions of forced prostitution and sexual exploitation (Muecke, 1992). In general, commercial sex work is a direct result of economic pressures, not choice. When sex workers rely on a client for money to pay for food, housing, or drugs, they are not in a position to be adamant about demanding that condoms be used (Mann, Tarantola, &

Netter, 1992). Once sex workers have contracted HIV, which is virtually inevitable in high-prevalence areas, survival for themselves and their children becomes an immediate and all-consuming problem.

In Mumbai (formerly Bombay), police commonly raid brothels, forcibly testing women for HIV and putting those found to be HIV+ in detention centers, where, according to an August 1996 newswire report, they are treated not as victims but as criminals. The sudden raids mean that women often leave behind money, belongings, even children. Tuberculosis (TB) is common in the detention centers, and HIV-infected women easily contract the disease. Many of these women, kidnaped from Nepal or otherwise forced into prostitution, are unable to return home to obtain support from their families and communities.

These problems are exacerbated for very young girls, who are often sold into prostitution by their families and thus, in a very real sense, are sex slaves with no rights and no one to whom to appeal for help. Younger females are especially vulnerable to HIV infection because their greater susceptibility to tearing and immature cervical cells allows the virus easier access to the bloodstream. Fear of AIDS is primarily responsible for "the spiraling demand for younger and younger children," according to Ofelia Calcetas-Santos, United Nations (UN) Special Rapporteur on Human Rights, in a study on children prostitution released November 1996 by the UN.

What It Means to Be Infected with HIV in India

HIV infection in India carries with it stigma, isolation, and discrimination. It is considered a "dirty disease," and a result of bad behavior. Family members often consider it a disgrace to have an HIV-infected person in the family. In such a context, HIV and AIDS are often associated with shame, guilt, and a feeling of having sinned (Bharat, 1995). Despite the increasing prevalence of HIV infection in India, knowledge regarding how HIV is spread is still very poor. HIV infection carries with it connotations of being contagious, incurable, and untreatable—similar to how leprosy was viewed in the past. Added to this is the prevalent attitude that PLWHA are immoral, and hence deserving of the suffering they experience as a result of HIV/AIDS (Bharat, 1995; Ahuja, Parkar, & Yeolakar, 1998).

HIV-Related Stressors Associated with Medical Needs and the Healthcare System

In a country where resources are meager, access to health care is poor, and lack of knowledge regarding the illness begets negative attitudes, even among health care providers, PLWHA have to deal with multiple stressors (Chandra & Prasadarao, in press). One significant set of stressors comprises poor physical health and the depletion of financial resources because of difficulty carrying out normal work and family care, as well as treatment costs.

Another source of stress is widespread inaccessibility of adequate health care. A number of barriers to quality care have been identified, including patient-related barriers (e.g., the perception that HIV/AIDS is incurable, and the reluctance of families to disclose that they have an infected family member), and barriers related to the health care delivery system (e.g., a person with AIDS seeking help in a rural clinic is usually referred to a specialized center in an urban area, which is inaccessible because of distance and cost) (Chandra & Prasadarao, in press).

Few patients can afford the expensive combination HIV medications that have made such a dramatic difference in reducing HIV mortality in the United States and Western Europe since 1997. The lack of access to these medications may be part of the reason for the increasing interest in alternative ("traditional" or unconventional) treatment methods. P. S. Chandra has observed that nearly 65% of HIV patients attending the counseling and care clinic in Bangalore have at some point tried some alternative treatment. Unfortunately, few of these treatments have proven efficacy, many have serious side effects, and most do no more than further deplete a family's resources (Chandra & Prasadarao, in press).

Psychological Reactions to Having HIV Infection

Prominent among the psychosocial problems with which PLWHA struggle are stigma, discrimination, and isolation, which in turn lead to feelings of alienation, guilt, and hopelessness. People who learn they are seropositive often become acutely depressed and may exhibit suicidal ideation (Ahuja et al., 1998; Chandra, Ravi, Desai, & Subbakrishna, 1998). Anxiety and depression related to fear of impending death and the social stigma associated with HIV/AIDS were reported in 33% of HIV patients attending a clinic in Mumbai (Ahuja et al., 1998). In a study of defense personnel, overall psychiatric morbidity was 50% among HIV-infected personnel compared to 10% among uninfected controls; depression was the most frequently observed condition (23%) (Madan, Singh, & Golechha, 1997). Depression is often related to a feeling of having done something wrong and of being irrevocably contaminated, as well as to stigma and isolation (Chandra & Prasadarao, in press).

HIV centers in South India have reported that suicidal thoughts occur in nearly 25% of PLWHA across the disease trajectory (Jacob, Eapen, John, & John, 1991). Suicidal ideas and attempts are most commonly seen soon after a person is informed of his or her seropositive status, in the context of social stigma and isolation, and when he or she experiences uncontrollable pain (Chandra et al., 1998).

Individuals forced to cope with these multiple stressors in the absence of organized counseling and social services often resort to familial support or spiritual methods of coping.

Dealing with HIV within the Family

The family plays a central role in Indian society. A person is often known as part of his or her family, and individual self-esteem is usually linked to family esteem and acceptance. Under these circumstances, the family's level of forgiveness and acceptance has a major influence on a person's sense of self worth. Among families in India, HIV infection is considered a stigma that can lead to ostracization of the family. Families often verbalize their anger at the HIV-infected individual for having disgraced the family, and blame that person. This attitude is often introjected by the PLWHA, who then feels responsible and guilty for all the problems that befall family members.

Discrimination and isolation of the PLWHA also occurs within the family. Common misperceptions and fear of transmitting infection through casual contact often result in self and/or family-imposed isolation of the PLWHA from spouse and children (e.g., eating, bathing, and sleeping separately) (Chandra & Prasadarao, in press). Even when families do not overtly desert HIV-infected members and continue to provide shelter and care, the infected individuals often feel emotionally isolated.

Although the family can be a source of stress to PLWHA, it can also be a source of strength and solace. A study of quality of life among HIV-infected men in India revealed a strong correlation between the quality of the marital relationship and subjective well-being (Krishna, 1996). A (subjectively) better quality of life was particularly related to affectional needs being met. Most of the respondents reported poor marital relationships; however, it was unclear whether this preceded their HIV infection or was a consequence of informing (and possibly infecting) their wives. In any case, these findings are relevant to planning psychosocial intervention programs for families with HIV-infected members.

Gender-Related Stressors within Families

Guilt is a major source of stress, particularly for men in the common situation of having acquired their infection through non-normative, multi-partner sex and/or sex workers. Men's guilt over having acquired HIV in these ways is greatly amplified if they subsequently transmit their infection to their spouses (Chandra & Prasadarao, in press).

Among women, anger is a frequent reaction to being infected through no fault of their own, a feeling of being victims of a situation that renders them vulnerable to HIV infection, and a reflection of being powerless in preventing the infection (Radhakrishnan, 1995). An October 1996 newswire report described the following, tragically, not uncommon situation in India: A husband becomes HIV-infected from an extramarital relationship with a sex worker and subsequently infects his wife, who is then blamed by in-laws for infecting the husband. The HIV+ wife is then thrown out on the streets to fend for herself and her HIV+ children, who become vulnerable to disease, violence, and, if girls, to sexual exploitation, with the consequent risk of HIV infection.

Having children and continuing the family lineage is an important aspect of Indian culture, even more so in women than in men. The majority of HIV-infected women are young and widowed, because their husbands have already died of the disease. Widowed women are seldom allowed to remarry; thus, the HIV-infected woman often carries the burden of multiple severe stressors: being HIV-infected, widowed, unable to remarry, and unable to have (more) children. Because treatments to prevent HIV infection during pregnancy are unavailable to the vast majority of women in developing countries, including India, if an HIV-infected woman becomes pregnant, she is usually advised to terminate the pregnancy (Chandra & Prasadarao, 2000).

RELIGION IN INDIA AND ITS ROLE IN FORGIVENESS

The condemnatory connotations of HIV infection as resulting from "sin" of one kind or another lead many PLWHA to internalize societal blame, which is then transformed into intrapunitive states of shame and guilt. In trying to cope with the internal as well as external suffering associated with HIV infection and AIDS, PLWHA may turn to religion and spirituality in an effort to find comfort, understanding, and a sense of meaning in their illness (cf. Pargament, 1997, for a discussion of religious coping). Forgiveness can be a major component of such coping (Pargament & Rye, 1998). For example, a sense of blame can be diminished when one forgives the self, or when God or another Spiritual Being or Force is forgiven for not remedying the situation of illness (Winiarski, 1991).

Hindu Philosophy and the Theory of Karma

Although a number of religions are represented in India, the vast majority of Indians are Hindus (83%), followed by Muslims (11%), Christians (2%), Sikhs (2%), Buddhists (0.7%), and Jains (0.5%) (Microsoft Corporation, 1996). Thus, we limit our discussion to Hinduism (cf. Chapter 2, this volume, for a discussion of forgiveness in other religions). Among Hindus, the theory of karma is often used to explain suffering and bad fortune (Radhakrishnan, 1995). According to this theory, this life, with all its pains and pleasures, is determined by the accumulated merit and demerits that result from all the actions committed in past lives ("As ye sow, thus shall ye reap"). Accrued karma can be counteracted by expiations and rituals, by "working out" through punishment or reward, or by renouncing all worldly desires (O'Flaherty, 1996). Every action is thought to lead to two results, a directly observable result of pain or pleasure, and the establishment of a disposition (i.e., a tendency to repeat the same action through the cycle of activity and rebirth). Tendencies are both acquired and hereditary, and are carried forward from previous births. Although they may be changed or modified, the direct result cannot be escaped.

In the theory of karma, the individual is responsible and accountable for everything in his or her life, even though something may have originated as a problem in a previous life. There is an acceptance of both pleasant and unpleasant happenings as being of one's own making. Thus, in Hindu philosophy, an individual is responsible for his or her actions but not to blame for misfortune. To the extent that misery is seen as a greater teacher than happiness, even misery can offer a kind of solace.

Forgiveness

In Hindu philosophy, forgiveness has been defined as the unaffected condition of the mind of a person, even while being reviled or chastised. Forgiveness has also been described as tolerance and as absence of agitation of the mind even though there is cause for agitation. The state of forgiveness is considered an important step in achieving equanimity or tolerance, both of which are considered virtues. Forgiveness is thought to be both verbal and mental, and manifests itself in attitudes and feelings, and through actions (Radhakrishnan, 1995; Sinha, 1985). Forgiveness has been distinguished from *non-anger*. When no change is produced in the mind of an abused or persecuted person, he or she has forgiveness. In forgiveness, there is, genuinely, no anger. In *non-anger*, however, the anger is suppressed but still exists in the mind, where it leaks out like a slow poison.

HIV and Forgiveness

Although Hindu philosophy and teachings in Indian culture emphasize the value of forgiveness and tolerance, conflicts related to these concepts are quite evident among individuals with afflictions such as HIV/AIDS. The first question an Indian affected with any illness would ask is, "Have I done anything wrong to have suffered from this illness, or is it a punishment for past sins?" The person would then use the theory of karma to find meaning in the situation. Before achieving that stage of equanimity, however, the person often goes through a process of anger, decrying the unfairness of the situation, and feeling unforgiving of the persons or situations perceived as responsible for the condition.

A PILOT STUDY OF ATTITUDES RELATED TO FORGIVENESS IN FAMILIES OF PLWHA

P. S. Chandra has been conducting an ongoing study through the HIV counseling and care clinic at the National Institute of Mental Health and Neurosciences in Bangalore of the attitudes of families that include someone living with HIV/AIDS. Interviews that included a special focus on the issue of forgiveness were conducted with 52 PLWHA, 25 women and 27 men.

Attitudes of Family Members

A striking observation was that 67% of family members blamed HIV-infected members for their condition, and 45% felt they would never be able to forgive them for this. Men appeared to be more unforgiving than women. For example, the father of a 26-year-old man who died of AIDS said soon after his son's death: "He should not have been born into our family, and I can never forgive him for what he did to us. We did not perform any funeral rites for him, and we feel he should suffer the way he has made us all suffer." This father also blamed the son for other negative events in the family, even those that were not directly related to the son's illness.

Attitudes of PLWHA toward Other Family Members

PLWHA are often unable to forgive family members for circumstances that led to their acquiring HIV infection. This is particularly true among infected women, who blame family and societal traditions for their vulnerability. For example, a 28-year-old widowed, HIV-infected woman said, "It is my parents whom I cannot forgive. They should not have made me marry a person with these bad habits. Instead, they should have educated me and helped me to become independent. More than my husband, I blame my parents for my current state, and will not be able to forgive them."

The women were asked who they felt was responsible for their current situation (multiple responses were allowed). Seventy percent felt God was responsible, 80% felt their family of origin was responsible, while 40% held their sexual partner responsible. Only three women felt that they were in some way responsible for their infection. All those who felt their families were responsible indicated that they could not forgive them easily.

Interview Findings on the Issue of Forgiveness in Men versus Women

In the interviews, women appeared to be unforgiving of the situations that rendered them vulnerable to infection in the first place and power-less to change these situations. They were, however, able to reconcile some of these unforgiving feelings by accepting their HIV infection as "fate." Among men, a key issue was forgiving the self. This is probably be-cause HIV infection among Indian men is most often a consequence of risk taking, while among women, the infection is acquired through a spouse or partner (Chandra, 1996).

Most of the women interviewed were in sex work because of difficult life situations and were unable to forgive the men who transmitted the in-fection to them. Not forgiving, therefore, appeared to stem from anger. They were also unable to forgive others and society in general for isolat-ing them and holding them responsible for spreading HIV infection. Given these circumstances, it is understandable that HIV-infected sex workers had difficulty resolving their unforgiving feelings through reli-gion.

Observations Regarding Emotional State

While recording the narratives about forgiveness, it was observed that the level and type of forgiveness varied as a function of the individual's mood state and immediate events. If the person was found to be depressed or angry, the level of forgiveness was lower. Anger was usually associated with not forgiving the person or persons perceived as the cause of infec-tion, and not forgiving God. Sadness and depression were evident when the person felt unforgiven, usually in an interpersonal context. There ap-peared to be a strong relationship between the state of well-being and the state of forgiveness, although it would be difficult to designate which is the cause and which the effect.

Working through the Issue of Forgiveness

Different methods of dealing with the issue of forgiveness were evident among the PLWHA interviewed. Those individuals with unforgiving atti-tudes tended to alienate themselves from their families as well as the health care system. These individuals also tended to persist in transmis-sion risk behaviors and frequent substance use. On the other hand, those who were able to forgive God and others were found to be more spiritu-ally inclined, adhered more to health care recommendations, and were more accepting of their circumstances, including suffering. These individ-uals also had fewer fears of death. Most study participants felt that God had or would forgive them, or that the suffering they were currently en-during was sufficient punishment to ensure better circumstances later or in their next lives.

These and other observations from this ongoing study suggested that it would be important to articulate a theoretical framework that would encompass the complexity of forgiveness for people both infected and affected by HIV/AIDS. Considering the global nature of the HIV pan-demic, it would be useful to apply such a framework in developing meth-odology appropriate for the kind of cross-cultural research on HIV and quality of life that is being implemented by the WHO, as described below.

FOUNDATIONS FOR STUDYING FORGIVENESS AS A DIMENSION OF QUALITY OF LIFE FOR PLWHA

Quality of Life, Forgiveness, and HIV/AIDS

To the extent that *forgiveness* is an inextricable component of *quality of life,* a concept that incorporates, but is broader than, health, it is important to bring these two concepts to bear in order better to understand the biopsy-chosocial impact of HIV/AIDS. Quality of life needs to be understood as a multidimensional construct incorporating the complex interrelation-ships among physical health, spiritual well-being, psychological state, cop-ing, work/role functioning, social relationships, cultural values, as well as personal goals, beliefs, and concerns (e.g., Testa & Simonson, 1996).

The WHO's Work on Assessing Quality of Life

Because our focus in this chapter is on India, we restrict our discussion of quality-of-life instruments to the international arena and the seminal work of the WHO in developing a Quality of Life Assessment Instrument (the WHOQOL) appropriate for international and cross-cultural studies. This instrument consists of six broad domains (physical, psychological, level of independence, social relationships, environment, and spirituality), each containing a number of subdomains or facets (WHOQOL Group, 1993, 1994). Results of international pilot testing in 15 collaborating centers throughout the world have attested to the instrument's reliability and cross-cultural validity (WHOQOL Group, 1995).

Assessing Quality of Life for PLWHA

With the rapid spread of HIV worldwide, WHO recognized the necessity of developing an international quality-of-life assessment module specifi-cally focused on HIV/AIDS (Temoshok & the WHOQOL Group, 1997).

The conceptual and methodological work described in this chapter were stimulated by a 1997 expert consultation to the WHO Division of Mental Health, which included Temoshok and Chandra. The WHOQOL was examined for its relevance and global applicability to PLWHA. The consultation concluded that the least elaborated of the existing domains, and thus the one requiring the most work to make it relevant to concerns of PLWHA, was that dealing with spirituality, religion, and personal beliefs (WHO/Division of Mental Health/Temoshok, 1997). It is within this domain that the concept of *forgiveness* plays a key role.

In the WHO consultation, the facet of forgiveness was conceptualized as two dimensional—forgiving and being forgiven (WHO/Division of Mental Health/Temoshok, 1997). This conceptualization suggested four separate areas of inquiry: (1) whether people forgive themselves (in the case of PLWHA, forgiving themselves for getting infected); (2) whether they forgive others—family, partners, caregivers, "God," Divine being or spiritual forces (e.g., others who they believe have let them down, failed to protect them, led them into situations that resulted in infection, or caused them other misfortune); (3) whether others forgive them (e.g., for being a burden, an embarrassment, or for having violated their trust); and (4) whether "God" or spiritual forces forgive them.

A Theoretical Framework for Research on Forgiveness and HIV/AIDS

In considering how these concepts could be elaborated into a more systematic model and method for assessing forgiveness (separate from other aspects of quality of life), Temoshok developed a theoretical framework, presented in Table 3.1, based largely upon her experience working with PLWHA in the United States and Europe over the past 16 years (e.g., Temoshok & Moulton, 1991; Straits, Temoshok, & Zich, 1990). This framework depicts a widening series of relevant contexts—biological, self, interpersonal, health care, community, and spiritual. For each context, specific emotional, cognitive, psychosocial, and behavioral consequences relevant to quality of life are hypothesized to be associated with forgiveness on the one hand, and with lack of forgiveness on the other. There is also the implicit hypothesis that forgiveness, across contexts, will be associated with "better" health outcomes, while lack of forgiveness will be result in "worse" health outcomes; that is, within each stage of disease, people who are able to forgive and to feel forgiven on multiple levels will have a better overall health status than those who are not.

A number of hypotheses concerning the relationships between forgiveness, quality of life, and health outcomes in HIV/AIDS can be generated on the basis of this theoretical framework. For example, considering the interpersonal context, one could hypothesize that PLWHA who have been able to forgive others and let go of unproductive feelings of anger, bitterness, resentment, or disappointment will probably be able to seek and receive social support more effectively from others. Feeling forgiven is associated with feeling loved, connected with others in a positive way, and feeling higher self-esteem—all states associated with more positive health outcomes in contradistinction to states of guilt, isolation, and self-blame (e.g., Benson, 1996; Pert, 1997). To the extent that social support is especially important for PLWHA, who often face stigma, isolation, and discrimination from multiple sources, forgiveness in this context would be hypothesized to be related to enhanced quality of life (Zich & Temoshok, 1987).

At the biological level, lack of forgiveness is hypothesized to engender negative states such as stress, fear, and anger, which decrease homeostasis and result in physiological and psychological dysfunction. Elsewhere, Temoshok has described the psychoneuroimmunological linkages by which psychosocial phenomena (including forgiveness) are hypothesized to influence homeostasis and immune functioning, and thus, health outcomes in HIV disease (Solomon, Kemeny, & Temoshok, 1991; Temoshok, 1993, 1997).

DEVELOPING AN APPROPRIATE METHOD FOR ASSESSING MULTIPLE CONTEXTS OF FORGIVENESS

Most measures of forgiveness in the psychological literature have concentrated on the interpersonal context (e.g., McCullough, Worthington, & Rachal, 1997), although some measures have subscales concerned with the self and/or spiritual context (e.g., Wade, 1989). To our knowledge, none have assessed forgiveness in the community or health care contexts that are of particular relevance for PLWHA. In order to measure or assess levels of forgiveness or lack of forgiveness across the contexts set forth in Table 3.1, we decided to adapt a methodology used by Temoshok to assess three types of general patterns of reactions to stressful life circumstances, including health status (Temoshok & Dreher, 1992; Temoshok, 1997).

The Vignette Similarity Assessment Method

In the Temoshok coping vignettes, respondents are asked to read several vignettes or paragraphs, each describing a person reacting to a stressful situation (e.g., a diagnosis of HIV or cancer, worsening disease symptoms, or a natural disaster). The person in each vignette is described as thinking, feeling, and behaving in ways that are consistent with a specific and distinct pattern of coping (i.e., "adaptive," "helpless/hopeless," or "Type C"

TABLE 3.1. Hypothesized Consequences and Outcomes for Different Contexts of Forgiveness

	Forgiveness			
Relevant contexts	Positive emotional and cognitive consequences	Psychosocial consequences	Behavioral consequences	Health outcomes
Spiritual	Love, hope, compassion	Hope, redemption	Spiritual integration	
Community	Caring, responsibility	Social integration	Ethical, responsible, altruistic behavior	
Health care	Trust, empowerment	Encouraged, partnership	↑ Adherence, ↑ Participation	
Interpersonal	Conciliation, acceptance	Relationship restored	↑ Intimacy, ↑ Social support	
Self	Acceptance, affirmation	Self-esteem	↑ Coping behaviors, better self-care	Better health outcomes
Biological	Letting go, relaxation	Coherence, balance	↑ Homeostasis	↑ Functioning
	Lack of forgiveness			
Relevant contexts	Negative emotional and cognitive consequences	Psychosocial consequences	Behavioral consequences	Health outcomes
Biological	Anger, fear, stress	Imbalance, incoherence, self-hatred	↓ Homeostasis	Dysfunction
Self	Anxiety, depression, feels victimized		Self-destructive behaviors	Worse health outcomes
Interpersonal	Bitterness, rumination	Conflict, discord	Divorce, abuse, revenge, violence	
Health care	Distrust, disempowerment	Discouragement	↓ Adherence, more avoidance behavior	
Community	Holding grudge, feelings of revenge	Social isolation	Irresponsible, antisocial behaviors	
Spiritual	Hopelessness	Despair	Suicide, homicide	

coping; Temoshok & Dreher, 1992). Respondents are asked to rate (on a scale of 1 to 10) how much they are similar or dissimilar to the person in each vignette, where the gender of the person in the vignette is matched to that of the respondent.

Because the vignettes are about other people, being asked to rate similarity to the emotions and behaviors *of others* (rather than rating one's own emotions and behaviors on a series of items in a scale) appears to circumvent or minimize defensiveness about reporting socially less desirable states and behaviors. Thus, the method is particularly useful for assessing complex coping patterns such as "Type C," which is defined as being less able to express or even be aware of so-called negative emotions (anger, sadness, fear), and presenting instead a socially pleasant facade to the world (Temoshok & Dreher, 1992).

This vignette method for assessing general patterns of coping has been adapted for use in several studies involving PLWHA (Solano et al., 1993), people who have recently experienced traumatic events (Temoshok & Moulton, 1991), and people with cancer (Temoshok & Dreher, 1992). The general experience with these different populations in the United States and Europe has been that this vignette method is well accepted and even liked by study participants (good face validity), and is a strong and significant predictor of health outcomes (high predictive validity) (cf. Messick, 1995).

Adapting the Vignette Similarity Method for Assessing Forgiveness

This approach to assessing complex concepts, such as patterns of coping, appears to be well-suited for assessing the complex multiple meanings and contexts of *forgiveness*. Within each context depicted in Table 3.1 (and following the general consensus of the 1997 WHO consultation on developing methods to assess quality of life for PLWHA), the state of forgiveness can be assessed along two dimensions: Forgiving versus Not forgiving, and Feeling forgiven versus Unforgiven. Vignettes describing individuals at the more extreme ends of these dimensions were developed by Temoshok for two of the contexts in Table 3.1: self and spiritual (cf. Appendix 3.1).

Chandra translated the vignettes from English into Kannada (the local language in Bangalore, India), with modifications to make them culturally appropriate. In addition, she developed two vignettes for the interpersonal context based on her work with HIV patients in Bangalore, and particularly the ongoing pilot study described earlier. These vignettes, back-translated into English, are presented in Appendix 3.2.

An Alpha Test of the Forgiveness Vignettes

Although the contexts of "health care" and "community" were included in the theoretical framework of forgiveness contexts (Table 3.1), the authors have not yet developed vignettes pertaining to these contexts. When Chandra conducted an alpha test of the vignettes in Appendix 3.2 on the HIV patients who participated in the interviews focused on forgiveness issues (described earlier), it was clear that the "health care" context, in particular, was a critical one to include. Interviewees expressed feelings reflecting lack of forgiveness related to health care professionals, particularly if the health care encounter had been a negative experience. In the interviews, some PLWHA reported being unable to forgive the person in the health care system who first informed them of their HIV infection. Reacting with understandable anger to the absence of effective treatment modalities or access to combination treatments available in developed countries, PLWHA often have an unforgiving attitude toward those who provide care perceived as inadequate.

The alpha test also suggested that the health care context for forgiveness could be widened conceptually to include counseling and psychosocial/psychiatric care, in addition to medical treatment. In the experience of Chandra, forgiveness issues often emerge in psychotherapy or counseling when the client is unable to forgive the therapist for not making things better, or is concerned about whether the therapist has forgiven the client for past behaviors (including those that may have contributed to the individual becoming infected with HIV). After knowledge of HIV infection, substance use or behavior that poses a risk of HIV transmission to others also raises issues of forgiveness in the psychotherapy situation.

Finally, the alpha test suggested that additional vignettes are probably needed to assess the complexity of forgiveness in the interpersonal context. This context includes not only marital relationships but also family and friends. For example, forgiveness is a prominent issue not only in the interpersonal context of how the infection was acquired but also in relation to subsequent relationships, especially in response to negative attitudes of family or friends who may be perceived as abandoning the PLWHA. Because there may be different degrees of forgiveness in each of these interpersonal situations, more accurate assessment would depend upon having specific vignettes for each relevant interpersonal situation. Obviously, the need to include relevant and significant contexts of forgiveness in order to understand the large and complex picture of forgiveness for PLWHA must be balanced by the exigencies of time for assessment and the cooperation of study participants.

CONCLUDING COMMENTS

We have attempted to explore as comprehensively as possible the meaning of forgiveness for the specific health status situation of being a PLWHA in the cultural context of India. The complexity of this task becomes apparent when one realizes the background required even to embark upon this exploratory journey. The first set of factors introduced into the discussion included the scope and nature of the HIV/AIDS epidemic in India, and more importantly, what it means to be infected with HIV in India, and the stressors associated with culturally interpreted gender differences, familial reactions, and the health care system. Another set of factors concerned religion in India, the role of religion in forgiveness, and how these are experienced by PLWHA in India.

Chandra's clinical experience in Bangalore, India, and her pilot study of PLWHA concerns and attitudes related to forgiveness were used to adapt, elaborate, and alpha test a flexible approach (the vignette similarity method) for assessing different contexts of forgiveness for PLWHA in India. Our approach to assessing forgiveness was also based on several converging bodies of work: Temoshok's experience in working with PLWHA in the United States and Europe, her work using the method to assess other complex constructs in research on the impact of psychosocial factors on health status, and the WHO initiatives on developing and testing a quality-of-life assessment module for cross-cultural studies of PLWHA.

Since it was first proposed by Engel (1977), the biopsychosocial model of health and illness has stimulated some important changes in medicine and clinical care, but its impact on research has been more in terms of supporting an approach rather than providing a framework for generating and testing hypotheses. It is clear that the usefulness of the biopsychosocial model—particularly its capacity to live and function in the real world—depends upon its translation and adaptation to fit the characteristics of specific diseases such as HIV/AIDS (e.g., Temoshok, 1990). In this chapter, we have outlined a theoretical framework for studying forgiveness as a dimension of quality of life for PLWHA. We have also described the application of the vignette similarity method, used in previous biopsychosocial research, to the challenge of assessing forgiveness among PLWHA in India. Our purpose in providing details of our exploratory journey was to illustrate the *process* of developing the framework and tools to conduct meaningful biopsychosocial research on an important psychosocial factor (forgiveness) in a specific situational and cultural context (having HIV/AIDS in India). We hope that in describing our journey, we have offered some ideas for kindred biopsychosocial researchers embarking on their own forays down other research paths, in other situational and cultural contexts.

APPENDIX 3.1. EXAMPLES OF FORGIVENESS VIGNETTES APPROPRIATE FOR NORTH AMERICA, EUROPE, AUSTRALIA

Spiritual Context: Feeling Forgiven

John's first reaction to being told he had HIV was one of shock. Gradually, however, he had come to feel that getting HIV was, in a way, a blessing and a reflection of his redemption by God. There were things he had done—and not done—in his life that John wasn't proud about. But for all John's imperfections, God loved

John so much that He had sent HIV as a "wake up call. " To save him. The call had worked: John was seeing his family, his friends, and what he was doing with his life in a whole new light. God had seen fit to include him in His plan. John's life now had a new purpose that was one with God's. He was filled with hope.

How similar do you think you are to John here? (Please circle ONE number on the scale below).

Extremely Different 1 2 3 4 5 6 7 8 9 10 Extremely Similar

Spiritual Context: Forgiving

Mary recognized that HIV was a very serious and life-threatening disease. It hadn't been easy for her to come to terms with this, and with the fact that God either willed or allowed her to get infected. But then she realized that her having HIV was part of God's plan, and a reflection of His all-knowing wisdom. She might not understand everything about this plan yet, but she accepted that God had a good reason for this and a purpose for her. Mary realized that she no longer felt any anger at God for HIV. In her heart and her mind, she embraced God.

How similar do you think you are to Mary here? (Please circle ONE number on the scale below).

Extremely Different 1 2 3 4 5 6 7 8 9 10 Extremely Similar

Spiritual Context: Feeling Unforgiven

Learning he had HIV hit John like a ton of bricks. His sins had finally caught up with him. Getting HIV was God's just punishment for what he had done—and not done—in his life. A righteous God was seeking vengeance against him—using HIV as his sword. John deserved this, and probably more. He was sure things were going to get even worse when God eventually just abandoned him, and left him to his miserable fate. God was cutting John out of the fabric of life and wanted nothing more to do with him. John felt hopeless.

How similar do you think you are to John here? (Please circle ONE number on the scale below).

Extremely Different 1 2 3 4 5 6 7 8 9 10 Extremely Similar

Spiritual Context: Not Forgiving

Why had God done this to her? Mary wondered. What kind of a God would heap the misery of AIDS on her, or on anyone for that matter? The world was filled with unhappiness, hate, and now the scourge of a terrible disease like AIDS. God had done all this or at least allowed this to happen. Was it because He wasn't so great and good, or because He just didn't care about human beings? The other possibility was that He didn't exist. But HIV and AIDS exist.

Mary hardened her heart and turned her back against a God that could inflict such a disease on her.

How similar do you think you are to Mary here? (Please circle ONE number on the scale below).

Extremely Different 1 2 3 4 5 6 7 8 9 10 Extremely Similar

Self Context: Forgiving

Mary now accepted the fact that she had HIV, much as she accepted the fact that some of her physical features weren't exactly perfect. Yes, probably some of her actions had contributed to her getting HIV in the first place. But she had stopped blaming herself for these past mistakes. Whatever happened, whatever she had done or not done—there was no way to change those things. She accepted this, and felt a kind of peace about it now. Anyway, Mary thought, her imperfections were a part of herself, and who she was as a person. What matters is the whole picture, imperfections and all, and what you do with that. Mary felt good about the whole picture of herself.

How similar do you think you are to Mary here? (Please circle ONE number on the scale below).

Extremely Different 1 2 3 4 5 6 7 8 9 10 Extremely Similar

Self Context: Not Forgiving

Mary thought constantly about what she could have done differently so that she didn't end up getting HIV. "If only I had not done this . . . if only I had done that . . . " were thoughts that ran through her head, especially at night. She blamed herself for what she did—and didn't do. She also blamed herself for who she was. If she had been a different person, this wouldn't have happened to her. But deep down, Mary felt that she could never change who she was, and that basically, she wasn't a very good person. No wonder she got HIV—she deserved this terrible disease, much as she deserved the other bad things that had happened to her in life.

How similar do you think you are to Mary here? (Please circle ONE number on the scale below).

Extremely Different 1 2 3 4 5 6 7 8 9 10 Extremely Similar

APPENDIX 3.2. INDIAN ADAPTATIONS OF FORGIVENESS VIGNETTES, BACK-TRANSLATED INTO ENGLISH

Spiritual Context: Feeling Forgiven

Raju was shocked when he came to know about his HIV status, but gradually he has been feeling that, in a way, it is good that he acquired the infection. He has been repenting for some of his acts in life. He thinks that whatever happens, God loves him, and He has sent this as a caution to him. Because of this, he sees new meaning in his family and friends, as well as himself. Now there is an aim in his life and also some hope.

Spiritual Context: Forgiving

Saroja has understood that HIV is a severe and life-threatening disease. She had initially found it difficult to accept, but she feels now that it is a part of God's creation. If God has given this infection to her, He may have some reason or purpose behind it. She is not angry with God. In fact, she prays to God more than before.

Spiritual Context: Feeling Unforgiven

Mohan felt a heavy burden on his head when he became aware that he was HIV positive. The mistakes that he committed finally had caused problems for him. He thinks that HIV infection is a punishment for certain deeds that he did or did not do in his life. He has the feeling that God is taking revenge on him. He anticipates more problems. God will not help him in any way with his infection. God will remove him from life itself. Mohan is very sad and feels that there is no hope for him at all.

Spiritual Context: Not Forgiving

Why had God done this to her? Saroja wondered. What kind of a God would put her, or anyone, into this misery of AIDS? The world was filled with unhappiness, hate, and now a terrible disease like AIDS had also come into the world. God had done all this, or at least allowed this to happen. Was it because God wasn't so great and good, or because He just doesn't care about human beings? The other possibility was that there was no God. But HIV and AIDS exist. Saroja's heart was hardened, and she stopped praying to a God that could inflict such a disease on her.

Self Context: Forgiving

Radha now accepted the fact that she had HIV, in the same way as she accepted the fact that some of her physical features were not perfect. Yes, probably some of her actions had resulted in her getting HIV in the first place. But she had stopped blaming herself for these past mistakes. Whatever happened, whatever she had done or not done—there was no way to change those things. She accepted this and felt a kind of peace about it now. Anyway, Radha thought, her weaknesses were a part of herself, and who she is as a person. What matters is who she is as a whole person, with all her weaknesses. Radha felt good about herself as a whole.

Self Context: Not Forgiving

Radha thought constantly about what she could have done differently so that she didn't end up getting HIV. "If only I had not done this . . . if only I had done that . . . " were the thoughts she had, especially at night. She blamed herself for what she did—and didn't do. She also blamed herself for who she was. If she had been a different person, this wouldn't have happened to her. But in her heart, Radha felt that she could never change who she was, and that basically, she wasn't a very good person. No wonder she got HIV—she deserved this terrible disease, much as she deserved the other bad things that had happened to her in life.

Self in Interpersonal Context: Not Forgiving

Radha has now accepted the fact that she has HIV, but cannot forgive her spouse who caused this. She feels sad because she had to got through all this. She often feels that it was her fault that she was not more careful. Being aware of her husband's habits, she should have been more careful about her well-being and health. She should have taken precautions for herself and for the sake of her children, and she feels extremely guilty for having let this happen to her.

Interpersonal Context: Feeling Forgiven

Madan was very sad when he learned that he had HIV infection. He is more worried about his family than himself and is very sad because he feels that his family has had to face the insult of his infection. His family, including his parents, brothers and sisters, have, however, accepted him the way he is. They do not blame him for the infection and look after him in the best way they can. He feels they have forgiven him despite all the problems he has caused them.

Interpersonal Context: Feeling Unforgiven

Rakesh is extremely sad because of his HIV-positive status, and always broods about this. His family and friends were shocked when they came to know and have totally rejected him. His wife and family behave as if he does not exist and ignore him. They are very angry with him for what he has inflicted on them. Rakesh feels that they have not forgiven him, and will not forgive him, for the pain he has caused them.

Interpersonal Context: Not Forgiving

Jaya feels extremely depressed whenever she thinks of her HIV infection. She wonders why she has to suffer for no fault of her own. She feels she should not have gotten married, as that was the reason for her infection. She is very angry at her husband for giving her this suffering and feels that she can never forgive him. She is also angry with her parents for getting her married at a young age to a womanizer with a bad character. She feels they should have known better and been more careful. Jaya thinks she cannot forgive her family and her husband for putting her through this suffering.

Interpersonal Context: Forgiving

Radha is aware that she has got the infection from her husband. Initially, she was very angry with him for giving her the infection, but she has now accepted it and is not angry with him any longer. She feels he is trying to make things as easy for her as possible, and he is also suffering. She has been looking after him and does not have any negative feelings toward him.

REFERENCES

Agence France-Presse. (1998, September 14). India admits dramatic rise in number of HIV carriers. AFP with Globe Online. *News about India.*

Ahuja, A. S., Parkar, S. R., & Yeolaker, M. E. (1998). Psychosocial aspects of seropositive HIV patients. *Journal of the Association of Physicians of India, 46,* 277–280.

Benson, H. (1996). *Timeless healing: The power and biology of belief.* New York: Scribner's.

Bharat, S. (1995). HIV/AIDS and the family: Issues in care and support. *Indian Journal of Social Work, 56,* 177–193.

Bhatnagar, A. (1998, June). Why forgive? *Life Positive,* pp. 12–16.

Chandra, P. S. (1996, February). Sexual control and awareness of STDs among HIV-infected women. *Proceedings of the Third Asia Pacific Conference on Social Science and Medicine,* Perth, Western Australia.

Chandra, P. S., & Prasadarao, P. S. D. V. (2000). Stressors in HIV infection in a developing country. In K. H. Nott, & K. Vedhara (Eds.), *Psychosocial and biomedical interactions in HIV infection.* London: Harwood Academic Press.

Chandra, P. S., Ravi V., Desai, A., & Subbakrishna, D. K. (1998). Anxiety and depression among HIV-infected heterosexuals: A report from India. *Journal of Psychosomatic Research, 45,* 401–409.

d'Cruz-Grote, D. (1996). Prevention of HIV infection in developing countries. *Lancet, 348,* 1071–1074.

Engel, G. L. (1977). The need for a new medical model: A challenge for biomedicine. *Science, 196,* 19–136.

Goldschmidt, M., Temoshok, L., & Brown, G. R. (1993). Women and HIV/AIDS: Challenging a growing threat. In C. A. Niven & D. Carroll (Eds.), *The health psychology of women* (pp. 91–106). London: Harwood Academic Press.

Jacob, K. S., Eapen, V., John, J. K., & John, T. J. (1991). Psychiatric morbidity in HIV-infected individuals. *Indian Journal of Medical Research, 93,* 62–66.

Krishna, V. A. S. (1996). *A study on the subjective well-being and the quality of marital life among male HIV patients.* Unpublished masters of philosophy psychiatric social work dissertation. Bangalore, India: NIMHANS.

Madan, P. C., Singh, N., & Golechha, G. R. (1997). Sociodemographic profile and psychiatric morbidity in HIV-seropositive defense personnel. *Indian Journal of Psychiatry, 39,* 200–204.

Mann, J. M., & Tarantola, D. J. M. (Eds.). (1996). *AIDS in the World II: Global dimensions, social roots, and responses.* Oxford, UK: Oxford University Press.

Mann, J. M., Tarantola, D. J. M., & Netter, T. W. (Eds.). (1992). *AIDS in the world: A global report.* Cambridge, MA: Harvard University Press.

McCullough, M. E., Worthington, E. L., & Rachal, K. C. (1997). Interpersonal forgiving in close relationships. *Journal of Personality and Social Psychology, 73,* 321–336.

Messick, S. (1995). Validity of psychological assessment: Validation of inferences from persons' responses and performances as scientific inquiry into score meaning. *American Psychologist, 50,* 741–749.

Microsoft Corporation. (1996). India. In Microsoft, *Encarta 96 Encyclopedia.* Microsoft Corporation, Funk & Wagnalls.

Mueke, M. (1992). Mother sold food, daughter sells her body: The cultural continuity of prostitution. *Social Science and Medicine, 35,* 891–901.

O'Flaherty, W. D. (1996). Hinduism. In Microsoft, *Encarta 96 Encyclopedia.* Microsoft Corporation, Funk & Wagnalls.

Pargament, K. I. (1997). *The psychology of religion and coping: Theory, research, and practice.* New York: Guilford Press.

Pargament, K. I., & Rye, M. S. (1998). Forgiveness as a method of religious coping. In E. L. Worthington, Jr. (Ed.), *Dimensions of forgiveness: Psychological research and theological perspectives* (pp. 201–223). Radnor, PA: Templeton Press.

Pert, C. B. (1997). *Molecules of emotion.* New York: Scribner.

Radhakrishnan, S. (1995). *Religion and society.* Indus, India: HarperCollins.

Rao, K. S., Pilli, R. D., Rao, A. S., & Chalam, P. S. (1999). Sexual lifestyle of long distance lorry drivers in India: Questionnaire survey. *British Medical Journal, 318,* 162–163.

Sinha, J. (1985). *Indian psychology: Vol. 2. Emotion and will.* New Delhi: Motilal Banarsidass.

Solano, L., Costa, M., Salvati, S., Coda, R., Aiuti, F., Messaroma, I., & Bertini, M. (1993). Psychosocial factors and clinical evolution in HIV infection: A longitudinal study. *Journal of Psychosomatic Research, 37,* 39–51.

Solomon, G. F., Kemeny, M., & Temoshok, L. (1991). Psychoneuroimmunologic aspects of human immunodeficiency virus infection. In R. Ader, D. L. Felten, & N. Cohen (Eds.), *Psychoneuroimmunology* (2nd ed., pp. 1081–1113). New York: Academic Press.

Straits, K., Temoshok, L., & Zich, J. (1990). A cross-cultural comparison of psychosocial responses to having acquired immune deficiency syndrome and related conditions in London and San Francisco. In L. Temoshok, & A. Baum (Eds.), *Psychosocial perspectives on AIDS: Etiology, prevention, and treatment* (pp. 139–166). Englewood Cliffs, NJ: Erlbaum.

Temoshok, L. R. (1990). Applying the biopsychosocial model to research on HIV/AIDS. In B. Bennett, J. Weinman, & P. Spurgeon (Eds.), *Current developments in health psychology* (pp. 129–158). London: Harwood Academic.

Temoshok, L. R. (1993). HIV/AIDS, psychoneuroimmunology, and beyond: A commentary and review. *Advances in Neuroimmunology, 3,* 87–95.

Temoshok, L. R. (1997). The complexity of cause: Linking emotional dynamics to health outcomes in cancer and HIV/AIDS. In A. Vingerhoets, F. van Bussel, & J. Boelhouwer (Eds.), *The (non) expression of emotions in health and disease* (pp. 15–24). Tilburg, The Netherlands: Tilburg University Press.

Temoshok, L. R. (1998). HIV/AIDS. In H. S. Friedman (Ed.), *Encyclopedia of mental health* (Vol. 2, pp. 375–392). San Diego: Academic Press.

Temoshok, L., & Dreher, H. (1992). *The Type C connection: The behavioral links to cancer and your health.* New York: Random House.

Temoshok, L., & Moulton, J. M. (1991). Dimensions of biopsychosocial research on HIV disease: Perspectives from the UCSF Biopsychosocial AIDS Project. In P. M. McCabe, N. Schneiderman, T. Field, & J. Skyler (Eds.), *Stress, coping and disease* (pp. 211–236). Englewood Cliffs, NJ: Erlbaum.

Temoshok, L. R., & the WHOQOL Group. (1997). *HIV/AIDS and quality of life: An international perspective.* Geneva: WHO Division of Mental Health and Prevention of Substance Abuse.

Testa, M. A., & Simonson, D. C. (1996). Assessment of quality-of-life outcomes. *New England Journal of Medicine, 334,* 835–840.

UNAIDS. (1998). *Epidemiological fact sheet on HIV/AIDS and sexually transmitted diseases.* Geneva: UNAIDS/WHO Working Group on Global HIV/AIDS and STD Surveillance.

Wade, S. H. (1989). *The development of a scale to measure forgiveness.* Unpublished doctoral dissertation, Fuller Graduate School of Psychology, Pasadena, CA.

WHOQOL Group. (1993). Study protocol for the World Health Organization project to develop a Quality of Life Assessment Instrument (WHOQOL). *Quality of Life Research, 2,* 153–159.

WHOQOL Group. (1994). The development of the World Health Organization Quality of Life Assessment Instrument (the WHOQOL). In J. Orley & W. Kuyken (Eds.), *Quality of life assessment: International perspectives* (pp. 41–57). Berlin: Springer-Verlag.

WHOQOL Group. (1995). The World Health Organization Quality of Life Assessment (WHOQOL): Position paper from the World Health Organization. *Social Science and Medicine, 41,* 1403–1409.

WHO/Division of Mental Health/Temoshok, L. R. (1997). *Report on the consultation regarding quality of life and HIV/AIDS.* Geneva: WHO.

WHO/UNAIDS. (1998). *Report on the global HIV/AIDS epidemic, June 1998.* Geneva: WHO Working Group on Global HIV/AIDS and STD Surveillance.

Winiarski, M. G. (1991). Spiritual issues in AIDS-related psychotherapy. In M. G. Winiarski (Ed.), *AIDS-related psychotherapy* (pp. 183–187). New York: Pergamon Press.

Zich, J., & Temoshok, L. (1987). Perceptions of social support in persons with AIDS and ARC. *Journal of Applied Social Psychology, 17,* 193–215.

CHAPTER 4

What We Know (and Need to Know) about Assessing Forgiveness Constructs

Michael E. McCullough, William T. Hoyt, and K. Chris Rachal

Improving the measures available for assessing forgiveness is one of the most important tasks necessary for creating a sustainable future for the psychology of forgiveness (McCullough & Worthington, 1995; McCullough, Worthington, & Rachal, 1997; McCullough, Sandage, Rachal, & Worthington, 1997). Currently, many aspects of forgiveness appear to be adequately assessed by existing measures. However, many aspects of forgiveness still cannot be studied properly because instruments for assessing them have not yet been developed. As well, many questions remain about how to use the existing measures in ways that optimize their performance.

In the present chapter, we set out to review what we know about assessing forgiveness-related constructs. As well, we address several of the most pressing issues in future psychometric work on forgiveness-related constructs.

A 3 × 2 × 4 FRAMEWORK

We have developed a taxonomy for categorizing the existent prima facie measures of forgiveness. All of the measurements included in this taxonomy consider the individual as the unit of analysis, although forgiveness might also be observed and assessed at the level of the dyad, the family, the neighborhood, or larger population aggregates. Such considerations, however, are beyond the scope of this chapter.

Our 3 × 2 × 4 taxonomy categorizes the available instruments along three dimensions. The first dimension refers to the level of *specificity* with which forgiveness is assessed. McCullough and Worthington (1999) classified the existing measures of forgiveness into three levels of specificity; offense-specific, dyadic, and dispositional.

Offense-specific measures are assessments of the extent to which a person has forgiven a specific offender for a specific offense. Ostensibly, an offense-specific measure of forgiveness would represent the extent to which a person has forgiven (or sought forgiveness) in the context of a single, circumscribed interpersonal offense. *Dyadic* measures of forgiveness ostensibly represent an aggregate of the extent to which an individual forgives (or seeks forgiveness) in a single relationship across multiple offenses. Such dyadic measures are more general than offense-specific measures, as they are aggregating (at least in theory) people's forgiveness responses across many offenses occurring within a single relationship. In a sense, dyadic measures loosely might be considered as a sort of weighted mean of a person's offense-specific forgiveness responses summed across multiple offenses within a single relationship. *Dispositional* measures of forgiveness ostensibly represent a person's tendency to grant (or seek) forgiveness across a variety of interpersonal offenses occurring in a variety of relationships. Thus, dispositional measures of forgiveness represent (at least in theory) a sort of weighted mean of a person's offense-specific forgiveness responses summed across multiple offenses *and* multiple relationships.

The second dimension along which existing forgiveness measures may be categorized is their *direction* of measurement. Most measures assess forgiveness in the direction of granting forgiveness (i.e., from the perspective of the forgiver). A few others also measure forgiveness in the direction of seeking or accepting forgiveness (i.e., from the perspective of the transgressor). Because fairly little research has examined the contours of seeking or accepting forgiveness from others (Gassin, 1998; Meek, Allbright, & McMinn, 1995), the measurement of forgiveness from the perspective of the person who seeks or accepts forgiveness is similarly undeveloped.

A third dimension on which the existing measures of forgiveness may be categorized refers to the *method* with which forgiveness is assessed. Offense-specific forgiveness (i.e., both granting forgiveness and receiving forgiveness) might ostensibly be assessed through at least four methods. First, using self-report methods, an offended person can report the extent to which he or she has forgiven the offending partner (or the offender can report the extent to which he or she has sought forgiveness from the offended partner). Second, using partner-report methods, the offending relationship partner can report the extent to which the offended relationship partner has granted forgiveness (or the offended relationship partner can report the extent to which the offending partner appears to feels forgiven). Third, an outside observer (e.g., a clinician or other third party) can assess the extent to which a partner has forgiven the offending relationship partner (or appears to have sought the offended partner's forgiveness). Fourth, measures of constructive or destructive behaviors toward an offending relationship partner, which do not rely on verbal or written reports, can be used to infer the extent to which an offended partner has forgiven an offending relationship partner, or to which the offender has sought the forgiveness of the offended partner.[1] In the section of the chapter that follows, we use the $3 \times 2 \times 4$ taxonomy to review the existing measures for assessing forgiveness constructs.

A REVIEW OF THE EXISTING MEASURES OF FORGIVENESS

Offense-Specific Measures of Forgiveness

At the offense-specific level, a measure of forgiveness assesses the extent to which a person has forgiven (or sought forgiveness) for a single interpersonal offense. Offense-specific measures are used to answer questions such as, "Did this person forgive her father for abandoning her and her mother?" or "Did this person seek forgiveness from his wife for his extramarital affair?" Most of the existing measures of forgiveness have assessed forgiveness at this level of specificity (McCullough & Worthington, 1999).

Offense-Specific Measures of Granting Forgiveness

Self-Report Measures. For nearly 20 years, social psychologists have assessed offense-specific granting of forgiveness with single-item self-report measures (e.g., Darby & Schlenker, 1982). Even today, correlation with such a face-valid, single-item measure of forgiveness remains something of a litmus test for making the case for the validity of a more complex measure (e.g., Subkoviak et al., 1995; McCullough et al., 1998).

As early as 1981, researchers also began to develop offense-specific, multi-item measures that assessed granting forgiveness by self-report. Trainer (1981) developed a nine-item self-report measure of offense-specific forgiveness that she called "general forgiveness" (i.e., absence of hostility, grudge-holding; presence of positive feelings and hopes for the offender's well-being). Along with this general measure of offense-specific forgiving, she also developed three self-report measures that ostensibly measure motivations for forgiving: intrinsic motivation (14 items), expedient motivation (10 items), and role-expected motivation (10 items). The four scales manifested internal consistency reliabilities ranging from .77 to .89 (Trainer, 1981). Park and Enright (1997) used seven of the nine items from Trainer's (1981) general forgiveness scale, added three new items, and used the 10-item total score (with an internal consistency reliability of alpha = .87) as a measure of general forgiveness.

In Trainer's (1981) work, the four forgiveness subscales were correlated with the extent to which offended persons blamed their offenders, experienced empathic attributions for their offenders' behavior, and maintained bitter/hostile feelings toward the offender. Moreover, there were important differences in the correlates of the four subscales, suggesting that they might be assessing different aspects of forgiveness.

However, factor analyses disputed the validity of a four-factor model for describing the interrelationships of the items on these four scales. Most of the general forgiveness and intrinsic items loaded on a first factor that explained approximately 18% of the total item variance. This factor seemed to represent forgiveness most adequately (indeed, we can be comforted that the item that loaded most strongly with this first factor was a single item assessing the extent to which the respondent had forgiven his or her offender). A second factor seemed to represent an angry, pragmatic, unempathic view of forgiveness that reflected respondents' use of forgiveness as a way of getting revenge or propping up a damaged self-image. A third factor appeared to represent a form of forgiveness that was motivated by a sense of hopelessness about the viability of other options, a sense of duty, and religious convictions. Nevertheless, given the encouraging initial work conducted with these scales, they might possibly merit greater attention in future research.

A variety of other self-report measures of granting forgiveness have been developed in the nearly 20 years since Trainer's (1981) work. More than 10 years ago, Wade (1987, 1989) developed an 81-item self-report pencil-and-paper measure that purports to assess nine dimensions of forgiveness. The measure has been used in several research efforts (Dreelin, 1993; Davidson & Jurkovic, 1993; McCullough & Worthington, 1995; Rhode, 1990). The subscales of Wade's Forgiveness Scale have demonstrated "known groups validity," successfully discriminating between people who report having forgiven an offender and those who report not having forgiven an offender (Wade, 1989). Subscales also appear to be correlated with spiritual well-being (Dreelin, 1993), and narcissism (Davidson & Jurkovic, 1994).

McCullough et al. (1998) reported the results of four studies in which they developed a 12-item measure based on items from Wade's (1989) Forgiveness Scale. Their 12-item scale—the Transgression-Related Interpersonal Motivations (TRIM) Inventory—is designed to assess the two negative motivational elements that are outlined in McCullough et al.'s (1997, 1998) theorizing about the nature of interpersonal forgiving: (1) the motivation to avoid the offender (Avoidance) and (2) the motivation to seek revenge (Revenge). The essence of forgiving, according to McCullough et al. (1998), is relative reductions in these two interpersonal motivations; thus, reductions in avoidance and revenge motivations are considered to be equivalent to "forgiving." The two TRIM subscales are correlated highly with many of the constructs that are central to McCullough et al.'s theorizing regarding the determinants of forgiving, including relational satisfaction, and commitment, and closeness, apology, empathy, and rumination. Confirmatory factor analyses also demonstrated that the TRIM subscale scores are distinct from these other constructs. As well, the two subscales predict approximately 50% of the variance (multiple $R = .70$) in a single-item measure of forgiveness and predict the reestablishment of relational closeness following an interpersonal offense.

Another important self-report measure has been developed by Enright and his colleagues at the University of Wisconsin–Madison (Subkoviak et al., 1995; Subkoviak, Enright, & Wu, 1992). The 60-item Enright Forgiveness Inventory (EFI) has been used in several studies and has a variety of desirable psychometric properties. It is intended to assess six aspects of forgiving another person: presence of positive affect, cognition, and behavior, and the absence of negative affect, cognition, and behavior. Internal consistency reliabilities for all six subscales are high, and internal consistency reliability for the total scale score is in the high .90s (Subkoviak et al., 1995, McCullough, 1995). In some subsamples, the EFI also was correlated negatively with measures of depression and anxiety (Subkoviak et al., 1995). Moreover, it is sensitive to experimental manipulations designed to facilitate forgiveness (Coyle & Enright, 1997).

Prior to the advent of the EFI Hebl and Enright (1993), Al-Mabuk, Enright, and Cardis (1995), and Freedman and Enright (1996) used a 30-item measure that they called the Psychological Profile of Forgiveness Scale. This scale was designed to assess the same six constructs as does the EFI. Internal consistency reliabilities for the total score on this 30-item measure tend to be above .90 (Al-Mabuk et al., 1995; Freedman & Enright, 1996; Hebl & Enright, 1993). Despite that fact that the 30-item Psychological Profile of Forgiveness Scale appears to be sensitive to experimental manipulations designed to facilitate forgiveness (e.g., Freedman & Enright, 1996), the 60-item EFI has been used in the stead of the 30-item Psychological Profile of Forgiveness Scale in more recent intervention studies by Enright and his colleagues (Coyle & Enright, 1997).[2]

Partner-Report Measures. We are aware of no measure that assesses the extent to which an offender perceives that an offended relationship partner has forgiven him or her for the offense. Given the essentially interpersonal nature of the concept of forgiveness, this seems like a tremendous oversight in the development of measures of forgiveness. Such measures would be relevant to (1) understanding the impact of forgiveness on the offender and (2) necessary for studying offense-specific forgiveness at the dyadic rather than simply the individual level (see Exline & Baumeister, Chapter 7, this volume).

Observer-Report Measures. Observer-report measures of forgiveness would be analogous to other interview-based measures for assessing psychological constructs, such as the Hamilton Depression Rating Scale for assessing depressive symptoms (Hamilton, 1960), and the Type A Structured Interview for assessing the Type A Behavior Pattern (Rosenman et al., 1964). Such measurement approaches have also lagged behind the development of self-report measures.

Along with developing the first multi-item self-report measure of granting forgiveness for a specific offense, Trainer (1981) also developed the first measure (see Trainer's Table E) of granting forgiveness to be completed by a trained rater. This measure was used only for validating the other scales that Trainer developed, but the approach deserves mention. Using this tool, trained raters categorize a person's degree of forgiveness for a specific offender as high, moderate, or low based on the relative presence or absence of several affective, cognitive, and behavioral qualities thought to reflect forgiveness (e.g., "relative absence of hostility and bitterness," "presence of gestures of good will," etc.).

In Chapter 9, this volume, Malcolm and Greenberg present a rating system for measuring offense-specific instances of forgiveness through analyzing psychotherapy process videotapes. This measurement system involves applying rating scales to videotapes of psychotherapy sessions during which the client and therapist discuss an interpersonal offense that the client has suffered. Though preliminary, Malcolm and Greenberg's approach is innovative and potentially quite useful—particularly for examining the unfolding of forgiveness in psychotherapy.

Behavioral Measures. Behavioral approaches whose scores might be interpreted as "forgiveness" have been explored in a variety of experimental settings. The Prisoner's Dilemma Game, for example, is a mixed-motive simulation in which two players are repeatedly faced with choosing either a cooperative or competitive strategy. The object is to win as many points as possible. If both partners cooperate in any given turn, each partner wins 3 points. If one partner cooperates while the other defects from cooperation, the "defector" wins 5 points, while the cooperator receives nothing. If both partners defect from cooperation, each wins 1 point. In this game, "forgiveness" has been operationalized as a cooperative move in response to the other player's competitive move (e.g., Axelrod, 1980a,

1980b). Rather than reciprocating a competitive move with another competitive move, the "forgiving" partner chooses to respond to the defection with a reassertion of his or her willingness to play the game in a cooperative mode.

Other behavioral measures should be considered also. Laboratory manipulations often present self-esteem threats or insults to participants and then give respondents the opportunity to behave in some way toward the person who is the source of the self-esteem threat or insult. In such laboratory settings, inhibition of aggressive responses to the transgressor may be considered an important aspect of forgiveness. Some aggressive responses that have been examined include (1) unfavorable evaluations of a transgressor that are believed to influence the transgressor's chances of winning a job or assistantship (e.g., Bushman & Baumeister, 1998; Caprara, Coluzzi, Mazzotti, Renzi, & Zelli, 1985; Kremer & Stevens, 1983; Zillman & Cantor, 1976); (2) delivery of shocks or other noxious stimuli (Caprara et al., 1985, 1987; Collins & Bell, 1997); and (3) making choices that cost the transgressor time, money, or some other resource (e.g., Brown, 1968; Caprara et al., 1987). In most instances, researchers would be interested in generalizing from participants' responses in such laboratory scenarios to interpersonal transgressions outside of the laboratory. Fortunately, it does appear that such laboratory-based measures of retaliatory aggression generalize well to nonlaboratory situations (Anderson & Bushman, 1997). Whether such behaviors in mixed-motive games or contrived laboratory scenarios actually correspond to forgiveness as measured using more conventional self-report, other-report, or observer-report measures, of course, remains to be investigated and would be substantively interesting for forgiveness theory.

Offense-Specific Measures of Seeking and Receiving Forgiveness

To date, we are aware of little research on how people seek or receive forgiveness for specific offenses (Meek et al., 1995). Meek et al. assessed (with single-item, Likert-type measures) the extent to which respondents would feel forgiven after confessing to the commission of certain transgressions. Little other published work has been completed in this domain.

Dyadic Measures of Forgiveness

At the dyadic level, a measure of forgiveness would assess a person's general tendency to forgive a particular relationship partner for interpersonal offenses that occur in the relationship. Relationship-specific assessments address questions such as the following: "Does this husband tend to seek forgiveness when he offends his wife?" "Does this employee tend to forgive his boss?" Thus, relationship-level measurements are less specific than offense-specific measurements in that they attempt to assess a person's tendency to forgive (or seek forgiveness from) a specific relationship partner generally, rather than for a specific offense.

Currently, we are aware of only one tool that assesses forgiveness at the dyadic level. This is the Hargrave and Sells (1997) Interpersonal Relationship Resolution Scale (IRRS). This scale consists of 44 yes–no items designed to assess the extent to which a person who has received serious hurts from a specific family member (1) continues to feel pain as a result of the offenses and (2) has forgiven the offending family member for the offenses that occurred in the past. The Pain scale consists of four subscales labeled Shame, Rage, Control, and Chaos. The Forgiveness scale consists of four subscales labeled Insight, Understanding, Giving the Opportunity for Compensation, and the Overt Act of Forgiving. Internal consistencies for the eight subscales ranged from .63 to .87, and internal consistencies for the Pain and Forgiveness scales exceeded .90 (Hargrave & Sells, 1997). Individuals in a sample of outpatient psychotherapy clients with family-of-origin issues scored significantly lower on all four Forgiveness subscales (and higher on all four Pain subscales) than did a sample graduate and undergraduate students who had received no prior counseling or psychotherapy. The Forgiveness and Pain subscales also demonstrated a complex pattern of correlations with a variety of other clinically relevant self-report measures.

Further exploration of dyadic measures of forgiveness would facilitate greatly the study of forgiveness from the perspective of marital/family relationships and other close relationships. Such measures could potentially be developed in the same fashion as have other relationship-specific measures, such as the Long and Andrews (1990) dyadic perspective-taking measures, which assess partners' capacity to take the perspective of their spouse, as well as perceptions that the spouse is capable of taking the partners' perspective. Observer-report and behavioral measures of forgiveness at the relationship-specific level should be developed also.

Dispositional Measures of Forgiveness

At the dispositional level, a measure of forgiveness ostensibly assesses a person's general disposition or tendency to forgive others (or to seek forgiveness after having harmed someone else). Measures that assess forgiveness at this level are attempts to assess a general response style that transcends individual offenses, or even individual relationships.

Dispositional Measures of Granting Forgiveness

Self-Ratings. A variety of self-report measures exist that are useful for assessing the disposition to forgive others. The most widely used is a measure of the dissipation–rumination construct that Caprara and colleagues have investigated for many years (Caprara, 1986; Caprara, Barbaranelli, & Comrey, 1992; Caprara, Manzi, & Perugini, 1992; Caprara et al., 1985). Dissipation, according to Caprara, is the capacity to overcome ill feelings or the desire to retaliate after being provoked. Rumination is the tendency to maintain or even nurture one's emotional distress and desire for vengeance after being damaged by another person (Caprara & Pastorelli, 1989). The Dissipation–Rumination scale consists of 15 Likert-type items (e.g., "When somebody offends me, sooner or later I retaliate" and "I do not forgive easily once I am offended") and appears to have adequate internal consistency (alpha = .79 for the Italian version and .89 for the English version). Dissipation–rumination scores appear to be positively correlated with the degree to which people retaliate against someone following a transgression or other self-esteem threat (Caprara, 1986; Caprara et al., 1985; Collins & Bell, 1997). In the last decade, similar scales have been developed as well. Mauger et al. (1992) developed a measure of the disposition to forgive other people, which they called the Forgiveness of Others Scale (FOS). Like the Dissipation–Rumination Scale, this measure consists of 15 items (in this case, in a true–false format) that assess people's desire to retaliate, hold grudges, and forgive following an interpersonal offense. Scores show adequate internal consistency. Two other dispositional scales that appear to draw from the same universe of items are the Emmons (1992) Beliefs about Revenge Questionnaire (BARQ) and the Stuckless and Goranson (1992) Vengeance Scale. The Dissipation–Rumination Scale, FOS, BARQ, and Vengeance Scale appear to have a variety of important correlates, including empathy, interpersonal trust, agreeableness, and social conformity. As well, people who are on the more "forgiving" end of scores for these measures appear to have lower irritability and emotional distress, and lower levels of anger and hostility.

The empirical relations among scores on the Dissipation–Rumination Scale, FOS, BARQ, and Vengeance Scale need to be examined empirically. Judging from the semantic similarity of their item content, it is likely that these measures share a large proportion of common variance. Intensive comparisons of the psychometric properties of these scales would help to broaden considerably researchers' and clinicians' tools for assessing the disposition to forgive.

An important measurement of self-reported disposition to grant forgiveness was developed by Hebl and Enright (1993). Their Willingness to Forgive Scale is a 16-item measure that instructs respondents to read 16 scenarios in which they imagine themselves to have been damaged by another person. Respondents choose one of 10 hypothetical responses to each offense to indicate how they (1) expect that they would respond to the offense, and how they (2) would prefer to respond to the offense, even if they do not believe that they would choose that particular mode of responding. One of the 10 response options to each scenario is to "forgive." Scores represent the number of times that respondents choose the "forgiveness" response to the scenarios. Internal consistency reliability for this measure was estimated at alpha = .70 (Hebl & Enright, 1993). Al-Mabuk, Enright, and Cardis (1995), using a 12-item form of this scale, demonstrated internal consistency coefficients in the .47–.75 range. Subjects' scores on this measure appear to increase after participation in interventions focused on encouraging forgiveness (Al-Mabuk, Enright, & Cardis, 1995; Hebl & Enright, 1993).

Aside from these measures, other approaches to assessing dispositional aspects of granting forgiveness have been developed through the years. The value that people ascribe to being "forgiving" is assessed with Rokeach's (1967) Value Survey. This scale requires respondents to place 18 terminal values and 18 instrumental values (including the value of being "forgiving") in rank order according to their relative priority in respondents' value systems. People who tend to be more religious, lower in Machiavellianism, and more traditional tend to place the value of being "forgiving" higher in their value systems than do people who are lower on each of those respective traits (for reviews see McCullough & Worthington, 1995, 1999).

Finally, Gorsuch and Hao (1993) examined a series of self-report items regarding people's tendencies to forgive and retaliate when they have been intentionally hurt by others. Gorsuch and Hao reported that a variety of measures of religious involvement differentiated between people scoring high and low on these measures of forgiveness. Because these items have been administered to a nationally representative sample, they should be looked at seriously for developing standardized measures of dispositional forgiveness.

Partner Ratings. Currently, no psychometric tools are available for assessing the disposition to forgive from the perspective of a significant other.

Observer-Report Measures. As well, no observer-report measures have been developed for assessing the disposition to forgive.

Behavioral Measures. Finally, no behavioral measures have been developed to assess dispositional forgiveness by observing and summing people's behavioral responses across a variety of real-life situations.

Dispositional Measures of Seeking–Receiving Forgiveness

We are not aware of any psychometric instruments to date that have attempted to measure people's tendencies to seek forgiveness (or receive forgiveness) from others when they have committed an interpersonal transgression.

Summary

Clearly, the measurement of forgiveness has been progressing for nearly two decades. The energy that has been devoted to developing self-report measures of offense-specific forgiveness probably reflects the fact that most theorizing about forgiveness has focused on granting forgiveness in the aftermath of transgression or victimization. The relative emphasis on measures of granting forgiveness might also be due to the fact that research to date has not focused on the interpersonal aspects as much as the intrapersonal or mental health aspects of forgiveness. Nevertheless, the scientific study of forgiveness would benefit a great deal from research efforts devoted to increasing the breadth of available measurement methods. Whereas many self-report instruments exist for assessing transgression-specific forgiveness, few instruments exist for measuring forgiveness at the dyadic level. Development of behavioral measures has been almost completely ignored. No dispositional measures of seeking–receiving forgiveness exist. We hope that these assessment gaps will be filled in years to come.

OTHER AREAS FOR PSYCHOMETRIC DEVELOPMENT

In addition to increasing the breadth of measures available for assessing forgiveness, the entire field of research on forgiveness would be much improved if procedural changes were made in how measures of forgiveness were developed and employed in research. First and foremost, we recommend that researchers begin to augment the use of classical measurement theory with generalizability theory, which can address the complexities of forgiveness assessment in a more elegant and informative way.

Four subsidiary psychometric issues emerge from a generalizability approach to thinking about the measurement of forgiveness constructs. First, we recommend that forgiveness constructs routinely be assessed using more than one method. Second, we recommend that researchers think hard about the appropriate level of specificity at which forgiveness should be assessed to address a particular research question adequately. Third, we recommend that researchers begin to explore (and exercise care in controlling) sources of variability that can influence forgiveness scores. Fourth, we recommend that researchers specify the nomological networks underlying the assessment of forgiveness prior to collecting construct validity data. We explore each of these themes in the remainder of the present chapter.

Generalizability Theory as an Adjunct to Classical Measurement Theory

Classical measurement theory would conceptualize people's scores on a measure of forgiveness as the additive combination of a true score component and an error component. The true score reflects the people's actual standing on the construct of interest (e.g., the extent to which persons "really" forgive the transgressor they are rating, the extent to which they "really" have a forgiving disposition, etc.). The error component refers to variance in the measure that is unstable across replications, thereby making the assessment procedure an imperfect measure of people's actual standing on the construct. Reliability coefficients (e.g., coefficient alpha) are interpreted under the assumptions of classical measurement theory as the proportion of the total variance in a measure that is attributable to true scores.

In classical measurement theory, psychometricians have typically been concerned with three sources of error variance because of their impact on the reliability of measures: (1) error due to temporal instability, (2) error due to heterogeneity among items, and (3) error due to inconsistencies in how two raters might apply a rating scale to the same stimulus. These sources of error are estimated, respectively, with test–retest coefficients (e.g., interclass r), internal consistency reliability coefficients (e.g., Cronbach's α), and interrater reliability coefficients (e.g., intraclass r, see Shrout & Fleiss, 1979). The major limitation of classical measurement theory for estimating a measure's dependability is that it does not allow one to consider multiple sources of error variance simultaneously. When two or more sources of error contribute to measurement variance, classical reliability tests always overestimate the proportion of variance that is attributable to true scores (Hoyt, 1998).

Generalizability theory (GT; Cronbach, Gleser, Nanda, & Rajaratnam, 1972) is an expanded psychometric approach that is not limited to the examination of a single source of extraneous variance at any given time. GT is to classical reliability theory what factorial analysis of variance is to one-way analysis of variance (ANOVA) (Hoyt & Melby, 1999). Although GT is not a new psychometric approach, it would be a new approach for use in developing measures of forgiveness constructs. Using a GT approach, a researcher would attempt to identify all of the facets (or dimensions along which observations might be classified) that might influence scores on a forgiveness measure in a given application, and examine their relative contributions to score variance simultaneously.

In the case of a self-report, offense-specific measure of granting forgiveness (e.g., Wade's Forgiveness Scale), for example, such facets would almost certainly include items (the facet for which internal consistency reliability estimates in classical measurement theory are conducted) and time (the facet for which test–retest reliability estimates in classical measurement theory are conducted). Such facets can be specified and estimated explicitly and simultaneously in a GT approach to scale development. As well, the interaction of these effects can be specified and examined. What matters most, from a GT point of view, is not a participant's "true score," but, rather, the universe of conditions (or levels of facets) to which a given score might generalize.

Although facets are commonly equated with sources of error in generalizability studies, an aspect of measurement that is error in one application may be substantively important when the construct of interest is considered from another point of view (Cronbach, 1995). By advocating a flexible, context-sensitive approach to interpretation of the results of generalizability studies, GT blurs conventional distinctions between reliability and validity of measurement (Cronbach et al., 1972).

Table 4.1 illustrates a 4 (victims) × 3 (offenders) × 2 (offenses) fully crossed factorial design for a hypothetical generalizability study of forgiveness. The number of levels of each factor is small for illustrative purposes; to estimate variance components reliably, it would be important to include more victims and offenders, or to study multiple small groups of victims and offenders (Smith, 1978). For concreteness, readers can think of victims as students (or siblings) and offenders as teachers (or parents). All victims are assumed to be acquainted with all individuals in the group of offenders, and victims are asked to report the extent to which they forgave offenders for one major and one minor offense in the recent past. Cell entries X_{ijk} are ratings of the extent to which victim i forgave offender j following offense k (1 = major; 2 = minor).

This data set is a fully crossed factorial design, and the generalizability analysis uses the same procedures as factorial analysis of variance; thus, this generalizability study investigates seven sources of variance in ratings: three main effects, three two-way interactions, and one three-way interaction (confounded with error because, as is typical in generalizability studies, the design includes only one observation per cell). However, unlike ANOVA,

TABLE 4.1. Design for Generalizability Study of Forgiveness Behaviors

Partner (j)	1		2		3	
Offense (k)	Major	Minor	Major	Minor	Major	Minor
Actor (i) 1	X_{111}	X_{112}	X_{121}	X_{122}	X_{131}	X_{132}
2	X_{211}	X_{212}	X_{221}	X_{222}	X_{231}	X_{232}
3	X_{311}	X_{312}	X_{321}	X_{322}	X_{331}	X_{332}
4	X_{411}	X_{412}	X_{421}	X_{422}	X_{431}	X_{432}

which focuses on testing main effects and interactions for statistical significance, generalizability analyses focus on the magnitude of these effects, estimating the variance accounted for by each main effect and interaction in the
model. These variance components indicate the relative importance of each
of these seven sources in determining forgiveness.

Of special interest in connection with our concerns about determining the appropriate level of measurement of forgiveness (discussed earlier) are the victim (i), offender (j), and relationship (ij interaction)
variance components. Examination of the relative magnitude of these
components addresses the following issues (see Table 4.2):

1. To what extent is forgiveness a function of victim disposition (i.e.,
   to what extent do victims differ in their average willingness to forgive)?
2. To what extent is forgiveness a function of offender "forgivability"
   (i.e., to what extent do offenders differ in the average level of forgiveness they elicit from those they have offended)?
3. To what extent is forgiveness a function of unique characteristics
   of the victim–offender relationship (i.e., are some victims more
   likely to forgive a particular offender than others)? If forgiveness
   in a relationship is mediated by liking, for example, relationship
   variance in forgiveness would be expected to be large, because liking is largely a dyadic phenomenon (Kenny, 1994).

**TABLE 4.2. Interpretation of Variance Components
from Generalizability Study**

Component	Question/issue addressed
i	To what extent is forgiveness a function of actor characteristics (ac-tor variance in the Social Relations Model)?
j	To what extent is forgiveness a function of partner characteristics (partner variance in Social Relations Model)?
ij	To what extent is forgiveness a function of characteristics of the dyad (dyadic variance in Social Relations Model)?
k	To what extent is forgiveness a function of the magnitude of the of-fense?
ik	Do actors vary in their willingness to forgive minor versus major of-fenses?
jk	Do partners vary in their forgiveability for minor versus major of-fenses?
Residual	To what extent is forgiveness a function of systematic or random factors not modeled in this study?

Our hypothetical generalizability study partitions forgiveness variance into other components, including variance attributable to the severity of offense (k) and to the interaction of offense severity with victim and offender effects (ik and jk interactions, respectively), along with a residual component. These components also address questions of dependability of measurement, although they are substantively interesting as well, since researchers should be aware of the extent to which a given victim's forgiveness levels are likely to generalize across offenses, both within and between relationships.

The main effect of offense examines whether forgiveness levels vary by the severity of the offense, as might be expected (e.g., Girard & Mullet, 1997). The ik interaction examines whether the ordering of victims on forgiveness differs by level of offense. A relatively small ik variance component indicates that individuals who readily forgive a trivial slight are also most willing to forgive more severe transgressions. If ik variance in forgiveness is large, however, the victims who are most forgiving of a minor offense may not be most forgiving following a major hurt. If this is the case, theories of forgiveness must be careful to specify the magnitude of the offense in their predictions, and offense-specific measures of forgiveness must control for severity to assess a unified construct. The jk interaction addresses a similar issue with respect to offender forgiveability: Are those who are most forgivable following minor transgressions also the most forgivable when they have committed a major offense? If jk-related variance is negligible in the generalizability study, it suggests that the answer to this question is "yes"; if not, then offense severity should be a consideration in theories and research on individual differences in forgivability.

In addition to the facets that are specified in Tables 4.1 and 4.2, other sources of error that are of interest in the measurement of forgiveness could be investigated either separately or in conjunction with the sources considered here. Stability of forgiveness over time (i.e., test–retest reliability) is clearly an important consideration for researchers: To what extent does forgiving a relationship partner today predict relative standing on the same forgiveness construct in the future? When multi-item measures of forgiveness are used to assess this construct, generalizability of forgiveness across items (i.e., internal consistency reliability) is also of interest.

Exalting Multimethod Measurement as a Gold Standard

Recently, researchers have begun to lament the fact that most studies of forgiveness have relied almost exclusively on monomethod measurement of forgiveness based on the self-reports of only a single person: the putative forgiver. There has been very little study of the perpetrator's side of things (Baumeister, Exline, & Sommer, 1998; Exline & Baumeister, Chapter 7, this volume). A serious limitation imposed by exclusive reliance on forgivers' self-reports is the unknown extent to which individual differences on these measures are confounded with response biases or differences among respondents in their interpretations of rating scales (Hoyt, 1998; Kenny, 1994). Unfortunately, variance due to response biases is reliable (i.e., it is counted as "true score" variance in conventional reliability analyses). Thus, validity coefficients in studies using self-report measures of forgiveness are attenuated to an unknown extent due to this confound, and statistical power is correspondingly decreased by an unknown amount.

To remedy the shortcomings imposed by monomethod assessment, researchers should strive to complement self-reports of forgiveness from the "forgiver's" side of things with reports from other informants (including relationship partners), rating scales completed by third parties, or behavioral measures. This is not to suggest that such measures will necessarily converge; in fact, the expectation that they might *not* produce convergent findings is precisely the reason why multimethod measurement is used. If we find, for example, that self-reported empathic affect is correlated with self-reported forgiveness (e.g., McCullough et al., 1997, 1998), but not with behavioral measures that putatively assess forgiveness, or the transgressor's perceptions of the extent to which he or she has been forgiven; then we learn something important about the limits of the empathy–forgiveness connection.

Assessing Forgiveness at the Appropriate Level of Specificity

Assessing forgiveness at the appropriate level of specificity is likely to have important consequences for the development of stable and theoretically compelling research findings regarding forgiveness. According to the aggregation principle explored initially by Fishbein and Ajzen (1974), and later by Rushton, Brainerd, and Pressley (1983), Epstein (1983), and Gorsuch (1984, 1988), scores on psychometric instruments are most likely to correlate with scores on other psychometric instruments that aggregate behaviors to the same level of specificity. A corollary of this principle is that measures assessing a single behavioral instance are most likely to be correlated with other measures that are germane to that same single behavioral instance. Moreover, measures that assess a variable (such as forgiveness) at the level of a specific relationship are most likely to correlate with other measures that assess qualities of a specific relationship. Finally, measures that assess an overall personality trait or disposition are most likely to correlate with other measures that assess an overall personality trait or disposition.

The generalizability study summarized in Tables 4.1 and 4.2 can be used to illustrate the specificity principle in the context of GT. People may be inconsistent in their responses to multiple offenses within a single relationship (variance attributed to k, ik, or jk components in Table 4.1). The inconsistency may be systematically related to the severity of the offense, which was manipulated in this example, but may also be a function of other factors (e.g., qualities of the relationship between offender and offendee) not examined in this study. People may be consistent in their tendencies to forgive within a single relationship but vary across relationships (j and ij components in Table 4.1). Forgiveness behaviors are probably at least partly a function of one or more of these facets.

Failure to pay attention to the specificity principle in selecting appropriate measures of forgiveness puts researchers at risk of failing to find important relationships. It also creates conceptual confusion. For example, imagine the following scenario. Dr. A. was interested in assessing the association of forgiveness and marital adjustment. To test his hypothesis that "forgiving promotes marital adjustment," Dr. A. administered Wade's (1989) Forgiveness Scale and the Locke–Wallace (1959) Marital Adjustment Test to a sample of 300 married persons. Dr. A. found that participants' scores on Wade's Forgiveness Scale were correlated significantly with scores on the Locke–Wallace at $r = .16$, $p < .01$. On this basis, Dr. A. concluded that forgiveness was related to marital adjustment.

Such a conclusion could potentially be both conceptually and empirically problematic. It was not forgiveness in any general sense that was measured, but rather individuals' reports of the extent to which they had forgiven their spouses for a particular interpersonal offense (presumably, one that each respondent chose without guidance from the researcher). Thus, even though Dr. A. appeared to be interested in forgiveness at the dyadic (relationship) level (i.e., the extent to which a partner forgives his or her spouse), he used an occasion-specific measure of forgiveness (the extent to which a partner forgave his or her spouse for a *single, isolated offense*). In GT terms, Dr. A.'s implicit assumption was that offense-specific forgiveness would generalize to other offenses within the relationship, that is, would be highly correlated with a good dyadic measure of forgiveness. To the extent that forgiveness is consistent across offenses within a relationship, this assumption is unproblematic. However, if actors vary in their willingness to forgive multiple offenses by a single partner, then the forgiveness assessment would have been error laden in Dr. A.'s study. The likely consequence is attenuation of the observed effect size, and reduced statistical power.[3] Clearly, the obtained correlation of $r = .16$ was statistically significant, but what is the meaning of this modest correlation? Because the measure used to assess forgiveness was not at the appropriate level of specificity, Dr. A.'s hypothesis received a weak test (and was only vaguely supported). A better test of Dr. A.'s hypothesis would have been to use a less specific measure of forgiveness. To test whether forgiving marriages really are better quality marriages, Dr. A. could have aggregated several instances of forgiveness within each marriage or developed a measure that assessed forgiveness as a general relational quality.

We are not trying to say that it is never appropriate to examine the relations of variables with different levels of specificity. For example, it would be surprising if people's level of empathy for an individual who had damaged them was not related, in an empirical sense, to their dispositional capacity for empathy. As well, it is clear that narcissism—a dispositional variable—is a predictor of the extent to which people will engage in aggressive behavior toward an offender who threatens their self-esteem in a laboratory scenario (Bushman & Baumeister, 1998). Responses to such laboratory scenarios, of course, would be considered offense-specific measures in the $3 \times 2 \times 4$ taxonomy. What we *are* saying, however, is that without good theory to explain how constructs at one level of specificity are related to forgiveness constructs that are assessed at different levels of specificity, such empirical efforts (1) obscure the fact that forgiveness is likely to operate at different levels, (2) ignore the fact that adequate generalizability between levels is by no means assured, and (3) (to the extent that generalizability across levels is limited) lead to attenuated associations.

Controlling Sources of Variability in Forgiveness Ratings

Just as measuring forgiveness at the appropriate level of specificity is likely to produce pay-offs, so is the stringent control of measurement error. Usually, researchers think of controlling measurement error through random assignment to experimental conditions or through statistical controls. As well, it is likely that unintended sources of error creep into forgiveness ratings through weak control of the instructions given to research participants. In many studies (e.g., McCullough, Worthington, & Rachal, 1997, Study 1), researchers direct respondents to recall a transgression they had suffered at some point in the past, and then to indicate the extent to which they have forgiven their transgressor for this offense. This rating task probably introduces measurement error from a variety of sources.

When respondents are free to choose a transgression to rate in such a task, researchers have no idea what sorts of considerations inform respondents' choices. Certainly, some respondents will choose recent transgressions that are still salient because they are actively trying to figure out how to cope with them. Other respondents might choose long-standing sources of bitterness that are salient because they have been discussing them in psychotherapy. Still others might choose rather trivial offenses, because such offenses are the only ones that they are able to recall. Some people might choose the transgressions of a close relationship partner, while others might choose the transgression of a coworker, acquaintance, or stranger. Because factors such as the recency, salience, perceived severity, and identity of the perpetrator of the offense are likely to influence forgiveness ratings (and because these sources of error are difficult to

control even statistically), it is likely that they introduce error that inter-
feres with our ability to understand the psychological processes at work in
forgiveness.

Such sources of variation in forgiveness ratings can be controlled
through two design features. First, when the researcher's goal is to assess
a person's general tendency to forgive, but forgiveness is assessed in only
a single relationship for each actor, variance due to actor, partner, and
dyad effects are confounded, potentially creating large amounts of noise
in forgiveness scores (Hoyt, 1998). One method to reduce confounding is
to include multiple partners and offenses, as illustrated in Table 4.1.

Second, such sources of error can be controlled (at least in part) by
examining forgiveness in the context of specific interpersonal transgressions. The most recent intervention work from Enright and his colleagues
(e.g., Coyle & Enright, 1997; Freedman & Enright, 1996) exemplifies this
approach. In both of these studies, sample participants were selected precisely because they had suffered similar transgressions. In the Coyle and
Enright (1997) study, all the participants were men who felt that they had
been damaged by a sexual partner who had decided to abort a fetus that
they had helped to conceive. While the abortions had taken place at varying lengths of time in the past and probably had different levels of salience for each of the men in the study, focusing on a more or less
uniform transgression probably helped to eliminate error that might have
influenced the men's scores on a measure of the extent to which they had
forgiven the relationship partner. Similarly, Freedman and Enright (1996)
examined the extent to which adult women had forgiven male family
members who had sexually abused them as children. Again, focusing on a
specific type of transgression, perpetrated by people in a specific kind of
relationship to the participant, probably helped to control a variety of
sources of variance that otherwise would have contributed to error.

Specifying the Nomological Network Prior to Collecting "Construct Validity" Data

Construct validation is the process of determining what psychological constructs account for the performance of an instrument (Cronbach &
Meehl, 1955). In theory, scores on a measure that assesses forgiveness
should be related, at the proper magnitudes, to the variables that a particular theory of forgiveness specifies to be related to forgiveness. Thus, the
endeavor to develop measures for assessing forgiveness that have "construct validity" presupposes that existing theoretical treatments of forgiveness specify a set of probabilistic statements about how forgiveness is
related to other constructs of interest (and measures of those constructs).
Cronbach and Meehl called this set of probabilistic statements the construct's "nomological net."

In their landmark paper on construct validity, Cronbach and Meehl

(1955) pointed out that concepts with short scientific histories tend to have sparse nomological nets. Early in construct development, little will be known about how the construct is related to other constructs because (1) little solid theoretical work will exist; and (2) the existing psychometric studies will be preliminary. This describes the status of forgiveness research perfectly—the existing theoretical work has not stimulated very much empirical work, and most of the existing measures of forgiveness are only loosely tied to theoretical treatments of forgiveness. Of course, this is exactly what Cronbach and Meehl would lead us to expect. But that does not mean that all is as it should be.

To move beyond this current state of psychometric development, researchers should begin to tie their conceptualizations (and measures) of forgiveness into larger conceptual networks. Based on the best theory and research, what constructs (and operationalizations of them) and variables should explain variability in forgiveness? Which of these should be causally prior to forgiveness? Which should be concomitants of forgiveness? Which should be consequences? What should be the strength of these relationships? At what levels of specificity (offense-specific, dyadic, or dispositional) should measures of forgiveness constructs be related to measures of other constructs? Currently, no comprehensive nomological net has been laid out that would permit us to determine whether the correlations of forgiveness variables with other variables of interest (e.g., hostility, blame, empathy, spirituality, hope, anxiety, etc.) that have been obtained in research to date are actually evidence "for" or "against" the construct validity of such forgiveness measures.

Another element of construct validation is specifying and examining which constructs (and measures of those constructs) should be independent of forgiveness constructs (and measures of those forgiveness constructs). Such conceptual and empirical exercises—the tasks of exploring discriminant validity—have been mostly ignored in psychometric research on forgiveness to date. All of the issues raised here should be addressed in efforts to understand the construct validity of a psychometric instrument designed to measure a forgiveness construct.

CONCLUSION

In this chapter, we have tried to bring some clarity to the existing empirical work dedicated to the assessment of forgiveness. By organizing the existing measures along three dimensions (specificity of measurement, direction of measurement, and method of measurement) we see that some psychometric work is being done in certain areas, but other areas remain weak or completely unexplored. Each of the unexplored areas remains uncharted scientific territory.

In charting this new scientific territory—and in elaborating what we already know—we recommend that researchers treat future psychometric studies on forgiveness with the same forethought and methodological rigor that is extended in other areas of social-scientific research. A generalizability framework provides, to our way of thinking, the best conceptual bridge for matching psychometric research strategies to the complexities that might underlie forgiveness in particular research applications. As well, researchers should also begin to use multiple measures of forgiveness that are appropriate to particular research applications and should choose research designs that reduce extraneous score variance. Researchers should also continue to develop more explicitly a set of theoretically derived, probabilistic statements that link particular forgiveness constructs (and their measures) to other constructs (and measures). Addressing these psychometric concerns in future studies will help increase both the breadth and depth of what we know about this set of interesting and important constructs.

NOTES

1. This third "methods" dimension is obviously somewhat plastic. Forgiveness constructs could be assessed with many more than these four methods, including qualitative analysis, content analysis, diary methods, physiological methods, archival methods, and historiometric methods. Our neglect of these methods is not meant to suggest that we do not believe them to be valid; rather, it reflects the fact that no measures currently exist using these methods, and so to include such methods in our taxonomy would have been pointless. Clearly, all of these categories represent alternative "methods" through which forgiveness could be assessed, and each of them deserves to be explored in its own right.
2. McCullough, Worthington, and Rachal (1997) also used a 5-item self-report measure of forgiveness. These items and their instructions were adapted from the EFI (Subkoviak et al., 1995), although the McCullough et al. paper failed to attribute these items to Subkoviak et al. Enright has requested that researchers refrain from using this combination of items from the EFI in their own research. Rather, he requests that interested researchers use the complete, 60-item EFI.
3. Ironically, the effect size in Dr. A.'s study would also presumably have been inflated to some extent by correlated response bias, because the same person rated forgiveness and dyadic adjustment for each relationship. The net impact of these uncontrolled upward and downward biases in effect sizes can only be estimated by conducting a multivariate generalizability study (Hoyt, 1998).

REFERENCES

Al-Mabuk, R. H., Enright, R. D., & Cardis, P. A. (1995). Forgiveness education with parentally love-deprived late adolescents. *Journal of Moral Education, 24,* 427–444.

Anderson, C. A., & Bushman, B. J. (1997). External validity of "trivial" experiments: The case of laboratory aggression. *General Psychology Review, 1,* 19–41.

Axelrod, R. (1980a). Effective choice in the Prisoner's Dilemma. *Journal of Conflict Resolution,* 24(3), 3–25.

Axelrod, R. (1980b). More effective choice in the Prisoner's Dilemma. *Journal of Conflict Resolution,* 24(3), 379–403.

Baumeister, R. F., Exline, J. J., & Sommer, K. L. (1998). The victim role, grudge theory, and two dimensions of forgiveness. In E. L. Worthington (Ed.), *The foundation of forgiveness* (pp. 79–104). Philadelphia: Templeton Foundation Press.

Brown, B. R. (1968). The effects of need to maintain face on interpersonal bargaining. *Journal of Experimental Social Psychology, 4,* 107–122.

Bushman, B. J., & Baumeister, R. F. (1998). Threatened egotism, narcissism, self-esteem, and displaced aggression: Does self-love or self-hate lead to violence? *Journal of Personality and Social Psychology, 75,* 219–229.

Caprara, G. V. (1986). Indicators of aggression: The dissipation–rumination scale. *Personality and Individual Differences, 7,* 763–769.

Caprara, G. V., Barbaranelli, C., & Comrey, A. L. (1992). A personological approach to the study of aggression. *Personality and Individual Differences, 13,* 77–84.

Caprara, G. V., Coluzzi, M., Mazzotti, E., Renzi, P., & Zelli, A. (1985). Effect of insult and dissipation–rumination on delayed aggression and hostility. *Archivio di Psicologia, Neurologia e Psichiatria, 46,* 130–139.

Caprara, G. V., Gargaro, T., Pastorelli, C., Prezza, M., Renzi, P., & Zelli, A. (1987). Individual differences and measures of aggression in laboratory studies. *Personality and Individual Differences, 8*(6), 885–893.

Caprara, G. V., Manzi, J., & Perugini, M. (1992). Investigating guilt in relation to emotionality and aggression. *Personality and Individual Differences, 13,* 519–532.

Caprara, G. V., & Pastorelli, C. (1989). Toward a reorientation of research on aggression. *European Journal of Personality, 3,* 121–138.

Collins, K., & Bell, R. (1997). Personality and aggression: The dissipation–rumination scale. *Personality and Individual Differences, 22,* 751–755.

Coyle, C. T., & Enright, R. D. (1997). Forgiveness intervention with post-abortion men. *Journal of Consulting and Clinical Psychology, 65*(6), 1042–1046.

Cronbach, L. J. (1995). Giving method variance its due. In P. E. Shrout & S. T. Fiske (Eds.), *Personality research, methods, and theory: A festschrift in honor of Donald Fiske* (pp. 145–157). New York: Wiley.

Cronbach, L. J., Gleser, G. C., Nanda, H., & Rajaratnam, N. (1972). *The dependability of behavioral measurements: Theory of generalizability for scores and profiles.* New York: Wiley.

Cronbach, L. J., & Meehl, P. E. (1955). Construct validity in psychological tests. *Psychological Bulletin, 52,* 281–302.

Darby, B. W., & Schlenker, B. R. (1982). Children's reactions to apologies. *Journal of Personality and Social Psychology, 43,* 742–753.

Davidson, D. L., & Jurkovic, G. J. (1993, April). *Forgiveness and narcissism: Consistency in experience across real and hypothetical hurt scenarios.* Paper presented at the annual convention of the Christian Association for Psychological Studies, Kansas City, MO.

Dreelin, E. D. (1993). *Religious functioning and forgiveness.* Unpublished dissertation, Fuller Graduate School of Psychology, Pasadena, CA.

Epstein, S. (1983). Aggregation and beyond: Some issues on the aggregation of behavior. *Journal of Personality, 51*(3), 360–392.

Fishbein, M., & Ajzen, I. (1974). Attitudes toward objects as predictors of single and multiple behavioral criteria. *Psychological Review, 81,* 59–74.

Freedman, S. R., & Enright, R. D. (1996). Forgiveness as an intervention goal with incest survivors. *Journal of Consulting and Clinical Psychology, 64,* 510–517.

Gassin, E. A. (1998). Receiving forgiveness as moral education: A theoretical analysis and initial empirical investigation. *Journal of Moral Education, 27,* 71–87.

Girard, M., & Mullet, E. (1997). Forgiveness in adolescents, young, middle-aged, and older adults. *Journal of Adult Development, 4,* 209–220.

Gorsuch, R. L. (1984). Measurement: The boon and bane of investigating religion. *American Psychologist, 39,* 228–236.

Gorsuch, R. L. (1988). Psychology of religion. *Annual Review of Psychology, 39,* 201–221.

Gorsuch, R. L., & Hao, J. Y. (1993). Forgiveness: An exploratory factor analysis and its relationships to religious variables. *Review of Religious Research, 34*(4), 333–347.

Hamilton, M. (1960). A rating scale for depression. *Journal of Neurology, Neurosurgery and Psychiatry, 23,* 56–62.

Hargrave, T. D., & Sells, J. N. (1997). The development of a forgiveness scale. *Journal of Marital and Family Therapy, 23*(1), 41–62.

Hebl, J. H., & Enright, R. D. (1993). Forgiveness as a psychotherapeutic goal with elderly females. *Psychotherapy, 30,* 658–667.

Hoyt, W. T. (in press). Rater bias: When is it a problem and what can we do about it? *Psychological Methods.*

Hoyt, W. T., & Melby, J. N. (1999). Dependability of measurement in counseling psychology: An introduction to generalizability theory. *Counseling Psychologist, 27,* 325–352.

Kenny, D. A. (1994). *Interpersonal perception: A social relations analysis.* New York: Guilford Press.

Kremer, J. F., & Stephens, L. (1983). Attributions and arousal as mediators of mitigation's effect on retaliation. *Journal of Personality and Social Psychology, 45*(2), 335–343.

Locke, H. J., & Wallace, K. M. (1959). Short marital-adjustment and prediction tests: Their reliability and validity. *Marriage and Family Living, 21,* 251–255.

Long, E. C. J., & Andrews, D. W. (1990). Perspective taking as a predictor of marital adjustment. *Journal of Personality and Social Psychology, 59,* 126–131.

Mauger, P. A., Perry, J. E., Freeman, T., Grove, D. C., McBride, A. G., & McKinney, K. E. (1992). The measurement of forgiveness: Preliminary research. *Journal of Psychology and Christianity, 11*(2), 170–180.

McCullough, M. E. (1995). *Forgiveness as altruism: A social-psychological theory of forgiveness and tests of its validity.* Unpublished doctoral dissertation, Virginia Commonwealth University, Richmond.

McCullough, M. E., Rachal, K. C., Sandage, S. J., Worthington, E. L., Jr., Brown, S. W., & Hight, T. L. (1998). Interpersonal forgiving in close relationships II: Theoretical elaboration and measurement. *Journal of Personality and Social Psychology, 75,* 1586–1603.

McCullough, M. E., Sandage, S. J., Rachal, K. C., & Worthington, E. L., Jr. (1997, August). *A sustainable future for the psychology of forgiveness.* Paper presented at the annual meeting of the American Psychological Association, Chicago, IL.

McCullough, M. E., & Worthington, E. L., Jr. (1995). Promoting forgiveness: A comparison of two brief psychoeducational group interventions with a waiting-list control. *Counseling and Values, 40,* 55–68.

McCullough, M. E., & Worthington, E. L., Jr. (2000). Religion and the forgiving personality. *Journal of Personality.*

McCullough, M. E., Worthington, E. L., Jr., & Rachal, K. C. (1997). Interpersonal forgiving in close relationships. *Journal of Personality and Social Psychology, 73*(2), 321–336.

Meek, K. R., Albright, J. S., & McMinn, M. R. (1995). Religious orientation, guilt, confession, and forgiveness. *Journal of Psychology and Theology, 23*(3), 190–197.

Park, Y. O., & Enright, R. D. (1997). The development of forgiveness in the context of adolescent friendship conflict in Korea. *Journal of Adolescence, 20*(4), 393–402.

Rhode, M. G. (1990). *Forgiveness, power, and empathy.* Unpublished doctoral dissertation, Fuller Graduate School of Psychology, Pasadena, CA.

Rokeach, M. (1967). *Human Values Survey.* Sunnyvale, CA: Halgren Tests.

Rosenman, R. H., Friedman, M., Straus, R., Wurm, M., Kositchek, R., Hahn, W., & Werthessen,

N. T. (1964). A predictive study of coronary heart disease. *Journal of the American Medical Association, 189,* 113–124.

Rushton, J. P., Brainerd, C. J., & Pressley, M. (1983). Behavioral development and construct validity: The principle of aggregation. *Psychological Bulletin, 94*(1), 18–38.

Shrout, P. E., & Fliess, J. L. (1979). Intraclass correlations: Uses in assessing rater reliability. *Psychological Bulletin, 86,* 420–428.

Smith, P. (1978). Sampling errors of variance components in small sample generalizability studies. *Journal of Educational Measurement, 3,* 319–346.

Subkoviak, M. J., Enright, R. D., & Wu, C. (1992, October). *Current developments related to measuring forgiveness.* Paper presented at the annual meeting of the Midwestern Educational Research Association, Chicago, IL.

Subkoviak, M. J., Enright, R. D., Wu, C., Gassin, E. A., Freedman, S., Olson, L. M., & Sarinopoulos, I. (1995). Measuring interpersonal forgiveness in late adolescence and middle adulthood. *Journal of Adolescence, 18,* 641–655.

Trainer, M. F. (1981). *Forgiveness: Intrinsic, role-expected, expedient, in the context of divorce.* Unpublished doctoral dissertation, Boston University.

Wade, S. H. (1987). *A content analysis of forgiveness.* Unpublished master's project, Fuller Graduate School of Psychology, Pasadena, CA.

Wade, S. H. (1989). *The development of a scale to measure forgiveness.* Unpublished doctoral dissertation, Fuller Graduate School of Psychology, Pasadena, CA.

Zillman, D., & Cantor, J. R. (1976). Effect of timing of information about mitigating circumstances on emotional responses to provocation and retaliatory behavior. *Journal of Experimental Social Psychology, 12,* 38–55.

PART II

Basic Psychological Research

CHAPTER 5

The Neuropsychological Correlates of Forgiveness

Andrew B. Newberg, Eugene G. d'Aquili,
Stephanie K. Newberg, and Verushka deMarici

Forgiveness is a complex neurocognitive and affective process that has multiple facets and has been increasingly recognized as an important aspect of psychotherapy and behavior change. However, a complete understanding of forgiveness requires knowledge of its underlying neuropsychological mechanisms, particularly those of the sense of self, a recognition of harm to the self, and revenge behavior. This, in turn, requires a review of the forgiveness process and its phenomenology. It is also necessary to consider any possible evolutionary origins of forgiveness that might suggest neuropsychological as well as social mechanisms. Such an analysis then necessitates a review of the neurophysiology and overall brain function that may be related to the act of forgiveness. Finally, we consider an initial model for the mechanism of forgiveness, which we hope leads to empirical testing or, at least, the possibility of future directions for research into this concept.

THE NEUROEVOLUTIONARY BASIS OF INJURY PERCEPTION AND REVENGE

When considering the evolution of forgiveness behavior, it is important to examine how various human brain functions evolved from the brain functions of more "primitive" animals. This type of neuroevolutionary process has been called "encephalization" (Laughlin, McManus, & d'Aquili, 1992). Encephalization of brain functions in primate and human evolution allows primitive survival mechanisms to be represented in the newly developing brain, although in a highly modified form. Thus, new and "encephalized" functions can be quite different from the primitive function on which they are based, often being only structurally or formally similar. For example, the frontal and prefrontal lobes originally developed to direct simple motor behavior. With the advent of the genus *Homo*, the frontal and prefrontal lobes developed the additional ability for the animal to plan and prioritize motor behaviors, and to develop and organize goal-directed motor behavior (Pribram & McGuinness, 1975; Stuss & Benson, 1986). Eventually, not only did motor behaviors come under the auspices of the frontal and prefrontal lobes, but cognitive and emotional responses also were planned and priori-tized by these areas. Therefore, these frontal and prefrontal functions, while seeming to be far removed from simple movement, nevertheless represent a highly sophisticated and abstract evolution of function that is primarily based on motor behavior (Joseph, 1990). It is becoming clearer that to truly understand complex hominid behaviors, particularly those embedded in, and crucial to, culture, one must understand their homologues in pre-hominid behavior. It is this kind of approach that we must have if we are go-ing to arrive at any significant understanding of a complex human behavior such as forgiveness.

We must begin by exploring some of the more primitive behaviors among humans and other animals in order to derive an understanding of forgiveness. It must be mentioned here that there may be other mecha-nisms, separate from evolutionary ones (i.e., religious or social), that play a role in the development of the forgiveness process in human beings. However, for the purpose of this chapter and its focus on neuropsycho-logical mechanisms, we consider the possible evolutionary basis of such mechanisms.

Since forgiveness seems always to presuppose that an injury has been incurred to the self, one might begin by determining the nature of "injury to the self" and how this occurs neuropsychologically and evolutionarily. A perception of injury to the self has several substrates: (1) a sense of self; (2) an ability to evaluate the behavior of conspecifics as being injurious or beneficial (the notion of conspecific congruence); and (3) memory of the event in order to link that injury to the offending person. As we describe, these also appear to be substrates for forgiveness and can help toward an understanding of why forgiveness occurs at all.

Sense of Self

As Geschwind (1965), and especially Luria (1980), first demonstrated, the inferior parietal lobule, particularly on the dominant side, underlies the capacity for abstraction and reification. In other words, the ability to generate classes of objects from particulars and to turn relationships into "things," both of which are necessary conditions for language, arises from the development and elaboration of this area of the brain. The inferior parietal lobule probably begins to become functionally significant at the Australopithicene level in evolution if the interpretation of skull structures has any significance at all (LeGros Clark, 1963). Probably the most important development is that the input of the body's senses and functions, as well as mental functions, are formed into a unified sense of self, and indeed, even a self-reflecting self. We must note here that the inferior parietal lobule in both the dominant and nondominant hemispheres has rich interconnections with the limbic system, which is the part of the brain primarily involved in the modulation of emotion (Joseph, 1990; Kandel, Schwartz, & Jessell, 1993). It is the inferior parietal lobule on the dominant side that probably modulates the sense of self (Joseph, 1990). The self is therefore imbued, when it is vividly experiencing, with the emotional tone of the dominant hemisphere. Several investigators (Hommes & Panhuysen, 1971) neatly demonstrated that when the dominant hemisphere of the brain is put to sleep with a barbiturate, what is released on the nondominant side is depressive affect. When the nondominant hemisphere is put to sleep, what is released on the dominant side is elation or hypomania. Both of these emotional responses are mediated by the limbic system in their respective hemispheres (Joseph, 1990; Kandel et al., 1993). The sense of self therefore, which for the most part is a function of the inferior parietal lobule on the dominant side, tends to be associated with positive affect at the very least, and often with some degree of hypomania. This partially explains why patients in serious depression usually have a significant struggle with their sense of self and, most certainly, asserting their selves (Deitz, 1991; Jackson, 1991; Segal & Blatt, 1993; Mukherji, 1995).

The expansion of the perception of the ego or self is such that we tend to perceive ourselves in a grander manner than we perceive other individuals (Jackson, 1991). This makes sense, since it is the self that must perceive, analyze, and evaluate all input regarding the self (Laughlin et al., 1992). This process may involve both the posterior superior parietal lobe and the limbic system, since these areas are involved in providing a sense of self and the affective valence toward the self, respectively. From an evolutionary perspective, such a perception is necessary for the maintenance of the self above all other things. If such an expansion of the self did not occur, it would make a person less interested in protecting his or her self. However, this expansion of the perception of the self also arises because all of our perceptions of emotions and sensations are perceived as part of our self and not usually as part of someone else (with the possible exception of dissociative states). This naturally sets up a greater sense and perception of the self and all things that happen to it.

Conspecific Congruence

The second substrate for the perception of injury is the notion of "conspecific congruence," which refers to the perceived nonhierarchical relationship between a given individual and the other conspecifics (or individuals) in the group. Along with hierarchical ordering, conspecific congruence is one of the more powerful psychosocial forces creating and limiting the structure, relationships, and roles within human (and other) mammalian) social groups. Whereas hierarchical ordering is "vertical" within a society and represents, as it were, the "protoaristocratic" element in social organization, conspecific congruence is "horizontal" and represents the "protodemocratic" psychosocial element. Both always seem to be present to some degree, however, within all stable human social groups.

A dramatic example of the interweaving of these two psychosocial forces would be a medieval serf's physically attacking his lord when the latter came to claim his "right of the first night" (*ius primae noctis*) with the serf's new bride. Rare as such incidents may have been, they are known to have occurred. In such a case, the serf is "appealing" to conspecific congruence even in the face of well-established and extremely powerful hierarchical ordering. Thus, conspecific congruence helps create a balance within the social group such that all members understand their role and relationship with all the others in the group. Clearly, both hierarchical ordering and conspecific congruence have the evolutionary advantage of helping to maintain the integrity of the group's social structure. Social organization itself has clearly been an adaptive advantage in both the hominid line and in other species (d'Aquili, 1972). Behaviors that help support the social structure therefore have an adaptive advantage.

In considering the evolution and dynamics of forgiveness, both conspecific congruence and hierarchical ordering play a role; however, conspecific congruence is central to our understanding of this phenomenon at its core. Conspecific congruence among human beings probably developed out of the structures in the brain that underlie the ability to form classes of groups with perceived similarities in humans and other animals. In human beings, the higher order cognitive and emotional functions of the brain allowed for the perception of the class "human," but more importantly, perception of the class "our group" or "our tribe." This was the essential neuropsychological basis for the emergence of conspecific congruence. Conspecific congruence is asserted when all members behave to maintain social balance.

An individual utilizes conspecific congruence to evaluate the behaviors of conspecifics to determine if they may result in altering the congruence in either a positive or negative manner. It is interesting that the same area of the brain (the inferior parietal lobe), which we discussed earlier with relation to abstractive ability and reification, is the same area of the brain that provides a number of logical–grammatical categories and functions (Bruce, Desimone, & Gross, 1986; Burton & Jones, 1976; Geschwind, 1965; Jones & Powell, 1970; Seltzer & Pandya, 1978; Zeki, Symonds, & Kaas, 1982). Comparisons such as "greater than," "lesser than," and "equal to" are also formulated by this part of the brain. Such comparisons are also given emotional bias via the connections between the inferior parietal lobe and the limbic system. Obviously, this function is essential to the principle of conspecific congruence. A change in congruence, with the subject positively valenced, is perceived by the subject as a favor or kindness, with the consequent obligation to return it in some way in order to balance the incongruence. A change in the congruence that is negatively valenced is perceived by the subject as an injury, an attack on the self, with the likely consequent desire for revenge to restore the congruence.

We propose that the principle of conspecific congruence could not have evolved without the development of the inferior parietal lobule, allowing both the perception of the "equality" of conspecifics and the perception of incongruence. It is also important to add that as the notion of conspecific congruence became encephalized into the human brain, this function expanded to include not only conspecifics, but also, eventually, the entire world. Thus, human beings have a perception of the relationship of their self to the entire world (Jackson, 1991). Such a relationship may be termed "self–world congruence," because it implies that a person has a certain understanding of the self and the congruence that exists between that self and the rest of the external world. We will consider the self–world congruence later in this chapter, but for now, we continue with the association between congruence and the perception of harm and revenge.

It is in the face of a change in conspecific congruence with the subject negatively valanced, that the process of forgiveness or revenge may occur. Revenge appears to be a more active approach to restoring congruence (Berscheid, Boye, & Walster, 1968), whereas forgiveness seems to restore congruence in a different manner. The evolution of human revenge behavior is, at first, easier to understand than the evolution of forgiveness. It seems to be more clearly related to self-preservation. Its cultural and derivative manifestation, justice, is certainly central for the preservation of societies and cultures. The *Lex Talionis*, that is, the law of "an eye for an eye and a tooth for a tooth," seems to be present in all cultures in one form or another. It is both the most primitive manifestation of justice and the clearest manifestation of personal revenge. True revenge, as practiced within the genus *Homo*, is certainly a considerable elaboration of the self-preservation motif. Since revenge behavior is based upon a negative change in conspecific congruence, true revenge requires a sense of self and the internal drive to equalize incongruence between two conspecifics. Thus, when an individual is offended or hurt, there is a strong impulse to return the hurt and thus bring the imbalance into congruence. Although this may be the basis of revenge, it is not the only example of conspecific congruence. Generous gift giving or granting favors by socially dominant individuals, such as the Patlatch among the native Americans of the northwest during banquets and drinking fests of Anglo Saxon Aethelings, causes a disequilibrium in conspecific congruence, with the resulting obligation on the part of the receivers of the generosity to return it in one form or another. There are a number of examples of the necessity among humans to restore the equilibrium that is destroyed when conspecific congruence is contravened. Here, however, we are only concerned when the disequilibrium is caused by a perceived hurt or injury generating a desire in the injured party to restore the balance by getting revenge.

Long-Term Memory of Injurious Events

In addition to the sense of self, its inflation, and the principle of conspecific congruence, another element must be in place before full-blown human revenge behavior can take place. This is the final substrate that we mentioned earlier regarding perception of injury—the evolution of long-term memory of causal events. Obviously, an individual who cannot carry the injury in memory for any significant time cannot get revenge on the perpetrator of the injury. For example, Murphy (1988) has defined forgiveness as the forswearing of resentment, which is differentiated from forgetting, which, he states, just happens. Thus, forgiveness requires memory of the causal framework within which the injury to the self occurred, so that the offender and the events are remembered. Murphy sees forgiveness as something that helps one to avoid the painful consequences of holding onto the memory of negative emotions associated with resentment. We maintain that, at a more primitive level, forgiveness involves forswearing revenge (Enright & the Human Development Study Group, 1991; North, 1987). Forswearing revenge is already an extremely encephalized and highly developed version of the forgiveness phenomenon.

What are the neuroanatomical and neurophysiological structures and functions that must have evolved in order for these elements to be present and grafted upon the basic prehominid instinct for self-preservation? These elements in what we call the "revenge complex" are not based on any single neural structure within the brain but rather on a number of structures related to each other in complex neural networks. The evolution of long-term memory arose from the development of the hippocampal–amygdalar memory system (Milner, 1970; Mishkin, 1978; Rawlins, 1985; Sarter & Markowitsch, 1985). This involved the evolution of neural connections between the limbic system (especially the hippo-campus and amygdala) and various parts of the neocortex. It is hard to tell when this long-term memory system evolved, but it may have been in place among protohominids (Laughlin & d'Aquili, 1974).

In turning to the evolution of forgiveness, we can begin to under-stand how it neuropsychologically relates to the substrates of injury per-ception and revenge. One might intuitively understand the adaptive advantage of revenge-seeking behavior as related to conspecific congru-ence. Indeed, some studies suggest that individuals who, in one way or an another, retaliate when wronged tend to be wronged less frequently (Baron, 1973, 1974; Rogers, 1980). It is certainly far less intuitive to un-derstand the evolutionary advantage of forgiveness behavior. Forgiveness consists of persons "giving up" their right to redress a wrong, to restore equilibrium, and to reestablish conspecific congruence in the usual way. We might get a clue as to the nonhuman homologue of forgiveness by looking at the animal world around us. There are a number of recon-ciliatory behaviors, including submission gestures, that help to terminate fighting between conspecifics. It is likely that forgiveness is the neocortical homologue of these types of behaviors. However, future studies of such behaviors in animals will be necessary in order to substantiate any claim specifically relating animal behaviors with human forgiveness.

Why Forgiveness?

But why would forgiveness have evolved? What is its adaptive advantage? Let us return to that interesting characteristic of humans to exaggerate both the self and the degree of wrong done to that "exalted" or "grandi-ose" self (Lynch, 1991). This exaggerated misperception of the offense to the subject results in an attempt to redress the wrong. Since the person who initially committed the offense is human also, he or she will perceive the excessive redress as even more excessive. With this mechanism operat-ing, it is almost impossible to restore equilibrium neatly. Every attempt to restore equilibrium results in further disequilibrium. Such a neuropsycho-logical system, if unchecked, could lead to the social chaos it initially evolved to avoid. Forgiveness, curiously, often eliminates the bellicosity in one's opponent (Enright, 1996). Thus, although forgiveness does not al-ways eliminate hostilities, it usually does (Komorita, Hilty, & Parks, 1991).

Furthermore, forgiveness, or at least nonretaliation observed by oth-ers, may have the curious quality of generating empathy and warm feel-ings for the injured victim from observers who were usually in no way involved in the initial fight or confrontation (Kanekar & Kolsawalla, 1977; Kanekar & Merchant, 1982). This can have remarkably profound social consequences. For example, a huge number of converts were gained for Christianity during the 10 great persecutions by the Roman Empire because of the empathy and warm feelings generated in many spectators observing Christians suffering and forgiving their persecutors. A third-century Christian dictum was *sanguis martyrorum semen christianorum* (i.e., the blood of martyrs is the seed of Christians), illustrating the profound neuropsychological effect upon many individuals who simply observed acts of forgiveness. The effect on many observers is usually the same as the effect on the hostile opponent, namely, an upsurge of empathy and warm feelings for the forgiver. Although this is a general response, it is clearly not a universal one. Individuals diagnosed with antisocial personality disorder do not seem to have a genuinely empathic response to a forgiving person. Assorted other individuals, as well, may also lack this response. But generally speaking, an empathic response to a forgiving person may be a primary evolved complement to forgiveness.

To summarize, the evolution of forgiveness behavior is profitable for social groups in that it tends to cut off progressively escalating revenge behavior. Such escalating revenge behavior is based on an affective misperception of the importance of the self, with its consequent misjudgment of the amount of revenge necessary to restore conspecific congruence. Thus, if the revenge interactions are approaching a lethal level, forgiveness may literally save one's life. Furthermore, the forgiving individual may gain significant advantage in social support owing to the positive affective alignment toward the forgiver that is generated in observers. Overall, the social advantages of forgiveness, as well as the advantages for the individual forgiver, almost certainly outweigh the dangers that arise from forgiving the relatively rare, nonresponsive person. Furthermore, as we describe, the individual may benefit emotionally from the act of forgiving.

Another possibility is that forgiveness does not inherently have an adaptive advantage but is linked to another trait that does serve an adaptive advantage, such as the ability to form family or social groups (Buss, Haselton, Shackelford, Bleske, & Wakefield, 1998). While such a possibility cannot be excluded at this time, it is likely that forgiveness may have played a role in the behaviors with which it is linked. Therefore, if forgiveness evolved in people more likely to form social groups, forgiveness may have been a behavior that, at least, helped facilitate group cohesion, as described earlier.

One additional point to consider is what it means neuropsychologically to give up the right for revenge. To answer this question, one must first ask what it means neuropsychologically to give up anything, or more subtly, one's "rights" to anything. The neuropsychological model presented for this human behavior is more speculative than the neuropsychological substrates of injury perception and revenge. First of all, the inferior parietal lobule is necessary for conceiving the abstract concepts involved in revenge. Once these concepts exist, whether or not the brain's linguistic operators give them a name, they can be related to each other via subtle or not-so-subtle emotional valences. This, again, is where the functioning of the limbic system may be involved in order to help provide a valence for the relationship between the concept of the self and the concept of revenge. A positive valence means that revenge (a specific revenge towards a specific person) is part of the self. A negative valence means that this revenge is not part of the self, that it is other, and therefore does not draw the self into revenge behavior. We would hypothesize that forgiveness, or giving up revenge, involves a shift of affective valence between the self and a "specific revenge," from a positive valence to a negative valence. Such an explanation of forgiveness evokes a whole theory of "affective valencing" (for which space does not permit greater elaboration) as at least one possible way of relating conceptual entities.

SOCIAL CONTROLS OF REVENGE BEHAVIOR

We have seen how injury perception and revenge evolved as encephalized manifestations of the more primitive self-preservation function in order to restore and correct any disequilibrium in conspecific congruence. Its obvious "purpose" was the enhancement of social cohesion by discouraging violations of the rights of other individuals. We have also posited that revenge behavior is poorly modulated and can easily lapse into an excessive mutual retaliation owing to an excessive evaluation of the self, with the consequent miscalculation of what is needed to restore equilibrium. This somewhat grandiose evaluation of self may have had many evolutionarily adaptive advantages, but it resulted in revenge behavior often working in an uncontrolled and faulty way. We have seen "the attempt" of biological evolution to correct this by the coevolution of forgiveness, which may be the encephalized manifestation of primitive submission gestures.

Superimposed on revenge behavior, one can discern cultural evolution attempting both to modify this behavior directly and to shore up forgiveness behavior and its neural substrate to allow for better modulation and control of revenge. Some researchers have even identified a feeling of the "obligation" to forgive as one of the motivators of forgiveness (Rowe, Halling, Davies, Leifer, Powers, & van Bronkhorst, 1989).

Justice and Law

One cultural mechanism that attempts to control revenge was the concept of justice and, later, of law. Justice attempts to get around the overvaluation of self by the social attempt to define "objectively" the nature of the offense and precisely what is necessary to reestablish congruence. Whether it is the judgment of a tribal council, the decision of a sovereign, or the ruling of a court of law, we are dealing in all cases with the sociocultural attempt to correct the imperfect revenge behavior. In this case, we see a culturally developed concept, justice, arising out of the biologically evolved revenge behavior, which itself is an encephalized manifestation of self-preservation. This is a good example of three levels of the development of a single theme, two levels arising from biological evolution and one from cultural evolution.

Spiritual Meaning and Forgiveness

A second mechanism in the attempt to control revenge behavior is for many societies to positively sanction and powerfully reinforce forgiveness. Unlike the evolution of justice, at least in its most primitive form, the *Lex Talionis,* the positive sanctioning of forgiveness is not a cultural universal, although it is very common. It reaches a summit in the theoretical ethos of Christianity, more often honored in the breach than in the observance. Nevertheless, the cultural reinforcement of forgiveness is still a powerful help in the modulation of revenge.

It would seem that the most usual way for cultures positively to sanction forgiveness is by investing it with a transcendent or religious meaning. In other words, God (or the gods) is said to love and bless the forgiver. That cultures can do this, and that the transcendent exists at all as a cultural category, may possibly arise from the biological evolution of unitary experiences. In other works, we have presented a model of how this occurs, involving, among other things, partial or total blocking of input into the posterior superior parietal lobule (d'Aquili & Newberg, 1993a, 1993b). Blocking of input into this area may possibly result in progressively greater unitary experiences that can be arranged along a spectrum or continuum. At the lower end of the continuum are aesthetic experiences in which the perception of unity over diversity is only slightly greater than baseline. As one moves along this continuum, the unitary experiences are successively more powerful, such as romantic love, religious awe, various trance states, Cosmic Consciousness, and, ultimately, what we have termed Absolute Unitary Being (AUB). AUB is the ultimate unitary state in which the boundaries of discrete entities in the world are dissolved, the perception of space and time are obliterated, and even the self–other dichotomy dissolves (d'Aquili & Newberg, 1993a, 1993b). Experiences at the lower end of the aesthetic–religious continuum are common. Those at the upper end are extremely rare. However, what is important for a consideration of forgiveness is that the sense of the transcendent, now conceptualized in the form of God, the gods, or other power sources, can be used positively to sanction any behavior or institution that the culture considers important. This helps to provide the social control over conspecific congruence by utilizing the transcendent to sanction behaviors and emotions that support conspecific congruence.

But the association of the transcendent with forgiveness is a little more tricky than simply an issue of positive sanctioning by the culture. As noted earlier, forgiveness generates positive feelings in the forgiver and usually in the forgiven aggressive opponent. These positive feelings seem somehow to be related to a lessening of the sense of self of the forgiver, resulting from a diminution of ego assertiveness. This is precisely the sort of state that may be associated with a mild unitary experience (unlike the negative affect associated with the difficulty in obtaining a sense of self in depression), likely on the part of the forgiver and perhaps in others as well. As we have shown in other works, these unitary experiences, even mild ones, tend to be perceived as transcendent. Hence, the mild unitary experience of the forgiver may tend to reinforce the positive sanction of the culture, making it clear to the forgiver that in the act of forgiving, he or she has briefly entered into a transcendent world.

THE FORGIVENESS PROCESS

We have already described forgiveness as a complex neurocognitive process that has multiple components. In order to examine the possible neurophysiological mechanism underlying forgiveness, we must consider the phenomenology of the forgiveness process. This entails following forgiveness from its early stages through its final endpoint. Of course, for something as complex as forgiveness, it is difficult to adhere to a rigid description of its phenomenology. Forgiveness, as we will consider, can often occur via a number of different paths. However, by considering the most consistent aspects of the forgiveness process, we may be able to identify certain specific patterns and paths that form at least the minimum requirements for forgiveness to occur. Such analysis has already been performed by several investigators who have suggested more global models of the forgiveness process. These models have been based on psychological theories, moral development, and the actual phenomenological process of forgiveness (Fow, 1996). Based on such analyses, the underlying neuropsychological mechanisms can be superimposed upon the psychological phenomenology of forgiveness. Psychological models generally divide the forgiveness process into the following: (1) recognition of the injury to the self; (2) commitment to forgive; (3) cognitive and affective activity; and (4) behavioral action (McCullough & Worthington, 1994).

Recognition of Injury to the Self

Psychologists have argued that for forgiveness to be able to happen at all, there must be an initial harm or injury to the self that is recognized (Close, 1970; Enright, 1996; Rowe et al., 1989). The injury or harm may take many forms, which can be grouped into two basic categories that find their bases in the neurobiological substrates we described earlier. The first category is harm that occurs directly to the individual. This could be in the form of physical, mental, sexual, or verbal actions (this includes self-inflicted harm) that directly damage an individual. Harm can also be incurred via a secondary mechanism. For example, persons may perceive their self to be damaged as the result of harm being done to a friend or relative. Even more derivative is injury to the self because another person committed some act against other human beings in general. This may cause harm to the self because of newfound fear, mistrust, or disappointment in other people as a result of the inciting act. Thus, for forgiveness even to be a consideration, there must occur some form of damage that alters a person's existing conspecific congruence or, if the injuring event is caused by a nonhuman object in the world, a person's self–world congruence.

For damage to an individual to occur, there must be a sense of the self. After all, there must first exist a self that can be injured before it can actually be injured. Furthermore, this sense of self must be distinguished from the one causing the damage. Once the harm is identified as having occurred to the self, the source of that injury can be determined. The injury can be self-induced, in which the person injured is also causing the injury. Examples of self-caused injury might be found in people suffering from anxiety, depression, eating and personality disorders, and even those who have poor self-esteem. However, in these cases, there is often a distinction made between that part of the self that causes the damage and that part that receives the damage. The injury can also be perpetrated by something or someone other than the self. Examples of injury caused by others can be in the form of physical, mental, sexual, or verbal injury. Therefore, there is usually a subject–object relationship (resulting directly from either conspecific or self–world congruence) between the damaging agent and the self that is damaged. This relationship is considered in a causal framework and requires the ability to make the distinction between self and other.

That the injury requires placement in a causal framework also appears to be an important aspect of forgiveness. If one cannot "track" the causality of the injuring event to a particular person or object, then it will not be possible to forgive. In addition, it is important to be able to maintain long-term memory of the causal set of events that resulted in the injury as well as of the individual(s) responsible for causing the injury. The abilities to think causally and to maintain a memory of the injury and its perpetrators are necessary elements prior to the initiation of the forgiveness process. If either of these is lacking, it will not be possible to remember the event requiring forgiveness or to identify the object or individual to be forgiven. While these statements seem intuitive, they may be empirically tested in certain patient populations suffering from stroke or dementing illnesses in which the ability to experience causal sequences or to remember events is impaired. However, to date, there have been no such studies reported in the literature.

After the damage has been incurred, the injured self interprets the damage either with respect to conspecific congruence or the rest of the external world (i.e., self–world congruence) depending on the nature of the offender and the offense. The psychological basis for this interpretation may be defined by many factors. Experiences from the past with parents help to shape a persons sense of morals and norms regarding behavior (Bonar, 1989; Shontz & Rosenak, 1988). Lapsley (1966) has theorized that, as children, individuals develop concepts of good and evil, as well as rules and categories for normative behavior.

Neuropsychologically, the development of abstract concepts such as good and evil, right and wrong, and justice and injustice, likely arise with the development of the inferior parietal lobe. It is this structure, along with its connections with the limbic system, that allows for these opposing concepts to be utilized by the individual to establish a set of norms or rules by which to evaluate future events and injuries. When an injury occurs and is compared to the previous understanding of the relationship, there is an incongruency. This injury-induced incongruency is not only disturbing in and of itself, but also it is understood that the new relationship between self and other is now experienced as inferior. Furthermore, this inferior relationship to the world is associated with negative emotions such as anger, because the person perceives the self to be worse off that before the injuring event (Fow, 1996).

Cognitive and Affective Processing

Once all the ramifications of the injury are perceived, the incongruency must be rectified, which, as we described earlier, may occur either via revenge behavior or via forgiveness (Enright, 1996). The initial decision to commit to forgiveness may be based on a number of affective and cognitive considerations, including the social controls as well as the other advantages that we previously described.

Forgiveness requires a complex neurocognitive process such that the new understanding of the self and its relationship with the world is analyzed so that the new and old understanding eventually are reconciled (Enright, 1996; North, 1987; Fow, 1996). This can occur via many possible neurocognitive and affective processes. For example, one possible solution to any given problem is to invoke a higher being (i.e., God) that can subsume responsibility, or at least explain the causality for any given damaging act. Thus, a person might state that God caused the event to happen for reasons that cannot be explained without divine knowledge. Because of God's role in the injuring event, the previously identified person who was originally held accountable is now perceived to have a different relationship to the injuring event and is therefore in the position to be forgiven. There are probably an infinite number of approaches to resolving the internal and external incongruency related to an injuring event. For interpersonal forgiveness to occur, these mechanisms may involve mutuality, concern, and desire on both sides that a congruent relationship continue, a sense that reconciliation has to occur, and that the offender has to take responsibility for his or her actions (Martin, 1953). Intrapersonal aspects of forgiveness include concepts of trust, benevolence, and the absence of anger and need for revenge or retaliation. All of these aspects are likely to become involved as part of the affectual and cognitive process necessary for forgiveness to occur (Cunningham, 1985, 1992; the Enright & Human Development Study Group, 1991). Regardless of the approach for revising the conspecific or self–world congruence in relation to the incurred injury, there is eventually a restoration of some type of equilibrium in which the world is understood again in such a manner that the incurred injury is incorporated within it and no longer is causing an internal disturbance.

Part of the ability to forgive most likely comes from the injured person's ability to identify or empathize with the offending individual (Rowe et al., 1989). The injured person realizes that the offender is also human and capable of making mistakes, and might also perceive that the offender should be forgiven much the same way that the injured person would want to be forgiven if the situation were reversed. In this approach, one might even consider that there is a sense of unity (as described earlier in the section on social controls of revenge behavior) between the forgiver and the offender, because both are perceived as being human.

Therefore, there are many variables that enter into the forgiveness process regarding the restoration of the conspecific or self–world congruence, as well as the ability to alter the emotional response to the offending person. The ultimate result is a new conspecific or self–world congruence that includes the offending individual, the offense, and the resolution of that offense (Rowe et al., 1989). Once the incongruity is resolved, there is a revised understanding of the self and its relationship to conspecifics and the world. This alleviates the emotionally disturbing problem of the incongruity itself and results in a sense of "acceptance" of the injury (Bergin, 1988). It should also be noted that the offending individual is part of both the original and new understanding of the relationship between the self and world. This is why, for example, an injury caused by a spouse can be more damaging on the one hand because of the deep relationship, but also more easy to forgive on the other, because of the previous trust and love.

Behavioral Activity

The positive affective response from the resolution of the incongruity can be directed outward toward the offending individual via behavioral activity. Such behavior includes both motor and verbal changes and generally reflects the more positive affective state of the forgiver. In addition to the decrease in general anger and resentment, there is a concomitant increase in demonstrations of compassion and empathy toward the offender. This may even relate to the newly realized sense of unity between the forgiver and the offender (as part of the revised self–other or self–world congruence) such that both are now realized to be human and capable of mistakes, of inflicting pain, and so forth.

AN INTEGRATED NEUROPSYCHOLOGICAL MODEL OF FORGIVENESS

We are now ready to propose a neuropsychological model of the forgiveness process based upon both the previously described neurophysiology and the phenomenological analysis of forgiveness. Such a model (see Figure 5.1) is only meant to provide a basic understanding of the underlying neuropsychology of forgiveness. Since forgiveness is such a complex phenomenon, it is unlikely that any rigid, all-encompassing model can be developed. However, it is probable that the basic components of forgiveness follow a relatively prescribed pattern, with the details dependent on the injurious event, the relationship between the offender and the injured, and the injured person's conspecific or self–world congruence. To develop our model, we proceed through the major stages of the forgiveness process and propose particular brain structures that are operative in each part of forgiveness.

As described earlier, since forgiveness requires an injury to the self, the first requirement is to have a sense of the self. The sense of self most likely requires an intact posterior superior parietal lobe, especially in the dominant hemisphere, since, as described previously, this brain region helps distinguish self from other. Furthermore, this part of the brain identifies specific objects that can cause damage to the self. The interconnections between the parietal, frontal, and temporal lobes (with input from the sensorimotor system) help to form what might be called the "primary circuit" that connects the self with the external world, and the person's relationship with the offender. This relationship is what helps us to understand the existing conspecific or self–world congruence. This relationship can be "fixed" in the brain via the memory circuits of the hippocampal and possibly the amygdalar formation. The hippocampus maintains memory of previous sensory, cognitive, and affective experiences and coordinates them into an overall description of the self and its relation to conspecifics and the external world.

The initial damage, or injury to the self, necessarily enters the brain via one or more of the sensorimotor systems. This input is then compared to the existing memory of the self and its relationship with the world. When there is an incongruency, a stress response in the injured self may cause activation of the sympathetic nervous system via the limbic system and the hypothalamus (the latter of which regulates activity in the sympathetic nervous system). This causes a feeling of "upsetness" and discomfort, as well as generating more visceral feelings via alterations in heart rate, blood pressure, and various stress hormones. Further negative feelings derived from the hippocampus are a response to the realization of the injurious nature of the incongruency and the possibility that there is danger in the lack of conspecific congruence. This stress response, caused by activity in the sympathetic nervous system, with concomitant release of norepinephrine, may result in alterations in neuronal plasticity (Kolb & Whishaw, 1998). Should such stress responses occur frequently, and without intervening resolution, more permanent effects may result, such as to the cardiovascular, nervous, and immune systems (Newberg & Newberg,

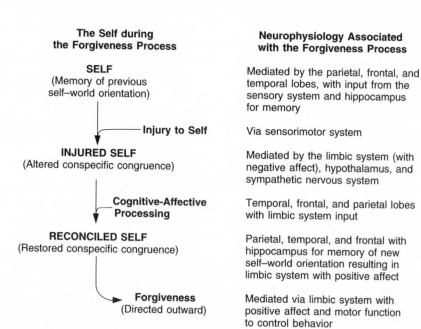

FIGURE 5.1. Simplified neurophysiological model of the forgiveness process.

1998). Thus, the negative emotional response to the injurious event could add to its impact and also provide a motivational force to help resolve the incongruency (Rowe et al., 1989).

This disturbance then causes the brain to begin to analyze the incongruency so that it can eventually be resolved. This resolution occurs via cognitive and affective processing within the temporal, frontal, and parietal lobes, which are responsible for higher order functioning as well as within the limbic system. Eventually, the cognitive and affective processes of the cerebral cortex, with help from neuronal alterations and plasticity, create the revised understanding of the self, or reconciled self, and its relation with conspecifics and/or the world. Part of this process likely involves concurrent activity in the right and left hemispheres of the brain. The right hemisphere is often used creatively to solve problems presented by the abstract and linguistic processes of the left hemisphere. When such a resolution to a problem occurs, there is a discharge from the right hemisphere (which helps in problem solving) that activates the parasympathetic nervous system, resulting in a feeling of happiness and relief that the problem is resolved. Phenomenologically, the act of forgiveness is often described as a revelation (Rowe et al., 1989), which is precisely the type of experience associated with the problem-solving ability of the right hemisphere with subsequent parasympathetic discharge. This also causes further activity in the limbic system such that the process of directing that positive feeling outward, toward the offending individual, may begin. Actually, strictly speaking, the positive feeling is not projected "outward" but is associated via a neural network with the imaginal representation of the offending individual in the sensorium, which is experienced phenomenologically as "external." In any case, this will eventually result in the establishment of positive feelings and behaviors directed out (via motor functions to control behavior) towards the offending individual as part of the revised understanding of the self and its relationship with the world. These positive feelings also have beneficial effects on the individual by decreasing the negative impact of the stress-induced changes that accompany the unresolved incongruity. Such beneficial effects may be mediated either through decreased sympathetic nervous system activity or increased parasympathetic activity. There are also the adaptive advantages to such a process (described earlier in the section on the neuroevolution of forgiveness).

CONCLUSION AND IMPLICATIONS

A neuropsychological analysis of forgiveness may also help us to understand the specific mechanisms by which forgiveness may contribute to improved psychological functioning. It is by utilizing autonomic and other neurophysiological parameters, in addition to more traditional psychological parameters, that some of the direct effects of forgiveness might be measured. Decreases in heart rate and respiratory rate, anxiety and depression, and feelings of hostility and anger, and improved self-esteem have been associated with various practices designed to augment parasympathetic activity such as meditation (d'Aquili & Newberg, 1993a; Newberg & Newberg, 1998). Such changes may therefore occur in patients undergoing the forgiveness process. One might also conceive of studies utilizing brain imaging techniques to measure various aspects of cerebral function as they relate to forgiveness. We have also indicated that forgiveness might improve a person's standing within a social group, which may improve interpersonal relationships. In addition, the forgiveness process itself is almost necessary for strong interpersonal bonds.

Encouraging forgiveness, therefore, might be a powerful therapeutic intervention with transforming consequences. A neuropsychological analysis of forgiveness helps to identify particular parts of the nervous system involved and points to future directions in research and clinical applications. Finally, a neuropsychological model suggests that forgiveness may ultimately have beneficial effects on the body, such as decreased levels of stress hormones and improvements in sleep patterns. In other words, forgiveness and healing might go hand in hand. It is difficult to accomplish one without the other, and a neuropsychological analysis of forgiveness can begin to delineate why forgiveness is such an important phenomenon psychologically, physically, and spiritually.

REFERENCES

Baron, R. A. (1973). Threatened retaliation from the victim as an inhibitor of physical aggression. *Journal of Personality Research, 7,* 103–115.

Baron, R. A. (1974). Threatened retaliation as an inhibitor of human aggression: Mediating effects of the instrumental value of aggression. *Bulletin of the Psychonomic Society, 3,* 217–219.

Bergin, A. E. (1988). Three contributions of a spiritual perspective to counseling, psychotherapy, and behavioral change. *Counseling and Values, 33,* 21–31.

Berscheid, E., Boye, D., & Walster, E. (1968). Retaliation as a means of restoring equity. *Journal of Personality and Social Psychology, 10,* 370–376.

Bonar, C. A. (1989). Personality theories and asking forgiveness. *Journal of Psychology and Christianity, 8,* 45–51.

Bruce, C. J., Desimone, R., & Gross, C. G. (1986). Both striate and superior colliculus contribute to visual properties of neurons in superior temporal polysensory area of Macaque monkey. *Journal of Neurophysiology, 58,* 1057–1076.

Burton, H., & Jones, E. G. (1976). The posterior thalamic region and its cortical projections in New World and Old World monkeys. *Journal Comparative Neurology, 168,* 249–302.

Buss, D. M., Haselton, M. G., Shackelford, T. K., Bleske, A. L., & Wakefield, J. C. (1998). Adaptations, exaptations, and spandrels. *American Psychologist, 53,* 533–548.

Close, H. T. (1970). Forgiveness and responsibility: A case study. *Pastoral Psychology, 21,* 19–25.

Cunningham, B. B. (1985). The will to forgive: A pastoral theological view of forgiving. *Journal of Pastoral Care, 39,* 141–149.

Cunningham, B. B. (1992). The healing work of forgiving: A pastoral care response to alienation and abandonment. *Review and Expositor, 89,* 373–386.

d'Aquili, E. G. (1972). *The biopsychological determinants of culture.* Reading, MA: Addison-Wesley Modular Publications.

d'Aquili, E. G. (1975). The biopsychological determinants of religious ritual behavior. *Zygon, 10*(1), 32–58.

d'Aquili, E. G., & Newberg, A. B. (1993a). Mystical states and the experience of God: A model of the neuropsychological substrate. *Zygon, 28*(2), 177–200.

d'Aquili, E. G., & Newberg, A. B. (1993b). Liminality, trance, and unitary states in ritual and meditation. *Studia Liturgica, 23*(1), 2–34.

Deitz, J. (1991). The psychodynamics and psychotherapy of depression: Contrasting the self-psychological and the classical psychoanalytic approaches. *American Journal of Psychoanalysis, 51,* 61–70.

Enright, R. D. (1996). Counseling within the forgiveness triad: On forgiving, receiving forgiveness, and self-forgiveness. *Counseling and Values, 40,* 107–126.

Enright, R. D., & the Human Development Study Group. (1991). The moral development of forgiveness. In W. Kurtines & J. Gewirtz (Eds.), *Handbook of moral behavior and development* (Vol. 1, pp. 123–152). Hillsdale, NJ: Erlbaum.

Fow, N. R. (1996). The phenomenology of forgiveness and reconciliation. *Journal of Phenomenological Psychology, 27,* 219–233.

Geschwind, N. (1965). Disconnexion syndromes in animals and man. *Brain, 88,* 585–644.

Hommes, O. R., & Panhuysen, H. H. M. (1971). Depression and cerebral dominance. *Psychiatria, Neurologia, Neurochirurgia, 74,* 259–270.

Jackson, H. (1991). *Using self psychology in psychotherapy.* Northvale, NJ: Jason Aronson.

Jones, E. G., & Powell, T. P. S. (1970). An anatomical study of converging sensory pathways within the cerebral cortex of the monkey. *Brain, 93,* 793–820.

Joseph, R. (1990). *Neuropsychology, neuropsychiatry, and behavioral neurology.* New York: Plenum Press.

Kandel, E. R., Schwartz, J. H., & Jessell, T. M. (Eds.). (1993). *Principles of neural science* (3rd ed.). Norwalk, CT: Appleton & Lange.

Kanekar, S., & Kolsawalla, M. B. (1977). The nobility of nonviolence: Person perception as a function of retaliation to aggression. *Journal of Social Psychology, 102,* 159–160.

Kanekar, S., & Merchant, S. M. (1982). Aggression, retaliation, and religious affiliation. *Journal of Social Psychology, 117,* 295–296.

Kolb, B., & Whishaw, I. Q. (1998). Brain plasticity and behavior. *Annual Review of Psychology, 49,* 43–64.

Komorita, S. S., Hilty, J. A., & Parks, C. D. (1991). Reciprocity and cooperation in social dilemmas. *Journal of Conflict Resolution, 35,* 494–518.

Lapsley, J. N. (1966). Reconciliation, forgiveness, lost contracts. *Theology Today, 22,* 44–59.

Laughlin, C., Jr., & d'Aquili, E. G. (1974). *Biogenetic structuralism.* New York: Columbia University Press.

Laughlin, C., Jr., McManus, J., & d'Aquili, E. G. (1992). *Brain, symbol, and experience* (2nd ed.). New York: Columbia University Press.

LeGros Clark, C. W. F. (1963). *The antecedents of man.* New York: Harper & Row.

Luria, A. R. (1980). *Higher cortical function in man.* New York: Basic Books.

Lynch, V. J. (1991). Basic concepts. In H. Jackson (Ed.), *Using self psychology in psychotherapy* (pp. 15–25). Northvale, NJ: Jason Aronson.

Martin, J. A. (1953). A realistic theory of forgiveness. In J. Wild (Ed.), *Return to reason* (pp. 313–332). Chicago: Henry Regenry.

McCullough, M. E., & Worthington, E. L. (1994). Models of interpersonal forgiveness and their applications to counseling: Review and critique. *Counseling and Values, 39,* 2–14.

Milner, B. (1970). Memory and the medial temporal regions of the brain. In K. Pribram & D. E. Broadbent (Eds.), *Biology of memory* (pp. 37–52). Orlando, FL: Academic Press.

Mishkin, M. (1978). Memory in monkeys severely impaired by combined but not by separate removal of amygdala and hippocampus. *Nature (London), 273*, 297–299.

Mukherji, B. R. (1995). Cross-cultural issues in illness and wellness: Implications for depression. *Journal of Social Distress and the Homeless, 4*, 203–217.

Murphy, J. (1988). *Forgiveness and mercy.* Cambridge, UK: Cambridge University Press.

Newberg, A. B., & Newberg, S. K. (1998). Incorporating stress management into clinical practice. *Hospital Physician, 34*(6), 52–58.

North, J. (1987). Wrongdoing and forgiveness. *Philosophy, 62*, 499–508.

Pribram, K. H., & McGuinness, D. (1975). Arousal, activation, and effort in the control of attention. *Psychological Review, 82*, 116–149.

Rawlins, J. N. P. (1985). Associations across time: The hippocampus as a temporary memory store. *Behavioral and Brain Sciences, 8*, 479–496.

Rogers, R. W. (1980). Expression of aggression: Aggression-inhibiting effects of anonymity to authority and threatened retaliation. *Personality and Social Psychology Bulletin, 6*, 315–320.

Rowe, J. O., Halling, S., Davies, E., Leifer, M., Powers, D., & van Bronkhorst, J. (1989). Exploring the breadth of human experience. In R. S. Valle & S. Halling (Eds.), *Existential–phenomenological perspectives in psychology* (pp. 233–244). New York: Plenum Press.

Sarter, M., & Markowitsch, J. J. (1985). The amygdala's role in human mnemonic processing. *Cortex, 21*, 7–24.

Segal, Z. V., & Blatt, J. (1993). *The self in emotional distress: Cognitive and psychodynamic perspectives.* New York: Guilford Press.

Seltzer, B., & Pandya, D. N. (1978). Afferent cortical connections and architectonics of the superior temporal sulcus and surround cortex in the rhesus monkey. *Brain Research, 149*, 1–24.

Shontz, F. C., & Rosenak, C. (1988). Psychological theories and the need for forgiveness: Assessment and critique. *Journal of Psychology and Christianity, 7*, 23–31.

Stuss, D. T., & Benson, D. F. (1986). *The frontal lobes.* New York: Raven Press.

Zeki, J. T., Symonds, L. L., & Kaas, J. H. (1982). Cortical and subcortical projections of the middle temporal area (MT) and adjacent cortex in galagos. *Journal of Comparative Neurology, 211*, 193–214.

Developmental and Cognitive Points of View on Forgiveness

Étienne Mullet and Michèle Girard

"**A**lthough the concept of forgiving has a rich history in philosophy . . . and Judeo-Christian theology, psychological treatments of forgiving have been rare until recently" (McCullough, Worthington, & Rachal, 1997, p. 321). The present chapter presents the existing studies devoted to the cognitive and developmental aspects of forgiveness. We review four lines of attack: (1) Piaget's views on forgiveness, (2) the early work on the effect of apologies and public confession, (3) Enright's theory on the development of reasoning concerning forgiveness, and (4) the recent work on the forgiveness schema.

PIAGET'S VIEWS ON FORGIVENESS

As far as we know, the first mention of forgiveness in the developmental psychology literature can be found in Piaget (1932). In *Le Jugement moral chez l'enfant*, Piaget devoted very little space to the concept of forgiveness: exactly three-fourths of a page (out of the 335-page volume). For this reason, it would be an exaggeration to speak of Piaget's position on forgiveness as if it were a strong one. Piaget essentially discussed the concept of forgiveness to contrast it with the concept of justice, the topic of his book.

Piaget stated that forgiveness implies more than a sense of "mathematical" reciprocity (in Piaget's words, *réciprocité de fait*). Forgiveness implies a sense of ideal reciprocity (*réciprocité de droit*), which can be

111

expressed as "Do unto others as you would have them do unto you." In Piaget's words, a complete understanding of forgiveness is attained "when the behaviors that are considered as right are the behaviors which demonstrate infinite reciprocity" (p. 258). The concept of infinite reciprocity— forgive because you have been forgiven in the past and in order to be forgiven in the future—is a complex one; for this reason, forgiveness cannot, according to Piaget, be understood before late childhood.

APOLOGIES, PUBLIC CONFESSION, AND FORGIVENESS

The Role of Apologies

As far as we know, the first experimental work on forgiveness was by Darby and Schlenker (1982). These authors were mainly interested in the effect of apologies on blame and punishment among children ages 6, 9, and 12, but they also included in their experiments a forgiveness scale. In one of their experiments, the participants were presented with vignettes depicting a central character, Pat, walking through the corridors of a school and inadvertently bumping into other children. Pat's responsibility for the incident, the amount of damage done, and Pat's response to the incident were systematically varied. Pat was described either as (1) simply walking away after the incident, without saying or doing anything; (2) simply saying "Excuse me"; (3) saying "I am sorry, I feel badly about this"; or (4) saying "I am sorry, I feel badly about this. Please let me help you." One of the questions asked of participants was the following: "Do you think Pat should be forgiven for what happened, and if so, how much do you think Pat should be forgiven?" A 10-point response scale, ranging from "None at all" to "A great deal," was provided. Mean responses observed showed that more elaborate apologies caused Pat to be forgiven more (M's = 4.3, 5.4, 6.4, and 7.3, respectively). No age × apologies interaction was found.

In another experiment, Pat was depicted as playing on a seesaw with a classmate. While playing, Pat caused the other child to be knocked to the ground and apparently to be hurt. Pat's intentionality for the incident, motives, and response to the incident (1–4) were systematically varied. Mean responses again showed that more elaborate apologies caused Pat to be forgiven more (M's = 4.8, 5.1, 6.3, 6.4) but an age × apologies interaction was found. The apologies effect was much more pronounced in 12-year-olds (3.3, 4.6, 6.7, 7.8) than in younger children (6.4, 5.5, 6.0, 6.2).

Public Confession and Forgiveness

Weiner, Graham, Peter, and Zmuidinas (1991) conducted a series of experiments to study whether public confession alters the perception of others regarding attributed blame, personal characteristics, and correlated consequences of these judgments, including forgiveness. In one of their experiments, the participants, college students, were presented with vignettes depicting a central character accused of having misused public funds. The status of the alleged transgressor (professional politician vs. student in government) and the response to the allegation were systematically varied. The alleged transgressor either (1) denied personal responsibility, (2) said nothing (control condition), or (3) acknowledged personal responsibility and gave a full and elaborate confession. Responses were given on various scales, including an 8-point forgiveness scale. Mean responses showed that acknowledgment of responsibility and public confession caused the alleged transgressor to be forgiven more (M's = 3.38, 4.00, 4.69; $p < .005$). No status × confession interaction was found.

In a second experiment, the participants were presented with similar vignettes depicting a senator accused of having misused campaign funds. The objective responsibility of the senator for the outcome and the response to the allegation were systematically varied. The senator was found to have been (1) personally negligent in the management of campaign funds, (2) the victim of his or her staff's dishonesty, or (3) both personally negligent and victim of his or her staff's dishonesty (an ambiguous case). Again, acknowledgment of responsibility and public confession caused the alleged transgressor to be forgiven more (M's = 4.20, 4.06, 5.37). No responsibility × confession interaction was found. In another experiment, the time of the confession was varied. The alleged transgressor (1) denied responsibility, (2) acknowledged personal responsibility and gave a full and elaborate confession after being accused, or (3) acknowledged personal responsibility and gave a full and elaborate confession before accusation. Spontaneous confession had more effect on propensity to forgive than confession after accusation (M's = 4.20, 5.03, 6.20).

ENRIGHT AND THE MORAL DEVELOPMENT OF FORGIVENESS

Enright and his developmental psychology group are credited for conducting the first experimental studies on the development of forgiveness (Enright, Santos, & Al-Mabuk, 1989; see also Enright, 1991, 1994; Enright, Gassin, & Wu, 1992). Enright's theory of the development of reasoning concerning forgiveness was modeled after Kohlberg's (1976) theory of the development of moral reasoning (see also Spidell & Liberman, 1981). As seen in Table 6.1, each stage in Kohlberg's model corresponds with one, and only one, stage in Enright's model. In the lowest stages—*Revengeful Forgiveness* and *Restitutional Forgiveness*—forgiveness can only occur after the wrongdoer has been subjected to revenge or appropriate punishment. In the middle stages—*Expectational Forgiveness* or *Forgiveness as Social Har-*

mony—forgiveness can be granted only if pressures from significant others are present.

It is only in the highest stage of the model—*Forgiveness as Love*—that forgiveness is conceived as an unconditional attitude and is seen as promoting positive regard and good will. This ultimate stage is the one that best illustrates the difference between the Piaget and Enright conceptions of forgiveness. According to Enright (1994), forgiveness, due to its gift-like character, does not entail any kind of reciprocity (even infinite reciprocity), as stated by Piaget (1932).

The procedure used in Enright's studies to test his model was also borrowed directly from Kohlberg (1976). Two of the dilemmas used by this author were taken and slightly altered in order to study reasoning about forgiveness. These were the well-known "Heinz dilemma" and the "Escaped Prisoner dilemma." The original Heinz dilemma reads as follows:

> A woman is near death from cancer. A druggist has discovered a drug that doctors believe might save her. The druggist is charging $2000 for a small dose—ten times what it costs him to make the drug. The sick woman's husband, Heinz, borrows from everyone he knows but can scrape only $1000. He begs the druggist to sell him the drug for less or let him pay later. The druggist refuses, saying, "I discovered the drug, and I am going to make money from it." Heinz, desperate, breaks into the man's store and steals the drug. Should Heinz have done that ? Why, or why not? (p. 40)

The alteration made by Enright concerned the final part of the dilemma:

> The druggist expected Heinz to steal the drug. So, the druggist hid the drug where no one could find it. Heinz's wife died. Heinz felt deeply sad toward and very angry with the druggist for hiding the drug and causing the death. (p. 102)

The end of the Escaped Prisoner dilemma was also altered. A set of questions devised to correspond with one and only one level of forgiveness development was presented to each participant ($n = 119$) in an interview format. Examples of questions from different levels are also given in Table 6.1. Three items, taken from the Defining Issue Test (DIT; Rest, 1979), were also presented.

The mean score observed in 9- to 10-year-old participants was close to 2 (Stage 2). This means that, on average, young participants were willing to consider that forgiveness can only occur after what had been taken away has been properly replaced or compensated. This corresponds with what Enright called a preforgiveness stage. The mean score observed in 15- to 16-year-old participants was close to 3 (Stage 3). This means that, on

TABLE 6.1. Stages of Justice and Stages of Forgiveness Development

Stages of justice	Corresponding stages of forgiveness	Example of questions tapping each forgiveness stage
	Stage 1	
Heteronomous Morality. I believe that justice should be decided by the authorities.	*Revengeful Forgiveness.* I can forgive someone who wrongs me only if I can punish him to a similar degree to my own pain.	If Heinz got even with the druggist by causing him to lose his business, would that make Heinz less sad than he is now?
	Stage 2	
Individualism. I have a sense of reciprocity that defines justice for me. If you help me, I must help you.	*Conditional or Restitutional Forgiveness.* If I can get back what was taken away from me, then I can forgive.	Suppose the druggist gives Heinz lots of money. Will this make Heinz feel better? Will this help him to forgive?
	Stage 3	
Mutual Interpersonal Expectations. Here, I reason that the group consensus should decide what is right and wrong.	*Expectational Forgiveness.* I can forgive if others put pressure on me to forgive. I forgive because other people expect it.	Suppose that all of Heinz's friends come to see him and say, "We want you to be friends with the druggist." Would this stop his sadness and anger and make him like the druggist?
	Stage 4	
Social System and Conscience. Societal laws are my guides to justice. I uphold laws to have an orderly society.	*Lawful Expectational Forgiveness.* I forgive because my philosophy of life or my religion demand it.	Suppose Heinz is a very religious man. His church leader points out that he must not stay so angry with the druggist. Would this help Heinz to forgive?
	Stage 5	
Social Contract. I am aware that people hold a variety of opinions. One usually should uphold the values and rules of one's group. Some nonrelative values must be upheld regardless of majority opinion.	*Forgiveness as Social Harmony.* I forgive because it restores harmony or good relations in society. It is a way of maintaining peaceful relations.	Are there benefits when an angry person like Heinz forgives the druggist?
	Stage 6	
Universal Ethical Principles. My sense of justice is based on maintaining the individual rights of all persons. People are ends in themselves and should be treated as such.	*Forgiveness as Love.* I forgive because it promotes a true sense of love. Because I must truly care for each person, a hurtful act on her part does not alter that sense of love. This kind of relationship keeps open the possibility of reconciliation and closes the door on revenge.	Suppose Heinz comes to bear no hard feelings toward the druggist and he even comes to love him. Now, the druggist hides another drug when Heinz is sick. Could Heinz forgive the druggist now?

Note. Adapted from Enright, Santos, and Al-Mabuk (1989). Copyright 1989 by *The Journal of Adolescence.* Adapted by permission.

average, young adolescents were willing to consider that forgiveness can occur as a consequence of favorable attitudes expressed by close others, even if what had been taken away has not been restored. (For 12- to 13-year-old participants, the mean score was located between the two.) Finally, the mean score observed in college students and in adults was close to 4 (Stage 4). This means that adults, young, or middle aged were willing to consider that forgiveness can occur as a consequence of religious or philosophical attitudes, without any intervention from the family or friends, even if restitution had not occurred. Few people can be classified in Stage 6, *Forgiveness as Love* (7 adults, for at least one dilemma).

Substantial individual differences were observed within age groups. The mean standard deviation obtained within age groups was around .70. This means that, at each age level, about 40% of the participants scored below or under the observed modal forgiveness level. No gender differences were observed. The correlation between age and forgiveness stage was strong (around .70). The correlation between DIT score and forgiveness stage was lower (around .50). The pattern of results obtained by Enright in U.S. samples has been subsequently replicated in a Taiwanese sample (Huang, 1990, quoted in Enright et al., 1992) and in a Korean sample, using one real-life dilemma as well as DIT dilemmas (Park & Enright, 1997).

Forgiveness in Late Adolescence and in Middle Adulthood

The dilemma technique is not the only one that has been used by Enright and his group to study the development of forgiveness. Subkoviak et al. (1995) used another technique, the Enright Forgiveness Inventory (EFI), to study the development of forgiveness from adolescence to middle adulthood. The EFI contains 60 items evenly divided among six areas: (1) absence of negative feelings (toward the offender), (2) presence of positive feelings, (3) absence of negative thoughts, (4) presence of positive thoughts, (5) absence of negative behavior, and (6) presence of positive behavior, these last two aspects referring to reconciliation as well as to forgiveness per se. Examples of statements relating to affect, cognition, and behavior items include the following: "I feel warm toward the other," "I think he or she is an annoyance," "Regarding the person, I do or would show friendship." The participants in the study were college students (mean age = 22.1) and their same-gender parents (mean age = 49.6). They were asked to think of the most recent experience of someone hurting them deeply and unfairly and then to describe their present feelings, thoughts, and behaviors toward the offender, using the EFI.

Results showed that adults' total scale scores were slightly but significantly higher than adolescents' scores (293 vs. 273, on a 60–360 scale, $p <$

.008). Another important result concerned the correlation between adolescents' and parents' scores when the degree of hurt was comparable. Among 21 parent–child dyads in which both child and parent indicated having experienced very deep hurt, the correlation was .54. This high value suggests that parents and children tend to forgive to similar degrees, as least in the case of very deep hurts.

INFORMATION INTEGRATION THEORY

The studies reported here are concerned with a central problem: How are multiple determinants integrated to form an overall judgment of forgiveness? The work reviewed earlier has demonstrated that multiple kinds of information are taken into account when people judge forgiveness. But none of that work has considered what rule governs this integration.

One hypothesis is that people use a configural rule: The impact of one piece of information (or informer) depends on other pieces of information with which it is combined. Each informer thus changes in value, depending on the other informers. For example, a harmful deed may be seen as less harmful if the person expresses remorse or makes some effort at atonement. In this configural view, the response to any set of informers depends on their interrelations and configuration. At the opposite extreme would be an additive rule: Each informer has a fixed value, regardless of the other informers with which it is combined; the person judges forgiveness by simply adding the separate values. There is no configurality.

How Can These Two Rules Be Distinguished?

A method to determine the rule has been developed in the theory of information integration (Anderson, 1996). The basic purpose of Anderson's information integration theory is to define the psychocognitive laws governing the processing of information and the integration of multiple stimuli, so as to accurately characterize the relationships between the stimulus values presented to subjects (here, intent to harm, apologies, etc.) and the ensuing judgments (here, propensity to forgive). Integration is the process by which information is combined into a judgment. The integration process can usually be described by simple algebraic operations (averaging, summing). Anderson's information integration theory is a very useful tool for researchers interested in studying the structure of the process by which separate items of information are combined into a single judgment. It has been successfully applied in many domains. Areas as varied as blame judgment (Przygodsky & Mullet, 1997), equity judgment (Anderson, 1997), and well-being judgment (Muñoz Sastre, 1999) have been the focus of numerous studies aimed at discovering the information-processing rules used by various kinds of people (children, adolescents, the elderly), and the way those rules change with development and maturation.

Anderson's functional theory of cognition offers the researcher a number of graphic techniques for analyzing this type of data. These techniques are generally used to characterize the main aspects of the information integration process in a simple fashion. Suppose that subjects are given two informers (presence or absence of intent to harm, and presence or absence of apologies) and asked to judge forgiveness.

An additive pattern of data is shown in the left panel of Figure 6.1. Hypothetical propensity to forgive judgments is plotted on the y-axis and apologies from the offender on the x-axis. Each curve represents a degree of intent to harm. The separation between the curves represents the effect of intent. The slope of the curves represents the effect of apologies. In this panel, the curves are steep, which means that the judgments are affected by information about the presence or absence of apologies from the offender. The curves are clearly separated, reflecting an impact of information about the intent to harm. Note, finally, that the curves are parallel, which indicates that in overall judgments of propensity to forgive, information items about apologies from the offender and intent to harm are combined in an additive way.

To illustrate, suppose a case in which each factor has two modalities, absence versus presence, where psychological forgiveness values are 1 and 4 for intent and 0 and 4 for apologies. The four responses corresponding to the four possible additive combinations of intent and apologies levels are $1 + 0 = 1$, $1 + 4 = 5$, $4 + 0 = 4$, and $4 + 4 = 8$. As seen in Figure 6.1, a factorial plot of these four values will show strict parallelism of the curves. An additive model predicts parallelism of the curves. Nonparallelism of the curves would eliminate the additive hypothesis.

A configural pattern of data is shown in the right panel of Figure 6.1. The slope of the higher curve is steeper than the slope of the lower curve. The curves are far apart. They diverge as we move to the right. The impact of the information about the presence or absence of apologies is greater in the absence of intent than in the presence of intent. There is configurality in information integration. A configural model predicts nonparallelism. Parallelism of curves would eliminate the configural hypothesis.

With a simple look at the curves, one can see (1) the relative impact of each piece of information that enters into the judgment process, (2) group differences (young, middle aged, elderly) in the impact of the same kind of information, and (3) the type of rule used to combine the information (additive, configural).

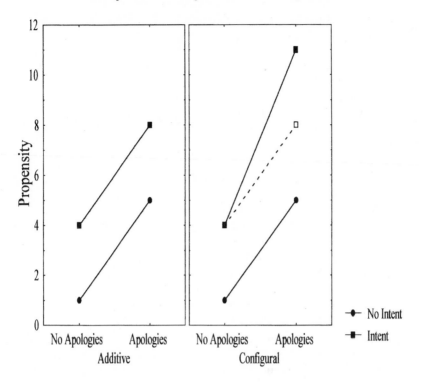

FIGURE 6.1. Additive and configural integration patterns.

Method Used in Girard and Mullet's Study

In Girard and Mullet's (1997) study, the sample comprised adolescents and young, middle-aged, and older adults (n = 236). The rationale for the inclusion of a broad range of adults of various ages was that, as shown by Subkoviak, Enright, et al. (1995), the likelihood that one will forgive may possibly evolve over the entire life span as a function of maturation and experience.

The material used consisted of 64 stories. One typical story is given below:

> Marie-Noelle and Josiane are sisters. They both worked in the same firm. Josiane, who had been working in the firm for several years, asked for a promotion. Marie-Noelle, who was very talkative but not mean, disclosed some information about Josiane's professional life. Josiane's section head heard about this information and began to doubt the working qualities of Josiane so he refused her promotion. Marie-Noelle, remorseful, felt really

sorry about what happened and asked Josiane to forgive her. Josiane's best friend, who knows Marie-Noelle well, also asked her to forgive her sister. Josiane asked another section head for a promotion, again, which she has got at the present time. Right now, do you think that you would forgive Marie-Noelle, if you were Josiane?

As can be seen in the example, each story contains six factors reflecting both reasons to forgive and conditions under which forgiving could be easier:

1. The degree of proximity to the target (brother or sister vs. colleague).
2. The degree of intent of the act (clear intent vs. no intent).
3. The severity of consequences of the act (moderate consequences vs. serious consequences).
4. Apologies/contrition for the act (apologies vs. no apologies).
5. Attitudes of others (favorable attitude vs. unfavorable attitude).
6. Cancellation of consequences (consequences still affecting the victim vs. consequences currently canceled).

The 64 stories were constructed by orthogonal crossing of the six factors: $2 \times 2 \times 2 \times 2 \times 2 \times 2 = 64$. Following each story was a 12-centimeter response scale, with "Absolutely not" on the left and "Definitely yes" on the right. Each participant responded individually, generally at home (at school for some young participants). Each rating by each participant in the experimental phase was then converted to a numerical value expressing the distance between the point on the response scale and the left anchor, serving as the origin. Three main findings emerged from this study.

Age Trends

Elderly people were clearly more likely to forgive than adolescents or young adults. In adolescents, the observed mean was close to 5.80. In middle-aged adults, it was close to 6.60. In elderly people, it was close to 7.90. The difference (more than 2 points on a 12-point scale, $p < .0002$) is impressive. This result was in line with those of Enright et al. (1989) and Subkoviak et al. (1995).

Effects of Variables

As shown in Figure 6.2, four factors had a strong impact: cancellation of consequences, intent, apologies, and proximity. In the left panel of Figure 6.2, the two curves show forgiveness for Intent to Harm and No Intent to harm, as listed. The vertical distance between these two curves shows that the intent variable was a substantial determinant of forgiveness. Even stronger was the effect of cancellation, which is measured by the slope of the curves.

In the center panel of Figure 6.2, the two curves show forgiveness for Sibling and Not Sibling. The vertical distance between these two curves shows that the intent variable was also a substantial determinant of forgiveness. About equivalent was the effect of apologies, which is measured by the slope of the curves. The effect of the apologies factor was in line with Darby and Schlenker's results (1982).

Finally, in the right panel of Figure 6.2, the two curves show forgiveness for Severe Consequences and Not Severe Consequences. The reduced vertical distance between these curves shows that the severity of consequences variable was not a substantial determinant of forgiveness. As shown by the slope of the curves, the attitude of others was no more substantial a determinant.

There were slight variations from adolescence to mature adulthood in the impact of some of the six factors: (1) the "attitude of others" factor had an impact only in adolescents, (2) the "proximity" factor appeared to have more of an impact in adolescents than in adults and elderly people,

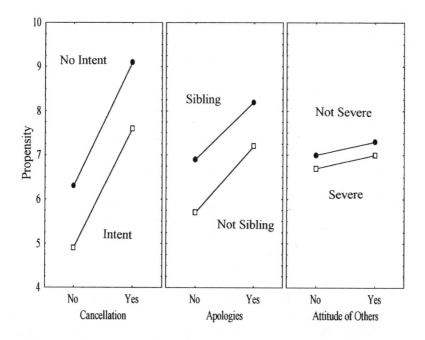

FIGURE 6.2. Effects of each of the six factors on propensity to forgive in Girard and Mullet's (1997) study (whole sample).

and (3) the "apologies" factor had more of an impact in adolescents and adults than in elderly people. These three observations are in line with the Enright et al. (1989) results.

Clusters of Individual Differences

A cluster analysis (complete linkage) conducted on the raw data showed evidence of at least eight different clusters. The first cluster was called the *Always Forgive* cluster. It was essentially composed of elderly people and 25- to 39-year-olds ($n = 33$). In these subjects, the information given did not make a difference, and the mean response was always close to the maximum. For each story, participants declared they would forgive, regardless of the circumstances of the offense. After the experiment, participants were invited to express their philosophy of forgiveness; they all insisted that it is always better to forgive than to remain resentful. However, they declared themselves very interested in the experiment despite the fact that they always responded in the same way. They were interested because the experiment allowed them, to a certain extent, to test their philosophy.

The second cluster, called the *Almost Never Forgive* cluster, was composed mainly of younger and middle-aged adults ($n = 11$). In these subjects, the mean response was close to the minimum and the only information that made a difference was the factor concerning intent. The effect of this factor, however, was very weak. These subjects expressed a philosophy exactly the opposite of the one expressed by the members of the first cluster.

The six remaining clusters are characterized by the relative dominance of the impact of one or another factor on the likelihood to forgive. More information about four of these six clusters is given in Figures 6.3 and 6.4. One of these clusters were labeled: *Social Harmony–Cancellation–Intent–Apologies* ($n = 65$). This cluster has been represented in the upper part of Figure 6.3. In the left panel, the two curves show forgiveness for Intent to Harm and No Intent to harm. The vertical distance between these two curves shows that the intent variable was a substantial determinant of forgiveness. About equivalent was the effect of cancellation, which is measured by the slope of the curves. In the center panel, the two curves show forgiveness for Sibling and Not Sibling. The vertical distance between these two curves shows that the intent variable was a substantial determinant of forgiveness. Lesser was the effect of apologies, which is measured by the slope of the curves. In the right panel of Figure 6.2, the two curves show forgiveness for Severe Consequences and Not Severe Consequences. The two curves are horizontal and tend to merge. Neither the "severity of consequences" variable nor the "attitude of others" variable was a substantial determinant of forgiveness. Only the four factors

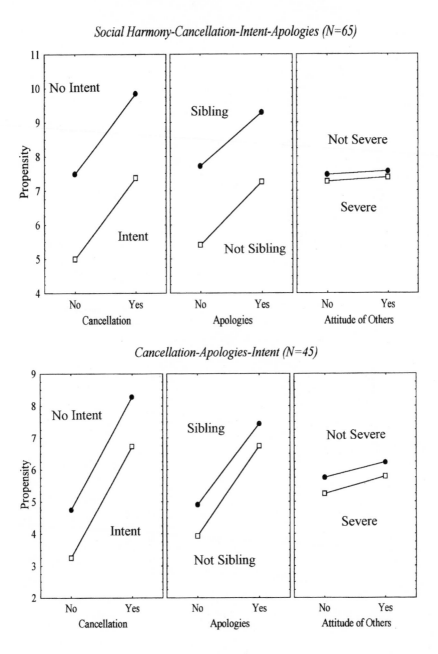

FIGURE 6.3. Effects of each of the six factors on propensity to forgive in Girard and Mullet's (1997) study (two main clusters).

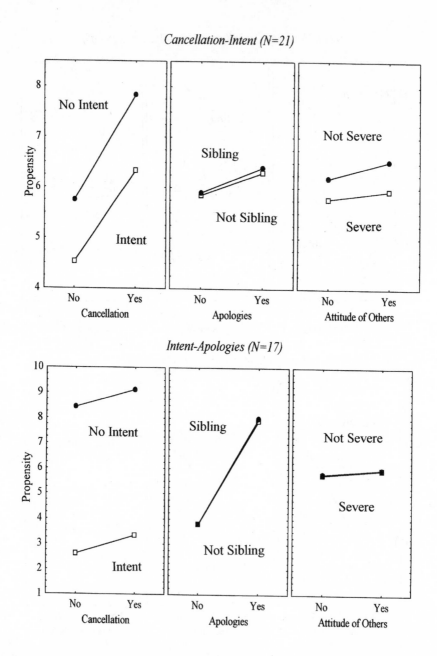

FIGURE 6.4. Effects of each of the six factors on propensity to forgive in Girard and Mullet's (1997) study (two secondary clusters).

mentioned in the title of the cluster have a strong impact on propensity to forgive.

Another of these clusters was labeled *Cancellation–Apologies–Intent* (*n* = 45). This cluster has been represented in the lower part of Figure 6.3. In the left panel, the curves are separated and their slope is very steep. In the center panel, the separation of the curves is lesser: The effect of the proximity factor was reduced compared with the previous cluster.

The *Cancellation–Intent* cluster (*n* = 21) is represented in the upper part of Figure 6.4. In the left panel, the curves are clearly separated and their slope is steep. In the center and right panels, the curves are more or less confounded and their slope is not steep. Finally, the *Intent–Apologies* cluster (*n* = 17) is represented in the lower part of Figure 6.4. In the left panel, the curves are clearly separated but their slope is not steep. In the center panel, the curves are more or less confounded but their slope is very steep. The two remaining clusters have been called *Cancellation–Social Harmony* (*n* = 15), and *Cancellation* (*n* = 18).

Sixth months after the end of the main study, 32 of the 33 members of the *Always Forgive* cluster were presented with a new set of eight scenarios, which included the same six factors as previously, but the values of three factors, "Proximity," "Others," and "Severity," were kept constant. Information load was thus considerably reduced. All 32 participants maintained that they would forgive unconditionally in each of the eight cases and rated the scenarios accordingly (i.e., using only the right anchor of the response scale).

Schema Structure

Girard and Mullet (1997) also tested the structure of the forgiveness schema. A schema is a cognitive organization that may be applied to more or less complex stimulus fields (Anderson, 1996, p. 23). In Girard and Mullet's study, each story constituted a complex stimulus field. Each of the clusters mentioned earlier represents a different schema (i.e., a different integration rule).

At least two kind of rules can be proposed: additive rules and configural rules (see Figure 6.1). If additive rules apply in the case of forgiveness judgment, this means that each element act independently in the production of the response. If configural rules apply, this means that each element does not act independently in the production of the response. There are interactions between the elements.

Results shown in Figure 6.2 for the whole set of data and in Figures 6.3 and 6.4 for different subsets of data support an additive forgiveness schema; each set of curves in each panel exhibits parallelism or near parallelism. Additivity is thus supported at the general level and at the cluster level, even though different groups of people appear to use different additive rules.

A powerful test between the additive and configural rules is available from analysis of variance. The configural rule implies that the analysis of variance (ANOVA) interactions should be generally significant; in sharp contrast, the additive rule predicts that these interactions should be generally nonsignificant.

ANOVAs conducted on the entire sample or on clusters showed that interactions of the kind Proximity × Intent, or Proximity × Intent × Apologies, or involving still more factors were not significant. In addition, high-order interactions including the Age or the Gender factor were not significant. The (additive) structure of the forgiveness schema did not vary as a function of age, gender, or cluster. The following formula—Propensity to forgive = Cancellation of consequences + Intent + Proximity + Apologies—indicates the structure that best suits a majority of participants. Possible formulae describing the information integration of other participants, except, of course, the one who does not integrate information (the members of the *Always Forgive* and *Almost Never Forgive* clusters), are probably only variations of this one. As shown in Figures 6.3 and 6.4, a majority of participants integrate at least four pieces of information, but some of them integrate only two or three pieces of information.

Averaging versus Summing

A more detailed analysis of the blame schema was conducted by Girard (1997) in a complementary study using only three factors: cancellation, intent, and apologies. The goal of this second study was to distinguish between an averaging rule and a summative rule, both of which are compatible with the aforementioned additive rule. Distinguishing between a summative rule and an averaging rule could appear futile. Both models are additive and at first glance seem identical. In fact, they have very different implications regarding the influence of the different factors specific to each case on propensity to forgive.

In a summative model, the impact of the different factors and the direction of the effects of the different factors (intent, apologies, cancellation of consequences) are constant, not alterable. The presence of apologies, for example, always constitutes a "positive" element even when these apologies assume a very weak form. Suppose that the present state of a person A and of a person B, expressed in terms of propensity to forgive toward an offender, is 2 (low) and 8 (high), respectively. Suppose the offender subsequently apologies and that forgiveness value of apologies for that person is 5. Suppose that the weight attached to the initial state and the apologies are equal. The final forgiveness value of person A can be estimated to 2 + 5 = 7. The final forgiveness value of person B can be estimated to 8 + 5 = 13. In both cases, the final value is higher than the initial one.

In an averaging model, by contrast, each new factor relevant to the problem at hand may alter the impact of the previous factors, and the direction of the effect of this factor depends on the values of the previous factors. The apologies can constitute either a "positive" or a "negative" element depending on the current level of propensity to forgive and on the form taken by the apologies. If the present level of propensity to forgive is very low and the value given to the newly offered apologies is moderate, the resulting new level of propensity to forgive will be somewhere between low and moderate, corresponding to a net increase in propensity to forgive. If the present level of propensity to forgive is high and the value given to the newly offered apologies is moderate, the resulting new level of propensity to forgive will be somewhere between moderate and high, thus corresponding to a net decrease. Suppose that, as in the previous example, the present state of a person A and of a person B, expressed in terms of propensity to forgive, is 2 (low) and 8 (high), respectively. Suppose, again, that the offender subsequently apologies and that the forgiveness value of apologies for these persons is 5. Suppose that the weight attached to the initial state and the apologies is equal. The final forgiveness value of person A can be estimated to $(2 + 5) / 2 = 3.5$. The final forgiveness value of person B can be estimated to $(8 + 5) / 2 = 6.5$. In person A, the final value is higher than the initial one, whereas in person B, the final value is lower than the initial one.

The observation of such unexpected effects is not a recent phenomenon, notably in personality impression (Anderson, 1981), where in some cases, communicating positive information about a person can lower the general attractiveness of that person. Consequently, distinguishing between the two forms of the general additive model has important implications for recommendations concerning reconciliation techniques following a "negative" act. If a summative model is at work, apologies can probably be counseled in all cases, but if an averaging model is at work, apologies can only be recommended under certain circumstances.

Girard (1997) presented her participants with scenarios describing several situations identical to the ones previously used in the main study, and several scenarios that contained a reduced set of factors. In some scenarios, intent information was missing. In other scenarios, cancellation information or apologies information was missing. The main design was Intent × Apologies × Cancellation, 2 × 3 × 3. The three subdesigns were Intent × Apologies, 2 × 3, Intent × Cancellation, 2 × 3, and Apologies × Cancellation, 3 × 3.

Figure 6.5 shows the main results of this complementary study. In the first panel (on the left), the two dotted curves are ascending (apologies effect), clearly separated (intent effect), and approximately parallel. The small deviation from parallelism is not significant. This pattern of results supports an additive rule. The solid curve is the test curve and corresponds with the values observed for the three levels of the apologies factor when intent information is missing. This curve is roughly parallel to the two dotted curves and does not intersect them. This means that the impact of the apologies factor (the slope) remains the same whether the intent information is present or absent. In the second and third panels, each test curve is parallel to the other curves. The impact of the cancellation factor also remained the same whether the apologies information (center) or the intent information (right) is present or absent.

This set of results can be interpreted as supporting a strict summative rule and ruling out an averaging rule. The rule shown in the Propensity to forgive = Cancellation of consequences + Intent + Social Harmony + Apologies equation can be taken at face value. Both the impact of each factor and the direction of its effect cannot be altered as a function of circumstances relevant to the offense.

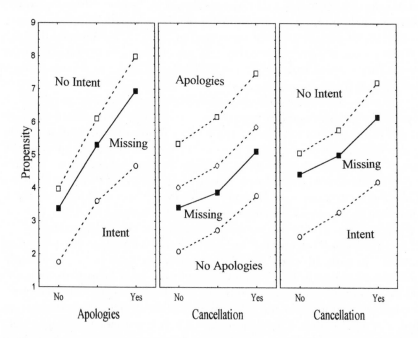

FIGURE 6.5. Averaging versus Summing Test. In each panel, the dotted curves are approximately parallel. This pattern of results supports an additive rule. The solid curve is the test curve and corresponds with the values observed for the three levels of the x-axis factor when one information piece is absent. This curve is roughly parallel to the two dotted curves and does not intersect them. This means that the impact of the x-axis factor remains the same whether all pieces of information are present or not.

LIMITATIONS OF THE PREVIOUS STUDIES
AND FUTURE ORIENTATIONS

The studies just summarized have many limitations. The same criticisms that apply to Kohlberg (Bègue, 1998) are also relevant for Enright's work. One major criticism made by many writers (Lickona, 1991) is that the moral dilemmas introduced by Kohlberg and adopted by Enright are very abstract. Children are rarely confronted with anything like the Heinz dilemma, nor would they be likely to comprehend it (Walker, Pitts, Hennig, & Matsuba, 1995; Wygant, 1997). Also children under age 12, say, cannot be well studied with the interview method. Note, however, that using one real-life dilemma, Park and Enright (1997) obtained, in adolescents a pattern of results similar to the one obtained in the Enright et al. (1989) study.

The criticisms of Kohlberg's work also concern the fact that his interview technique is effective for studying principled reasoning but not for studying everyday thinking and behavior (Burton, 1984). With such a technique, which consists of obtaining the verbalization of attitudes and the justification of action propositions, it remains difficult to distinguish between morality (forgiveness) development and mere linguistic development. Finally, with regard to another usual criticism of Kohlberg's model, the stage-like character of his theory, Enright's position is moderate (Enright et al., 1992, p. 106). In his latest papers, Enright presents each of the six proposed levels (see Table 6.1) as distinct forgiveness styles (or soft stages) and assumes that each style is possibly more or less frequently encountered at each age level.

The main criticism of Girard and Mullet's work is that only one kind of scenario has been studied: the section head scenario. One of the merits of this scenario is its real-life character, but it would also be prudent to gather information concerning other everyday-life situations, notably highly emotional situations, such as separation, divorce, and physical aggression. It would also be interesting to study the possibility of generalizing across situations. Would the members of the *Always Forgive* cluster in the work-problem situation also be members of a similar cluster in a different, romantic love-type situation? The numerous clusters encountered would gain much more significance if they could be generalized to other situations.

Another criticism is that all of the existing empirical studies are cross-sectional rather than longitudinal, and are thus confounded by the age–period–cohort problem. These is a need for longitudinal development research in the future.

Despite their numerous limitations, the studies analyzed above have uncovered a number of interesting results. First, the propensity to forgive has a developmental character, and this development extends over the entire life span. Adults are more likely to forgive than adolescents, and elderly people are more likely to forgive than younger adults. Moreover, a substantial proportion of elderly people are willing to forgive independently of the circumstances. Second, the development of forgiveness seems to follow the same paths in the United States and in Asian countries. Third, propensity to forgive appears strongly influenced by the presence of apologies and public confession—modifiable factors—and by the cancellation of consequences. Both factors are operative throughout one's entire life, with few exceptions. Fourth, the forgiveness schema is a true summative schema. Each factor *adds* its effect to the other factors, and this effect is largely independent of the level of these factors. Consequently, the presence of apologies, for example, is always a positive element, and the forgiveness value of this element remains constant.

One promising line of future research is to pursue the study of the relationship between blame and forgiveness (Boon & Sulsky, 1997; Darby & Schlenker, 1982). An obvious hypothesis is that they are essentially the same schema, with forgiveness an opposite or negative of blame. This makes sense in terms of the direction in which such determinants as apology, restitution, and so on, act on both (Hommers & Anderson, 1991). There is a difference in that forgiveness presupposes some degree of blame. Otherwise, there would be nothing to forgive. A natural line of attack in this view would be to get judgments of both blame and forgiveness from the same subjects. One might speculate that even the *Always Forgive* people would be able to blame in a differentiated manner.

Another promising line is the study of forgiveness in individuals and in populations that have been deeply hurt in international conflicts. To what extent are people in these countries willing to forgive each other? What factors could be introduced in order to facilitate forgiveness and reconciliation among people? Some studies of this kind are currently in progress (Enright, Gassin, Longinovic, & Loudon, 1994; Azar, Mullet, & Vinçonneau, 1999).

ACKNOWLEDGMENTS

This work was supported by the UPRES Vieillissement, Rythmicité et Développement Cognitif. We are grateful to Norman H. Anderson, Jolyon Barthorpe, Wilfried Hommers, Jennifer Marenberg, Michael E. McCullough, Ken Pargament, and Carl Thorensen for their thoughtful comments on earlier drafts of this chapter.

REFERENCES

Anderson, N. H. (1981). *Foundation of information integration theory.* New York: Academic Press.
Anderson, N. H. (1996). *A functional theory of cognition.* Hillsdale, NJ: Erlbaum.
Anderson, N. H. (1997). Moral algebra of fairness and unfairness. *European Review of Applied Psychology, 47,* 5–15.

Azar, F., Mullet, E., & Vinçonneau, G. (1999). The propensity to forgive: Findings from Lebanon. *Journal of Peace Research, 36,* 169–181.

Bègue, L. (1998). De la "cognition morale" à l'étude des stratégies du positionnement moral: Aperçu théorique et controverses actuelles en psychologie morale. *Année Psychologique, 98,* 295–352.

Boon, S. D., & Sulsky, L. M. (1997). Attributions of blame and forgiveness in romantic relationship. *Journal of Social Behavior and Personality, 12,* 19–44.

Burton, R. V. (1984). A paradox in theories and research in moral development. In W. M. Kurtines & J. L. Gewirtz (Eds.), *Morality, moral behavior and moral development* (pp. 74–106). New York: Wiley.

Darby, B. W., & Schlenker, B. R. (1982). Children's reaction to apologies. *Journal of Personality and Social Psychology, 43,* 742–753.

Enright, R. D. (1991). The moral development of forgiveness. In W. Kurtines & J. Gewirtz (Eds.), *Handbook of moral behavior and development* (Vol. 1, pp. 123–152). Hillsdale, NJ: Erlbaum.

Enright, R. D. (1994). Piaget on the moral development of forgiveness: Identity or reciprocity? *Human Development, 37,* 63–80.

Enright, R. D., Gassin, E. A., Longinovic, T., & Loudon, D. (1994, December). *Forgiveness as a solution to social crisis.* Paper presented at the conference, Moral and Social Crisis at the Institute for Educational Research, Beograd, Serbia.

Enright, R. D., Gassin, E. A., & Wu, C.-R. (1992). Forgiveness: A developmental view. *Journal of Moral Education, 21,* 99–114.

Enright, R. D., Santos, M. J. D., & Al-Mabuk, R. (1989). The adolescent as forgiver. *Journal of Adolescence, 12,* 95–110.

Girard, M. (1997). *Le pardon et ses déterminants chez les adolescents, les adultes et les personnes âgées.* Thèse de doctorat de l'Ecole Pratique des Hautes Etudes. Paris: EPHE.

Girard, M., & Mullet, E. (1997). Propensity to forgive in adolescents, young adults, older adults, and elderly people. *Journal of Adult Development, 4,* 209–220.

Hommers, W., & Anderson, N. H. (1991). Moral algebra of harm and recompense. In N. H. Anderson (Ed.), *Contributions to information integration theory* (Vol. II, pp. 101–141). Hillsdale, NJ: Erlbaum.

Huang, S. T. (1990). *Cross-cultural and real-life validations of the theory of forgiveness in Taiwan, the republic of China.* Unpublished doctoral dissertation, University of Wisconsin, Madison.

Kohlberg, L. (1976). Moral stages and moralization: The cognitive-developmental approach. In T. Lickona (Ed.), *Moral development and behavior: Theory, research and social issues* (pp. 31–53). New York: Holt, Rinehart & Winston.

Lickona, T. (1991). Moral development in the elementary school classroom. In W. M. Kurtines & J. L. Gewirtz (Eds.), *Handbook of moral behavior and development* (Vol. 3, pp. 143–161). Hillsdale, NJ: Erlbaum.

McCullough, M. E., Worthington, E. L., & Rachal, K. C. (1997). Interpersonal forgiving in close relationships. *Journal of Personality and Social Psychology, 73,* 321–336.

Muñoz Sastre, M. T. (1999). Perceived determinants of well-being among young adults, mature adults, and the elderly people. *Social Indicators Research, 47,* 203–231.

Piaget, J. (1932). *Le jugement moral chez l'enfant.* Paris: Alcan.

Park, Y. O., & Enright, R. D. (1997). The development of forgiveness in the context of adolescent friendship conflict in Korea. *Journal of Adolescence, 20,* 393–402.

Przygotzki, N., & Mullet, E. (1997). Moral judgment and aging. *European Review of Applied Psychology, 47,* 15–23.

Rest, R. R. (1979). *Revised manual for Defining Issue Test.* Minneapolis: Moral Research Project.

Spidell, S., & Liberman, D. (1981). Moral development and the forgiveness of sin. *Journal of Psychology and Theology, 9,* 159–163.

Subkoviak, M. J., Enright, R. D., Wu, C.-R., Gassin, E. A., Freedman, S., Olson, L. M., &

Sarinopoulos, I. (1995). Measuring interpersonal forgiveness in late adolescence and middle adulthood. *Journal of Adolescence, 18,* 641–655.

Walker, L. J., Pitts, R. C., Hennig, K. H., & Matsuba, M. K. (1995). Reasoning about morality and real-life moral problems. In M. Killen & D. Hart (Eds.), *Morality in everyday life: Developmental perspectives* (pp. 371–407). New York: Cambridge University Press.

Weiner, B., Graham, S., Peter, O., & Zmuidinas, M. (1991). Public confession and forgiveness. *Journal of Personality, 59,* 281–312.

Wygant, S. A. (1997). Moral reasoning about real-life dilemmas: Paradox in research using the Defining Issues Test. *Personality and Social Psychology Bulletin, 23,* 1022–1033.

CHAPTER 7

Expressing Forgiveness and Repentance

Benefits and Barriers

Julie Juola Exline and Roy F. Baumeister

How are people to respond in the wake of a damaging transgression? A wife continually lies to her husband about an ongoing extramarital affair. A woman humiliates a close friend by teasing her about a sensitive issue in front of a group. Caught up in a drunken rage, a man hits his 10-year-old son with a closed fist. In the worst case, conflicts can escalate and relationships can shatter. After an interpersonal wound has been created, what responses promise to be healing and constructive?

In the past 5 to 10 years, there has been an increasing focus on forgiveness as a response to transgression (for reviews, see Enright & the Human Development Study Group, 1991; Enright, Eastin, Golden, Sarinopoulos, & Freedman, 1992; McCullough, Exline, & Baumeister, 1998; McCullough, Sandage, & Worthington, 1997; McCullough & Worthington, 1994; Meek & McMinn, 1997; Sells & Hargrave, 1998; Worthington, 1998). When one person harms or transgresses against another, this action effectively creates an interpersonal debt. Forgiveness involves the canceling of this debt by the person who has been hurt or wronged. This cancellation could take place through multiple channels (e.g., Hebl & Enright, 1993; Wade, 1989), including those that are cognitive (e.g., deciding not to think about the debt; recalling one's own debts), affective (e.g., ceasing to feel angry about the debt), behavioral (e.g., deciding not to seek repayment or punishment for the debt), and/or spiritual (e.g., deciding to relinquish control of the debt to God) (see Meek & McMinn, 1997, for a discussion of religious aspects).

Recent research has suggested many benefits of forgiveness, including increased mental health (Al-Mabuk, Enright, & Cardis, 1995; Coyle & Enright, 1997; Freedman & Enright, 1996; Hargrave & Sells, 1997; Hebl & Enright, 1993) and marital satisfaction (Fenell, 1993). In contrast, defensive responses such as revenge fantasies and blaming have been associated with psychopathology (e.g., Greenwald & Harder, 1994; Zelin et al., 1983), criminality (Holbrook, White, & Hutt, 1995), poor recovery from bereavement (Weinberg, 1994), and poor health outcomes (e.g., Affleck, Tennen, Croog, & Levine, 1987; Tennen & Affleck, 1990; see also Williams & Williams, 1993). Less studied but equally important is the counterpart of forgiveness: repentance by the person who committed the transgression. As we discuss in detail later, repentance not only facilitates forgiveness but also may carry mental and even physical health benefits for the repentant person. Taken together, repentance and forgiveness form a cornerstone for the healing of emotional and relational wounds after transgression.

Depending on the level of analysis, forgiveness and repentance could be viewed as either *intrapsychic* or *interpersonal* processes. If one were to consider only the victim's perspective, forgiveness and repentance could appear to be purely intrapsychic processes that reflect psychological, emotional, and possibly spiritual changes within the individual. We might think of forgiveness as a private decision to let go of bitter or vengeful attitudes. Similarly, we might think of repentance as a private attitude of contrition accompanied by a motive to avoid repeating the transgression. In some situations, it may be appropriate to view forgiveness and repentance in these purely intrapsychic terms. For example, when interpersonal connections between victims and perpetrators are distant or absent, forgiveness and repentance may be confined to the private realm.

Yet in daily life, transgression incidents often involve people who have close or regular contact with one another, such as friends, work associates, family members, and romantic partners. In such contexts, it may be appropriate to move to a higher level of analysis, one that allows us to see not only intrapsychic processes but also interpersonal actions: How do people *behave* toward one another after incidents of transgression, and what are the sources and consequences of their choices? This is the central issue that we address in this chapter, and it requires taking an *interpersonal* perspective.

More specifically, our goal is to outline some of the difficult decisions that people can face when deciding whether to communicate forgiveness or repentance to one another. We first highlight some major benefits of expressing forgiveness and repentance. We then draw on psychological

research and theory to pinpoint some risks that might make people reluctant to engage in these actions, and we offer predictions about conditions
likely to heighten these risks. Finally, we use this cost–benefit analysis to
suggest some factors likely to foster the constructive expression of repentance and forgiveness.

DEFINITIONS AND DELINEATION OF SCOPE

We use the terms "victim" and "perpetrator" throughout this chapter to
refer to the parties involved in transgression incidents. For our purposes,
a "victim" is a person who suffers harm or wrongdoing or perceives this to
have happened. A "perpetrator" is a person who commits an immoral or
harmful act against another person or has been accused of doing so. For
simplicity, we use the terms "victim" and "perpetrator" as though we are
speaking of two distinct individuals, one in each role. Yet we acknowledge
that transgression is often mutual, whether in the form of a marital argument or a barroom brawl (see Baumeister, 1997). Thus, in many situations, a person could occupy both roles. In a sibling conflict, for example,
a girl might be both the victim of one transgression (being insulted by her
brother) and the perpetrator of another (breaking her brother's cassette
tape). Although we focus on dyadic exchanges, some of the ideas here
may also apply in group contexts.

This chapter focuses on the communication of forgiveness and repentance in the wake of transgression. Expressions of forgiveness and repentance may be either implicit or explicit, to use a distinction made in
the literature on reconciliation (Worthington & Drinkard, 1998). By our
definition, "explicit" expressions of forgiveness make direct reference to
the presence of a debt and to one's willingness to release the other person
from the debt. Sample statements might include "I forgive you for cheating on me" or "Yes, you did hurt me, but I'm willing to put it behind me
now." Note that a certain degree of confrontation is required in explicit
statements of forgiveness. By saying "I forgive you," victims imply that
they have suffered harm, that they view the other person as the source of
that harm, and that they are choosing to release him or her from the debt.
In fact, the words "I forgive you" may provoke outrage if they are unsolic-
ited, because recipients of the words may not believe that they have committed any offense warranting forgiveness. Some victims might thus be
reluctant to use explicit communication of forgiveness, perhaps because
they find it impolite or because they fear confrontation. Alternatively,
they might simply believe that their position is understood and requires
no clarification.

Perhaps more often, then, people *implicitly* express forgiveness; that
is, they do not make it clear that some harmful act was committed that

caused an interpersonal debt. In implicit forgiveness, one's statements or behaviors communicate either that no transgression was committed (thus, no debt exists) or that the transgression was so minor as to be of no consequence. Sample statements might include "That's okay," "No big deal," or "No problem." Implicit expressions do not always require the use of words. Instead, victims might communicate forgiveness by resuming contact with a perpetrator or by stopping themselves from making angry remarks about the offense. Similarly, expressions of repentance may also range from the very explicit ("I'm so sorry for the pain I caused by cheating on you. Please forgive me. How can I make it up to you?") to the more implicit (e.g., buying flowers, affectionate behavior).

The construct of forgiveness is often confused with reconciliation (Enright, Eastin, et al., 1992), and this distinction is likely to become especially blurred when we speak of forgiveness-related communication. Reconciliation is defined by Worthington and Drinkard (1998) as "the restoration of trust in an interpersonal relationship through mutual trustworthy behaviors" (p. 4). Reconciliation implies a willingness to come together to work, play, or live in an atmosphere of trust. Although intrapsychic forgiveness often co-occurs with attempts at reconciliation (Park & Enright, 1997), the two are independent constructs; forgiveness can occur independently of reconciliation and vice versa (Worthington & Drinkard, 1998). Expressions of both repentance and forgiveness might foster reconciliation, but they cannot be equated with it. Reconciliation requires a restoration of trust and a willingness to have ongoing contact. In some cases, people may want to apologize or extend forgiveness without seeking to build or restore a relationship.

POTENTIAL BENEFITS OF EXPRESSING REPENTANCE AND FORGIVENESS

Relationship Benefits

Sincere expressions of forgiveness and repentance are likely to have positive effects on relationships. When people behave in repentant or forgiving ways, their actions may intercept a downward spiral started by the transgression, replacing it with a cycle of positive intent and action (McCullough, 1997; see also Rusbult, Verette, Whitney, Slovik, & Lipkus, 1991).

Expressions of Repentance Promote Forgiveness

Victims are much more likely to forgive perpetrators who respond in repentant ways, as demonstrated in one of our recent studies (Exline, Yali, & Lobel, 1998b). We asked college students to recall an incident in which they were the victim of a transgression and to answer a series of questions about the incident. We found that people reported greater forgiveness toward those perpetrators who did the following: acknowledged that they committed the offense, offered sincere apologies, asked for forgiveness, expressed feelings of guilt or sadness, did something positive to "make up" for the offense, or forgave the participant for some other offense. Defensive responses by the perpetrator, such as insincere apologies, downplaying or covering up the offense, and blaming the victim, were associated with lower levels of forgiveness.

Our study corroborates other findings that suggest that people are more likely to forgive perpetrators who apologize (e.g., Darby & Schlenker, 1982; McCullough, Worthington, & Rachal, 1997; Ohbuchi, Kameda, & Agarie, 1989; O'Malley & Greenberg, 1983), confess wrongdoing (e.g., Weiner, Graham, Peter, & Zmuidinas, 1991), or cooperate in a subsequent interaction (Komorita, Hilty, & Parks, 1991). A perpetrator's efforts to maintain contact with the victim may also facilitate forgiveness (Gerber, 1987, 1990). A victim's anger might even be quelled simply by believing that the perpetrator feels guilty, as suggested by research on the "down-payment effect" (O'Malley & Greenberg, 1983) and by the fact that victims often try to induce guilt in perpetrators (Baumeister, Stillwell, & Heatherton, 1995). In contrast, defensive reactions such as self-justifications or refusal to accept responsibility generally lead to harsher judgments of perpetrators and a greater desire to punish them (Gonzales, Haugen, & Manning, 1994).

Might Expressions of Forgiveness Also Promote Repentance?

Although there are many studies suggesting that expressions of repentance lead to forgiveness, we are not aware of studies that directly test the inverse relationship: Could expressions of forgiveness make perpetrators more likely to repent? We could think of this as a "turn the other cheek" strategy in which a victim preempts the perpetrator by offering forgiveness before receiving repentance. If the expression of forgiveness is viewed as sincere, the perpetrator could note the victim's admirable behavior and feel inspired (or perhaps shamed) toward repentance. (Then again, expressions of forgiveness might obviate any perceived need for repentance.) At the very least, forgiving behaviors should avoid the escalation of conflict, as suggested in laboratory studies using the Prisoner's Dilemma paradigm (e.g., Axelrod, 1980a; Bendor, Kramer, & Stout, 1991).

Personal Benefits

In addition to relationship benefits, people who express forgiveness or repentance may reap private mental and physical health benefits from their actions. Some of these benefits can occur even if the other party does not respond in a positive way. Thus, even when reconciliation is not desired or possible—and sometimes in the absence of intrapsychic forgiveness or repentance—people may choose to express forgiveness or repentance and may even benefit from doing so.

Reduced Guilt and Increased Confidence Based on Constructive Action

As suggested in a recent review (Baumeister, Stillwell, & Heatherton, 1994), guilty feelings can prompt action to restore relationships, particularly those that are close. Thus, friendly overtures by both victims and perpetrators should decrease feelings of guilt while increasing feelings of confidence and well-being. In other words, either repentance or forgiveness can be a vital step toward restoring a relationship toward harmony and trust.

Another potential benefit is that expressions of forgiveness and repentance could symbolically erase the roles of victim and perpetrator, placing the involved parties on more equal footing. By communicating cancellation of a debt, people might remove feelings of weakness or failure engendered by the victim role. To the extent that the perpetrator role carries malign associations of cruelty or carelessness, acts of repentance are likely to mitigate these as well.

Mental and Physical Health Benefits of Disclosure

Research on emotional self-disclosure raises an additional possibility: Expressions of forgiveness or repentance—at least those that involve writing—might bring mental and physical health benefits (see Pennebaker, 1995; see also Kelly & McKillop, 1996). As demonstrated in a recent meta-analysis (Smyth, 1998), people who write about the emotional content of traumatic events often have short-term increases in physiological arousal followed by a long-term decrease in health problems. Although the mechanisms behind these physiological changes are not entirely clear, the benefits of disclosure might stem from an ability to find meaning in the incident (e.g., Pennebaker, Mayne, & Francis, 1997) or release from the burdens of inhibition (e.g., Pennebaker, 1993). Although the link to forgiveness and repentance remains speculative,[1] this body of research does raise the possibility that writing about painful transgression incidents might have benefits for both victims and perpetrators.

The Darker Side: Using Expressed Forgiveness or Repentance for Self-Protective Advantage

People might also use superficial communications of forgiveness or repentance in order to gain power or self-protection. Such communications could occur in the absence of intrapsychic forgiveness or repentance (Baumeister, Exline, & Sommer, 1998). For example, a victim might express forgiveness in order to appear noble or to have a ready weapon for later attempts at guilt induction ("Don't you remember that I forgave you even after you cheated on me twice?"). Likewise, a perpetrator could avoid retaliation through the strategic use of empty apologies, insincere promises, or superficial attempts at restitution. Such benefits, while not morally laudable, may be powerful motivators when self-protective concerns predominate.

Summary: Potential Benefits

Even in the complete absence of intrapsychic forgiveness or repentance, people can use superficial apologies, reparations, or expressions of forgiveness in order to gain short-term, self-protective benefits. In most cases, however, sincere communications of forgiveness and repentance can benefit both relationships and individuals. Acts of repentance clearly facilitate forgiveness, and the reverse might also be true. Persons who respond constructively to transgression could also benefit from reduced guilt, increased confidence, or relief at being released from a burden. Ideally, such communications promote a mutual perception that the debt is canceled and the victim and perpetrator roles are erased.

BARRIERS TO THE EXPRESSION
OF FORGIVENESS AND REPENTANCE

Given the benefits of expressing forgiveness and repentance, why would anyone ever fail to forgive or repent? Why is it often difficult to admit wrongdoing or to offer an apology, even if these actions carry the hope of obtaining forgiveness as well as peace of mind? And why might a victim be reluctant to forgive, when forgiving will foster reconciliation and help one escape the victim role?

One obvious possibility is that people do not express forgiveness or repentance because they simply do not want to. When people become consumed by anger and defensiveness, they may not want their adversaries to have the satisfaction of a confession or apology on one hand, or an assurance of forgiveness on the other. Yet, as we suggest later, bitterness and spite are not the only reasons that people fail to behave in forgiving and repentant ways. Regardless of how people manage their private feelings of hurt and anger, they may be reluctant to take the risks involved in communicating repentance or forgiveness. In this section, we draw on psychological research and theory to illuminate some of these risks and the conditions likely to intensify them. Rather than attempting to generate an exhaustive list, our aim is to highlight some of the major risks that victims and perpetrators can encounter.

Barriers to Expressing Repentance

When we refer to expressions of repentance, we include both confession (taking responsibility for an offense) and acts of apology and restitution. All of these actions require humility and a willingness to temporarily set aside pride. Barriers to expressing repentance are likely to center on people's reluctance to make themselves vulnerable in this way.

Disagreement with the Charge

One major barrier to expressing repentance is that perpetrators are likely to perceive the charge as inaccurate, excessive, or unfair. For example, in one study (Baumeister, Stillwell, & Wotman, 1990), college students were asked to write accounts of two real-life incidents: one in which they were the victim and another in which they were the perpetrator. Results suggested that, relative to victims, perpetrators were more likely to see an offense as stemming from causes that were impulsive, uncontrollable, justifiable, or due to mitigating circumstances. They downplayed the impact of their transgressions and were quick to remember their use of apologies. Perpetrators were also less likely than victims to see their offenses as part of an accumulating set of provocations, instead viewing them as isolated incidents. A study using similar methods (Exline, Yali, & Lobel, 1998a) corroborated and extended these findings. Relative to situations in which they were victims, participants portrayed their own offenses as less harmful, less repeated, less intentional, less malicious, more justifiable, and more reparable. They also portrayed their own subsequent responses, as perpetrators, as much more repentant than those of other perpetrators: Participants reported that, relative to those who had transgressed against them, they were much more likely to follow their own transgressions with acknowledgment of the offense, acceptance of responsibility, apologies, requests for forgiveness, restitution, expressions of guilt, and forgiveness of the victim for another offense. Participants also recalled that, relative to other perpetrators, they less frequently used the destructive responses of blaming the victim, downplaying the offense, and offering insincere apologies. Similar findings were obtained in a field study of business executives, who tended to view their conflict strategies as more reasonable and less antagonistic than those of their opponents (Thomas & Pondy, 1977).

In short, perpetrators tend to perceive their transgressions as less harmful and serious than victims do, creating what Baumeister (1997) has termed the *magnitude gap*. The magnitude gap appears to reflect self-serving distortions on the part of both victims and perpetrators, as demonstrated in a recent set of experiments (Stillwell & Baumeister, 1997). Because their perceptions of the transgression incident are likely to differ from those of the victim, perpetrators are likely to view victims as overreacting. This point, too, has found empirical support (Baumeister, Stillwell, & Heatherton, 1995; Baumeister et al., 1990; see also Baumeister & Wotman, 1992). Perpetrators may even see themselves as the true victims, even in the case of heinous crimes such as torture and serial murder (Baumeister, 1997). Rather than seeing themselves as intentionally harming others, perpetrators of violent crimes are likely to see themselves as responding to provocation by the victim. As such, they see their actions as justifiable. For example, both aggressive boys and abusive husbands tend to see self-esteem slights and aggressive overtones in social exchanges that others perceive as neutral in tone (Goldstein & Rosenbaum, 1985; Nasby, Hayden, & DePaulo, 1980). When perpetrators see themselves as victims, whether accurately or not, such perceptions will no doubt serve as major barriers to repentance.

In cases of mutual transgression, such as a marital argument that degenerates to the level of caustic remarks and name-calling by both parties, people are especially likely to disagree with charges against them. They are likely to focus on their victim status while overlooking their roles as perpetrators. Perpetrators are also more likely to protest when they are placed on the defensive by a victim who angrily confronts them in a blaming manner (Kubany, Bauer, Muraoka, Richard, & Read, 1995). Persons who tend to externalize blame and have difficulty empathizing with others should also be more likely to view themselves as innocent.

In general, then, people may be reluctant to repent because they do not want to accept the guilt that is implied by repentance. Some may regard themselves as thoroughly innocent. Even perpetrators who acknowledge some wrongdoing, however, may be reluctant to accept the full load of guilt that victims assign to them. Because victims typically perceive greater guilt than perpetrators, this discrepancy is likely to be common, and often some negotiation or mutual understanding may be required before a perpetrator becomes willing to take responsibility for wrongdoing.

Fear of Punishment or Restrictions Associated with Confession

Accepting responsibility for an offense may often carry severe pragmatic costs, and these can raise obstacles to confession and repentance. Perpetrators may be able to protect themselves from sanctions if they can conceal that they committed a certain act—or, alternatively, if they can convince others that the act was not damaging or morally wrong. Each of the problems discussed below becomes magnified if the transgression is highly damaging (e.g., a murder as opposed to breaking a curfew) or blameworthy (e.g., seeking out a married person for an illicit affair as opposed to dating a married person one believed to be single).

Perpetrators might be reluctant to confess if there is a chance that they can successfully hide or deny their role in a transgression. A series of experiments by Weiner et al. (1991) demonstrated the quandary that people face when debating about whether to confess a misdeed. Their results suggested that confession increased forgiveness and reduced negative inferences about perpetrators. Spontaneous confessions—those given in the absence of an accusation by another party—were viewed in an especially favorable light. However, spontaneous confessors were not viewed as favorably as their counterparts who never confessed and were never accused of a misdeed. Spontaneous confessions seemed to raise moral questions and issues that did some damage to the perpetrator's reputation. Thus, perpetrators who fear punishment might be tempted to avoid confession if there is a chance that others will never learn of their transgression.

Whether confession is spontaneous or solicited, perpetrators might also fear that admitting wrongdoing will lead to restrictions on their future behavior. When people admit that they have committed an act and concede that it was hurtful or wrong, such an acknowledgment will make it difficult to justify repeating the behavior in the future. If people gain pleasure or some other benefit from a given behavior, they may not be prepared to give up the option of performing it again. For example, even if an alcoholic privately knows that her drinking is harming not only herself but also her family, she may be reluctant to acknowledge its frequency or harmfulness for fear of being expected to stop. In contrast, if she refuses to label her behavior as wrong, she can avoid measuring her drinking against a moral standard that might require self-control (Baumeister, Heatherton, & Tice, 1994) and lead to feelings of failure if not met (e.g., Higgins, 1987).

Shame

Even in the absence of external punishment for confession, people may be reluctant to express repentance because they find it shameful to do so. The distinction between guilt and shame is an important one. According to Tangney (e.g., Tangney, Wagner, Fletcher, & Gramzow, 1992), guilt refers to negative affect that is focused on some specific action (or failure to act), often accompanied by a desire to repair the damage. Shame, in contrast, refers to a perception of the entire self as bad and a sense of being exposed, often accompanied by a desire to hide. In general, shame-prone persons are more susceptible to anger, suspiciousness, blaming others, and aggressive behavior than guilt-prone persons (Tangney et al., 1992; Tangney, Wagner, Hill-Barlow, Marschall, & Gramzow, 1996). Revenge may also be tied to a shame-based desire to save face, as suggested in laboratory experiments (e.g., Brown, 1968) and field studies in business settings (Bies & Tripp, 1996). Thus, whereas feelings of guilt often press a person toward confession and resolution, feelings of shame are more likely to prompt self-protective responses designed to hide the offense, to deflect responsibility, or to make the perpetrator appear innocent, competent, or powerful. Such responses would clearly serve as deterrents to the expression of repentance. There are at least two major areas where shame could arise for perpetrators: One centers on taking responsibility for a misdeed, while the other deals with taking on the role of a supplicant.

One problem arises at the level of confession. Because people are motivated to see themselves as morally good, they often find it shameful to admit that they committed an immoral act or caused pain to another person. Shame should be more intense if the transgression was severe and strongly implies blameworthiness for the perpetrator—that is, the action was deliberate and avoidable, not simply an accident (Boon & Sulsky, 1997; Gonzales et al., 1994; Hodgins, Liebeskind, & Schwartz, 1996; Lysak, Rule, & Dobbs, 1989). Clearly, having a damaging and willful act attributed to the self is likely to downgrade one's public and private images, prompting feelings of shame.

Shame might be especially likely to arise when a perpetrator must publicly take the stance of a supplicant, such as by apologizing, asking for forgiveness, or making reparations. People may view such acts as demeaning or humiliating, especially if the offense was serious and intentional. For persons who are highly susceptible to feelings of shame, the need to save face may be too great to warrant the risk of repenting. Perpetrators may also suspect that the victim is vigilant for any signs of weakness and is prepared to attack them or reject their attempts at concessions. Most people would naturally be reluctant to place themselves in such a vulnerable position. Fears of showing vulnerability should be especially salient for perpetrators who have a strong motive to maintain a dominant position in the relationship, either because of personal need for power or because they believe—accurately or not—that the other party will attack if given the opportunity.

Barriers to Expressing Forgiveness

By definition, forgiveness involves the cancellation of a debt. Very often this debt is one that, in strict terms of justice, the victim has a legitimate claim to collect (Enright & the Human Development Study Group, 1991). Whereas intrapsychic forgiveness involves mentally canceling this debt, interpersonal expressions of forgiveness communicate this cancellation to the other person. In one sense, then, forgiveness can carry substantial costs for victims: By giving up their claims to a debt, they relinquish something without the assurance that they will receive anything tangible in return.

Fear that the Transgression Will Be Repeated

One of the most common concerns raised about the wisdom of forgiveness is whether it opens the door for future transgression (see Enright, Eastin, et al., 1992, for a discussion). Although this issue is often raised in the context of severe, chronic patterns of transgression such as domestic violence or sexual abuse (e.g., Engel, 1989), it could apply to virtually any offense: If victims express cancellation of an interpersonal debt, are they simply leaving themselves vulnerable to being hurt again? Will perpetrators interpret forgiving responses as free license to repeat the transgression?

Before we address this question, we would like to note one potential pitfall of such logic: the assumption that a victim can control a perpetrator's subsequent behavior. Some victims may believe that if they refuse to communicate forgiveness, this gives them leverage in terms of influencing the perpetrator not to harm them again. Granted, in some cases, victims will indeed be able to wield some influence by withholding expressions of forgiveness (Baumeister et al., 1998), especially in close relationships, where they can successfully induce guilt (cf. Baumeister et al., 1995). Ultimately, however, the perpetrator's decision about whether to commit an act again will be based on many factors, such as his or her self-control, the extent to which the action is viewed as rewarding, and the strength of the desire to avoid hurting the victim. The victim's response, while potentially important, is only one factor among many. With this caveat in mind, what are some conditions that might make expressing forgiveness risky in terms of repeated transgression?

Repeated transgressions are especially likely in interpersonal environments characterized by hostility and mistrust. Guilt, a deterrent to future transgression (Meek, Albright, & McMinn, 1995), is more prevalent within close, communal relationships (Baumeister et al., 1994; Baumeister, Reis, & Delespaul, 1995). Thus, victims should legitimately fear being hurt again by people who are distant or not highly motivated to protect the victim's well-being. In general, people find it most difficult to forgive when offenses are severe, intentional, and repeated, and when perpetrators are unrepentant (e.g., Exline et al., 1998b). These criteria are likely to apply to the expression of forgiveness as well. Not only may victims be enraged with unrepentant perpetrators, but they could also have legitimate fears of being harmed again.

The benefits and risks of forgiving behavior emerged clearly in a series of contests (Axelrod, 1980a, 1980b) using the Prisoner's Dilemma

Game to simulate conflict situations in the laboratory. In the Prisoner's Dilemma, players have the option of cooperating or defecting in each of a series of turns. Cooperation works toward the greatest mutual good but leaves one vulnerable to exploitation by the other. Defection protects one against exploitation and can achieve maximum individual benefit by exploiting the other. Each player gains a few points for mutual cooperation but can win more points by betraying a cooperative opponent. In two contests, entrants submitted computer-programmed strategies and were then pitted against each other in a series of iterations. The strategy that scored the most points won the contest. In the Prisoner's Dilemma, a "forgiving" strategy is one that cooperates after a defection by the partner. In the first contest (Axelrod, 1980a), the winner was a somewhat forgiving, reciprocity-based strategy called TIT FOR TAT: The strategy would respond to defections with defections and to cooperation with cooperation. Based on the results of the contest, the author contended that a more forgiving strategy called TIT FOR TWO TATS would have fared even better. This strategy responded with a defection only after two defections by the opponent. However, for the second contest (Axelrod, 1980b), some entrants submitted strategies that were deliberately designed to take advantage of other players. The highly forgiving TIT FOR TWO TATS fared more poorly than the reciprocity-based TIT FOR TAT in this hostile environment. Although these findings deal with computer-based strategies rather than human exchanges, the results have important implications: If others are out to harm you deliberately and have the power to do so, you do risk some harm to your self-interest by repeatedly offering gestures that suggest trust and good will.

We might also predict that repeated transgression are more likely when victims use highly implicit means to express forgiveness. It is true that in intrapsychic terms, forgiveness can be distinguished from condoning (see McCullough, Sandage, & Worthington, 1997). Condoning involves refusal to label a given act objectionable; in terms of this discussion, condoning may be viewed as refusal to acknowledge that a debt exists. Forgiveness, in contrast, requires recognition that a debt did occur, along with a conscious decision to release the perpetrator from the debt. Yet when we begin to look closely at how people communicate forgiveness in daily life, the line between forgiving and condoning quickly becomes blurred (Baumeister et al., 1998). Because the expression of forgiveness is often implicit rather than explicit (cf. Worthington & Drinkard, 1998), forgivers may fail to communicate accurately or directly their private thoughts and feelings to perpetrators. Instead of openly discussing the transgression incident, framing it as a debt, and telling perpetrators that they are being released from the debt, victims may choose means of expression that are less confrontational or direct. Even if their private process is one of forgiveness, their responses might suggest condoning ("That's okay"), minimizing ("It's no big deal"), or justification ("I know you've been under a lot of stress lately"). Victims might also choose to express forgiveness without using any words at all, perhaps by resuming contact with a perpetrator or by stopping themselves from making cynical remarks about the transgression. No confrontation or limit setting is involved in these communications. Although research is needed to determine whether such implicit responses increase the risk of future transgression, it is easy to imagine how they might do so, especially if the perpetrator finds the behavior rewarding and faces few deterrents.

Regardless of the actual risk of repeated transgression, some victims are likely to fear it more than others. Because the fear of repeated transgression is largely based on mistrust, persons who generally have difficulty trusting others are more likely to have such fears. Those who have been deeply and repeatedly hurt by the perpetrator are also more likely to fear taking the interpersonal risks required to express forgiveness, especially if these expressions are considered attempts at reconciliation.

Fear of Appearing Weak

Another potential barrier is that those who express forgiveness might appear weak, timid, or vulnerable to others or to themselves. To communicate forgiveness is viewed as backing down, which prompts feelings of shame. When victims have a strong desire to "save face," they are more likely to seek revenge and respond in other angry ways. Face-saving needs may be situationally prompted (Brown, 1968), but they may also reflect a shame-prone personality (Tangney et al., 1992, 1996). Unless they can restore their sense of power using some other means, humiliated victims are likely to desire revenge rather than forgiveness (Fagenson & Cooper, 1987). At one level, it seems paradoxical that forgiveness could suggest weakness, since surrendering one's claim to a legitimate debt may require tremendous self-control. Yet forgiveness often implies a willingness to bypass immediate self-interest and loosen justice-oriented rules in favor of mercy (see below). Some people will equate such priorities with weakness. Finally, if a victim expects a perpetrator to respond in mocking or aggressive ways to any suggestion of "softness" (cf. Worthington & Drinkard, 1998), expressing forgiveness may seem a foolhardy prospect.

Belief that Justice Will Not Be Served

Some people might be reluctant to express forgiveness because they believe that pardoning a debt violates standards of justice (Enright, Gassin, & Wu, 1992; Enright, Santos, & Al-Mabuk, 1989). For example, standards of retributive justice dictate a reciprocity-based, eye-for-an-eye approach, with little, if any, room for mercy toward the perpetrator. Restitutional

justice also demands repayment in the form of apologies or other concessions. In contrast, forgiveness—whether intrapsychic or behavioral—often
requires the loosening of justice standards in order to permit mercy
(McCullough, Sandage, & Worthington, 1997). Thus, if retributive justice
concerns are very salient, victims might be reluctant to release a perpetrator from a crime without demanding punishment or repayment. In such
situations, expressions of forgiveness might be viewed as not only difficult
but also morally remiss.[2]

Releasing a perpetrator from a debt should raise more justice-related
protest when the victim suffers great harm and the perpetrator is clearly
blameworthy. If a perpetrator is totally unrepentant and has not suffered
any negative consequences for the offense, expressions of forgiveness that
remove the necessity of punishment or restitution may be deemed unjust
by some people: The scales are still unbalanced. Some individuals are
more likely than others to embrace standards of retributive and restitutional justice (Enright et al., 1989; Enright, Gassin, et al., 1992; Park &
Enright, 1997). Those who are more oriented toward justice concerns
(e.g., rules, fairness) than relational concerns (e.g., harmony, empathy,
mercy) are likely to resist expressing forgiveness if they are not satisfied
that justice has been served.

Loss of Benefits of Victim Status

In spite of the many emotional and motivational problems that go along
with victim status (see, e.g., Tice & Hastings, 1997), portraying the self as a
victim may bring substantial rewards. For example, people who receive the
label of victim may occupy a moral high ground by virtue of having been
wronged. Victim status may provide the power to induce guilt, to demand
apologies and reparations (in some cases, even millions of dollars), or to
seek punishment of the perpetrator. Such grudge-holding actions can provide the victim with substantial leverage within the relationship (Baumeister
et al., 1998).[3] Victims might also use the other's indebtedness as justification
for some countertransgression of their own, such as an illicit affair
(Mongeau, Hale, & Alles, 1994). They might believe that by expressing forgiveness, they will lose their excuse for engaging in the forbidden but appealing act. People who label themselves as victims can also justify ongoing
feelings of anger and righteous indignation—emotions that can make them
feel powerful. Finally, being seen as a victim may also be an effective tool for
eliciting support and sympathy from others, benefits that will be lost if victim status is relinquished. In fact, people with a character style of moral mas-
ochism may regularly portray themselves as victims in order to gain such
rewards (McWilliams, 1994). To forgive is to relinquish the victim role and
the rewards that go with it. As such, it is hardly surprising that some people
will find it very difficult to extend forgiveness.

Summary: Risks and Intensifying Conditions

According to our analysis, anger and defensiveness are clearly not the only reasons that people fail to express forgiveness and repentance. When people confess, make concessions, or extend forgiveness, they may do so at considerable risk to their self-interest. Perpetrators often fear the punishment and shame associated with confessing to a misdeed, and they may believe that the charges brought against them are more serious than the offense warrants. Meanwhile, many of the risks of expressing forgiveness stem from the erasure of the victim and perpetrator roles: Will the perpetrator, having been forgiven, use this as an excuse to transgress again? Will justice be served if the perpetrator is released from the debt, especially if punishment or repentance is not forthcoming? Must the benefits of victim status be sacrificed?

Certain risks, and the conditions likely to increase them, are common to expressions of both forgiveness and repentance. For example, both victims and perpetrators have strong motives to view themselves as innocent, kind, and reasonable, and both recall transgression incidents in self-serving ways that foster these perceptions. Unfortunately, when people view their own motives as pure and those of others as unreasonable or malicious, they erect significant barriers that interfere with mutual understanding. Issues of trust also appear central for both victims and perpetrators. If people believe that others will take advantage of their generosity and kindness, they will be reluctant to put themselves in a vulnerable position. Finally, considerable humility can be required for acts of forgiveness and repentance. Making a forgiving or repentant overture toward another person—especially an adversary—requires people temporarily to set aside their own needs to appear powerful or correct. Some people may find such actions intensely shaming, and their fear of being seen as weak or flawed may make them unwilling to take the risk.

We also predicted that certain conditions will intensify the risks of expressing repentance or forgiveness. For example, risks should be greater in hostile interpersonal environments, those in which relational bonds between the parties are weak or absent. Such environments should make it difficult for people to empathize, instead fueling their tendencies to vilify each other and lament the injustices done to them. In hostile contexts, people may legitimately fear that others will deliberately take advantage of any sign of gentleness (Axelrod, 1980b). Certain individuals should be especially likely to perceive interpersonal situations as dangerous, most notably persons who are prone to shame (cf. Tangney et al., 1996), chronically mistrustful, or seeking dominance. Finally, people may be reluctant to express repentance or forgiveness if they have not privately experienced these processes. In the absence of intrapsychic forgiveness, a victim may have no desire to remove the perpetrator's sense of indebtedness, instead preferring to retain the option of inducing guilt or demanding an apology. Similarly, a perpetrator who feels no private remorse may be unwilling to take the risk of making a sincere apology.

FUTURE RESEARCH ON FORGIVENESS AND REPENTANCE: FIVE KEY TOPICS FROM SOCIAL PSYCHOLOGY

In spite of growing interest in the topic of forgiveness in the past few years, the empirical study of forgiveness and repentance remains largely an uncharted area. The social-psychological perspective of this chapter suggests many avenues for basic research, any of which might then be used to inform applied studies and clinical interventions. Five broad areas for further study are briefly presented.

Responses of Victims and Perpetrators after Expressions of Forgiveness

We have proposed that expressing forgiveness may carry interpersonal risks, many of which are based on how perpetrators might respond after receiving an expression of forgiveness. However, more studies are needed that directly evaluate the responses of forgiven perpetrators (that is, those who have received interpersonal expressions of forgiveness). For example, are forgiven perpetrators, relative to those who are unforgiven, more or less likely to transgress again? After receiving forgiveness, are perpetrators more likely than their forgivers to forget the offense and to resume the relationship as though nothing had happened? An alternative (and more optimistic) hypothesis is that forgiveness will actually prompt perpetrators to repent rather than to commit more transgressions. Potential moderators of perpetrator responses might include relationship closeness and trust as well as the perpetrator's level of empathy or guilt-proneness (cf. Tangney et al., 1992).

A similar issue relates to the victim perspective: What psychological changes—either positive or negative—do victims experience after they express forgiveness? We have contended that it can be risky to communicate forgiveness if intrapsychic forgiveness has not actually (or completely) occurred. However, it is possible that by behaving in forgiving ways, victims might actually increase their odds of being able to intrapsychically forgive. Longitudinal and experimental data might prove especially useful in addressing this question.

Perceptions of Forgiving Persons: Positive or Negative?

One issue raised repeatedly in this chapter is the possibility that people who express forgiveness or repent may be viewed as weak—either by themselves or by others. Direct empirical tests of this question are needed. To what extent are persons who communicate forgiveness or repentance seen as weak versus strong? Because forgiveness and repentance can be expressed in many ways, the means of communication (e.g., implicit vs. explicit; spontaneous vs. coerced) might influence observer perceptions. Observer ratings might also depend on whether there is some clear objective to be gained by forgiving or repenting that makes it seem wise to transcend self-protective impulses in the immediate situation. Finally, certain people may be more likely than others to view forgiving and repentant behaviors as weak, perhaps based on their own needs for dominance or justice.

Effects of Grudges on Relationships

According to existing research, forgiveness can be an important step in restoring relationships that have been harmed through transgression. However, less attention has been devoted to the relationship effects of withholding forgiveness or maintaining grudges. If expressions of forgiveness help to restore relationships, does it naturally follow that grudges will damage a relationship? What sorts of damage are most likely to occur, and what factors predict the degree of distress that these rifts will cause for victims and perpetrators? Longitudinal data would prove especially useful in answering such questions. Another question is whether unforgiving behaviors (e.g., guilt induction, retribution, social withdrawal) can ever serve positive functions in relationships. For example, unforgiving behaviors might influence people to treat others with respect or to feel accountable for their actions. One possibility is that unforgiving behavior may bring some positive social effects, but that these effects might also be obtained through other, less punitive means.

The Roles of Offense Severity and Intentionality

Prior research clearly suggests that it is harder to forgive people for offenses that are severe, intentional, and blameworthy (e.g., Boon & Sulsky, 1997; Gonzales et al., 1994; Hodgins et al., 1996; Lysak et al., 1989). Much of the controversy about the appropriateness of forgiveness also focuses on severe offenses. Yet many questions remain regarding the roles of offense severity and intentionality. For example, does the process of intrapsychic forgiveness differ depending on whether the offense was mild or severe? Are people less likely to view apologies or concessions as genuine when an offense was severe and/or intentional? Is it possible that people might have greater increases in well-being when they forgive or repent for very severe transgressions as opposed to less severe ones? In such studies, it would be important either to use external ratings of offense severity and intentionality or experimentally manipulate these variables in order to avoid self-serving distortions about the gravity of the offense.

Mediators of the Associations between Forgiveness, Repentance, and Well-Being

A number of studies have suggested beneficial effects of forgiveness on well-being (e.g., Al-Mabuk et al., 1995; Hebl & Enright, 1993). These findings might also extend to repentance, although controlled studies would be needed to determine this. If robust links between forgiveness, repentance, and well-being can be established, a critical next step would be to identify moderators and mediators of these effects. Do changes in well-being stem primarily from affective or cognitive shifts, relationship improvements, spiritual transformations, or other factors? Are changes in well-being associated mainly with intrapsychic forms of forgiveness and repentance, or do their interpersonal expressions also play a role?

CONCLUSION

Research on forgiveness has focused primarily on three major themes: demonstrating its benefits, uncovering its predictors, and describing the intrapsychic process of forgiveness (for reviews, see McCullough, Sandage, & Worthington, 1997; McCullough & Worthington, 1994). Using this research as a starting point, we have addressed three different facets of forgiveness that have received less attention in the literature. First, we examined responses associated with repentance, the less-studied counterpart of forgiveness. In doing so, we considered the perspectives of both victims and perpetrators. Second, we focused on overt social behavior as opposed to purely private responses. Finally, we went beyond the demonstration of benefits to outline risks that might make people reluctant to express forgiveness or repentance.

Our analysis suggests that communications of repentance and forgiveness, while often beneficial, may carry substantial risks. For both victims and perpetrators, these risks often reflect shame, self-protective thought patterns, and an inability to trust the other party. Such concerns are likely to be especially salient in hostile interpersonal contexts or among persons who are prone to shame and mistrust. In short, it may be dangerous to assume that people who do not extend forgiveness or repentance are acting entirely out of anger or selfishness. Fear and shame may prove to be major obstacles, even for people who privately feel merciful or contrite.

NOTES

1.   We do not wish to imply that repentance or forgiveness, per se, are the operative factors in health improvement in these studies. The central focus was on writing about troubling events. There is some suggestion that the beneficial effects may be limited to writ-

ten communication rather than face-to-face communication (Pennebaker, Hughes, & O'Heeron, 1987), which raises another question: Would writers have different physiological responses if they believed that their accounts would be read by those with whom they were in conflict? In the existing studies, participants knew that their letters would not be read by people they had harmed or who had harmed them, eliminating the risk of social punishment (see Kelly & McKillop, 1996). One final caveat is that existing studies have focused on traumatic events in general rather than transgression in particular, although it is reasonable to assume that transgression plays a role in many traumatic events.

2. Note, however, that expressions of forgiveness do not always spare the perpetrator from punishment. For example, the family of a murder victim could tell the murderer that she is forgiven, but their actions may not stop her from being sentenced to the death penalty.

3. The act of expressing forgiveness can also provide leverage within a relationship. Because forgiveness is often viewed as a noble act, victims who express forgiveness might gain relationship power by virtue of having taken the moral "high road." However, the relationship power gained by expressing forgiveness seems more subtle than that gained by holding a grudge. Forgivers might feel powerful by virtue of having done something kind or good. If their action is noted and appreciated by the perpetrator, he or she might be motivated to repentance or improved behavior. Yet because those who express forgiveness are ostensibly relinquishing their claim to the debt, they may not feel free to wield their leverage directly by exacting confessions or reparations.

REFERENCES

Affleck, G., Tennen, H., Croog, S., & Levine, S. (1987). Causal attribution, perceived benefits, and morbidity after a heart attack: An 8-year study. *Journal of Consulting and Clinical Psychology, 55,* 29–35.

Al-Mabuk, R. H., Enright, R. D., & Cardis, P. A. (1995). Forgiveness education with parentally love-deprived late adolescents. *Journal of Moral Education, 24,* 427–444.

Axelrod, R. (1980a). Effective choice in the Prisoner's Dilemma. *Journal of Conflict Resolution, 24,* 3–25.

Axelrod, R. (1980b). More effective choice in the Prisoner's Dilemma. *Journal of Conflict Resolution, 24,* 379–403.

Baumeister, R. F. (1997). *Evil: Inside human violence and cruelty.* New York: W. H. Freeman.

Baumeister, R. F., Exline, J. J., & Sommer, K. L. (1998). The victim role, grudge theory, and two dimensions of forgiveness. In E. L. Worthington, Jr., (Ed.), *Dimensions of forgiveness: Psychological research and theological perspectives* (pp. 79–104). Philadelphia: Templeton Foundation Press.

Baumeister, R. F., Heatherton, T. F., & Tice, D. M. (1994). *Losing control: How and why people fail at self-regulation.* San Diego: Academic Press.

Baumeister, R. F., Reis, H. T., & Delespaul, P. A. E. G. (1995). Subjective and experiential correlates of guilt in daily life. *Personality and Social Psychology Bulletin, 21,* 1256–1268.

Baumeister, R. F., Stillwell, A. M., & Heatherton, T. F. (1994). Guilt: An interpersonal approach. *Psychological Bulletin, 115,* 243–267.

Baumeister, R. F., Stillwell, A. M., & Heatherton, T. F. (1995). Personal narratives about guilt: Roles in action control and interpersonal relationships. *Basic and Applied Social Psychology, 17,* 173–198.

Baumeister, R. F., Stillwell, A., & Wotman, S. R. (1990). Victim and perpetrator accounts of interpersonal conflict: Autobiographical narratives about anger. *Journal of Personality and Social Psychology, 59,* 994–1005.

Baumeister, R. F., & Wotman, S. R. (1992). *Breaking hearts: The two sides of unrequited love.* New York: Guilford Press.

Bendor, J., Kramer, R. M., & Stout, S. (1991). When in doubt . . . cooperation in a noisy prisoner's dilemma. *Journal of Conflict Resolution, 35,* 691–719.

Bies, R. J., & Tripp, T. M. (1996). Beyond distrust: "Getting even" and the need for revenge. In R. M. Kramer & T. R. Tyler (Eds.), *Trust in organizations: Frontiers of theory and research* (pp. 246–260). Thousand Oaks, CA: Sage.

Boon, S. D., & Sulsky, L. M. (1997). Attributions of blame and forgiveness in romantic relationships: A policy-capturing study. *Journal of Social Behavior and Personality, 12*(1), 19–44.

Brown, B. R. (1968). The effects of need to maintain face on interpersonal bargaining. *Journal of Experimental Social Psychology, 4,* 107–122.

Coyle, C. T., & Enright, R. D. (1997). Forgiveness intervention with post-abortion men. *Journal of Consulting and Clinical Psychology, 65,* 1042–1046.

Darby, B. W., & Schlenker, B. R. (1982). Children's reactions to apologies. *Journal of Personality and Social Psychology, 43,* 742–753.

Engel, B. (1989). *The right to innocence: Healing the trauma of childhood sexual abuse.* Los Angeles: Jeremy Tarcher.

Enright, R. D., Eastin, D. L., Golden, S., Sarinopoulos, I., & Freedman, S. R. (1992). Interpersonal forgiveness within the helping professions: An attempt to resolve differences of opinion. *Counseling and Values, 36,* 84–103.

Enright, R. D., Gassin, E. A., & Wu, C. (1992). Forgiveness: A developmental view. *Journal of Moral Education, 21,* 99–114.

Enright, R. D., & the Human Development Study Group. (1991). The moral development of forgiveness. In W. Kurtines & J. Gewirtz (Eds.), *Moral behavior and development* (Vol. 1, pp. 123–152). Hillsdale, NJ: Erlbaum.

Enright, R. D., Santos, M. J. D., & Al-Mabuk, R. (1989). The adolescent as forgiver. *Journal of Adolescence, 12,* 99–110.

Exline, J. J., Yali, A. M., & Lobel, M. (1998a, April). *Self-serving perceptions in victim and perpetrator accounts of transgression.* Poster presented at the annual meeting of the Midwestern Psychological Association, Chicago, IL.

Exline, J. J., Yali, A. M., & Lobel, M. (1998b). *Repentance promotes forgiveness.* Unpublished raw data.

Fagenson, E. A., & Cooper, J. (1987). When push comes to power: A test of power restoration theory's explanation for aggressive conflict escalation. *Basic and Applied Social Psychology, 8,* 273–293.

Fenell, D. L. (1993). Characteristics of long-term first marriages. *Journal of Mental Health Counseling, 15,* 446–460.

Freedman, S. R., & Enright, R. D. (1996). Forgiveness as an intervention goal with incest survivors. *Journal of Consulting and Clinical Psychology, 64,* 983–992.

Gerber, L. A. (1987). Experiences of forgiveness in physicians whose medical treatment was not successful. *Psychological Reports, 61,* 236.

Gerber, L. A. (1990). Transformations in self-understanding in surgeons whose treatment efforts were not successful. *American Journal of Psychotherapy, 44*(1), 75–84.

Goldstein, D., & Rosenbaum, A. (1985). An evaluation of the self-esteem of maritally violent men. *Family Relations, 34,* 425–428.

Gonzales, M. H., Haugen, J. A., & Manning, D. J. (1994). Victims as "narrative critics": Factors influencing rejoinders and evaluative responses to offenders' accounts. *Personality and Social Psychology Bulletin, 20,* 691–704.

Greenwald, D. F., & Harder, D. W. (1994). Sustaining fantasies and psychopathology in a normal sample. *Journal of Clinical Psychology, 50*(5), 707–710.

Hargrave, T. D., & Sells, J. N. (1997). The development of a forgiveness scale. *Journal of Marital and Family Therapy, 23*(1), 41–62.

Hebl, J. H., & Enright, R. D. (1993). Forgiveness as a psychotherapeutic goal with elderly females. *Psychotherapy, 30,* 658–667.

Higgins, E. T. (1987). Self-discrepancy: A theory relating self and affect. *Psychological Review, 94,* 319–340.

Hodgins, H. S., Liebeskind, E., & Schwartz, W. (1996). Getting out of hot water: Facework in social predicaments. *Journal of Personality and Social Psychology, 71,* 300–314.

Holbrook, M. I., White, M. H., & Hutt, M. J. (1995). The Vengeance Scale: Comparison of groups and an assessment of external validity. *Psychological Reports, 77,* 224–226.

Kelly, A. E., & McKillop, K. J. (1996). Consequences of revealing personal secrets. *Psychological Bulletin, 120,* 450–465.

Komorita, S. S., Hilty, J. A., & Parks, C. D. (1991). Reciprocity and cooperation in social dilemmas. *Journal of Conflict Resolution, 35,* 494–518.

Kubany, E. S., Bauer, G. B., Muraoka, M. Y., Richard, D. C., & Read, P. (1995). Impact of labeled anger and blame in intimate relationships. *Journal of Social and Clinical Psychology, 14*(1), 53–60.

Lysak, H., Rule, B. G., & Dobbs, A. R. (1989). Conceptions of aggression: Prototype or defining features? *Personality and Social Psychology Bulletin, 15,* 233–243.

McCullough, M. E. (1997). Marital forgiveness: Theoretical foundations and an approach to prevention. *Marriage and Family: A Christian Journal, 1*(1), 77–93.

McCullough, M. E., Exline, J. J., & Baumeister, R. F. (1998). An annotated bibliography of research and related concepts. In E. L. Worthington, Jr. (Ed.), *Dimensions of forgiveness: Psychological research and theological perspectives* (pp. 193–317). Philadelphia: Templeton Foundation Press.

McCullough, M. E., Sandage, S. J., & Worthington, E. L., Jr. (1997). *To forgive is human: How to put your past in the past.* Downers Grove, IL: Intervarsity Press.

McCullough, M. E., & Worthington, E. L., Jr. (1994). Encouraging clients to forgive people who have hurt them: Review, critique, and research prospectus. *Journal of Psychology and Theology, 22*(1), 3–20.

McCullough, M. E., Worthington, E. L., Jr., & Rachal, K. C. (1997). Interpersonal forgiving in close relationships. *Journal of Personality and Social Psychology, 73,* 321–336.

McWilliams, N. (1994). *Psychoanalytic diagnosis: Understanding personality structure in the clinical process.* New York: Guilford Press.

Meek, K. R., Albright, J. S., & McMinn, M. R. (1995). Religious orientation, guilt, confession, and forgiveness. *Journal of Psychology and Theology, 23,* 190–197.

Meek, K. R., & McMinn, M. R. (1997). Forgiveness: More than a therapeutic technique. *Journal of Psychology and Christianity, 16,* 51–61.

Mongeau, P. A., Hale, J. L., & Alles, M. (1994). An experimental investigation of accounts and attributions following sexual infidelity. *Communication Monographs, 61,* 326–344.

Nasby, W., Hayden, B., & DePaulo, B. (1980). Attributional bias among aggressive boys to interpret unambiguous social stimuli as displays of hostility. *Journal of Abnormal Psychology, 89,* 459–468.

Ohbuchi, K., Kameda, M., & Agarie, N. (1989). Apology as aggression control: Its role in mediating appraisal of and response to harm. *Journal of Personality and Social Psychology, 56,* 219–227.

O'Malley, M. N., & Greenberg, J. (1983). Sex differences in restoring justice: The down payment effect. *Journal of Research in Personality, 17,* 174–185.

Park, Y. O., & Enright, R. D. (1997). The development of forgiveness in the context of adolescent friendship conflict in Korea. *Journal of Adolescence, 20,* 393–402.

Pennebaker, J. W. (1993). Putting stress into words: Health, linguistic, and therapeutic implications. *Behaviour Research and Therapy, 31,* 539–548.

Pennebaker, J. W. (Ed.). (1995). *Emotion, disclosure, and health.* Washington, DC: American Psychological Association Press.

Pennebaker, J. W., Hughes, C. F., & O'Heeron, R. C. (1987). The psychophysiology of confession: Linking inhibitory and psychosomatic processes. *Journal of Personality and Social Psychology, 52,* 781–793.

Pennebaker, J. W., Mayne, T. J., & Francis, M. E. (1997). Linguistic predictors of adaptive bereavement. *Journal of Personality and Social Psychology, 72,* 863–871.

Rusbult, C. E., Verette, J., Whitney, G. A., Slovik, L. F., & Lipkus, I. (1991). Accommodation processes in close relationships: Theory and preliminary empirical evidence. *Journal of Personality and Social Psychology, 60,* 53–78.

Sells, J. N., & Hargrave, T. D. (1998). Forgiveness: A review of the theoretical and empirical literature. *Journal of Family Therapy, 20,* 21–36.

Smyth, J. M. (1998). Written emotional expression: Effect sizes, outcome types, and moderating variables. *Journal of Consulting and Clinical Psychology, 66,* 174–184.

Stillwell, A. M., & Baumeister, R. F. (1997). The construction of victim and perpetrator memories: Accuracy and distortion in role-based accounts. *Personality and Social Psychology Bulletin, 23,* 1157–1172.

Tangney, J. P., Wagner, P., Fletcher, C., & Gramzow, R. (1992). Shamed into anger? The relation of shame and guilt to anger and self-reported aggression. *Journal of Personality and Social Psychology, 62,* 669–675.

Tangney, J. P., Wagner, P. E., Hill-Barlow, D., Marschall, D. E., & Gramzow, R. (1996). Relation of shame and guilt to constructive versus destructive responses to anger across the lifespan. *Journal of Personality and Social Psychology, 70,* 797–809.

Tennen, H., & Affleck, G. (1990). Blaming others for threatening events. *Psychological Bulletin, 108,* 209–232.

Thomas, K. W., & Pondy, L. R. (1977). Toward an "intent" model of conflict management among principal parties. *Human Relations, 30,* 1089–1102.

Tice, D. M., & Hastings, S. (1997, April). *Performance and the victim role.* Paper presented at the annual meeting of the Midwestern Psychological Association, Chicago, IL.

Wade, S. H. (1989). *The development of a scale to measure forgiveness.* Unpublished doctoral dissertation, Fuller Theological Seminary, Pasadena, CA.

Weiner, B., Graham, S., Peter, O., & Zmuidinas, M. (1991). Public confession and forgiveness. *Journal of Personality, 59,* 281–312.

Williams, R., & Williams, V. (1993). *Anger kills.* New York: Random House.

Worthington, E. L., Jr. (Ed.). (1998). *Dimensions of forgiveness: Psychological research and theological perspectives.* Philadelphia: Templeton Foundation Press.

Worthington, E. L., Jr., & Drinkard, D. T. (in press). Promoting reconciliation through psychoeducational and therapeutic interventions. *Journal of Marital and Family Therapy.*

Zelin, M. L., Bernstein, S. B., Heijn, C., Jampel, R. M., Myerson, P. G., Adler, G., Buie, D. H., Jr., & Rizzuto, A. M. (1983). The Sustaining Fantasy Questionnaire: Measurement of sustaining functions of fantasies in psychiatric inpatients. *Journal of Personality Assessment, 47,* 427–439.

Personality and Forgiveness

Robert A. Emmons

Just as neurobiological approaches to forgiveness are based upon how we think about the brain (Newberg, d'Aquili, Newberg, & de Marici, Chapter 5, this volume), personality approaches to forgiveness are based on how we think about personality. Recent advances in the development of comprehensive frameworks for understanding persons suggest the possibility of advances in understanding the personality basis of forgiveness. This chapter reviews current research on personality and forgiveness from the standpoint of McAdams's comprehensive framework (1995, 1996) for understanding the person. The prospects for studying and understanding forgiveness within this framework are the primary focus of the chapter. Illustrating how the framework might lead to advances in the scientific understanding of forgiveness is another objective. The primary focus is to illustrate how this integrative model of personality description offers a helpful framework for guiding theoretical and empirical efforts on forgiveness within personality psychology. I argue that a comprehensive framework is needed to provide some conceptual tools and measurement guidelines for mapping forgiveness onto a broader personological framework.

LEVELS OF THE PERSON

I begin with the supposition that a complete understanding of the role of forgiveness within personality requires an extended discussion of how personality is conceptualized by contemporary personality psychologists. Only then can the interplay between personality and forgiveness, at both the level of theory and method, be effectively approached.

The history of personality psychology is synonymous with the search for appropriate units of analysis for studying the person. What units of analysis should be used to describe persons? A bewildering array of possibilities awaits the contemporary personologist. McAdams (1995, 1996) articulated a framework for the understanding of human individuality. He proposes that knowing a person requires being privy to information at three distinct levels or domains of personality description: (1) comparative dispositional traits, (2) contextualized personal concerns, and (3) integrative life stories. Each level contains different constructs and a different focus, and is accessed through different measurement operations. The three levels are relatively orthogonal realms of functioning, unfolding independently of each other and differing in their accessibility to consciousness. They provide different vantage points or perspectives from which to approach the scientific study of persons, and, of more immediate concern, the study of forgiveness and personality.

The first level, Level I, comprises relatively nonconditional, decontextualized, and comparative dimensions of personality called "traits." Characteristics at this level are essential in describing the most general and observable aspects of a person's typical behavioral patterns. Personality trait psychology has recently culminated in what many have argued is a consensus around the five factor model of personality traits (Bradlee & Emmons, 1992). Five traits—openness to experience, conscientiousness, extraversion, agreeableness, and neuroticism (or OCEAN, for short)—offer a unifying frame of reference that seems to have been readily adopted by many researchers inside and outside the field of personality psychology proper. OCEAN has proven to be a powerful framework for organizing existing trait questionnaire measures and for predicting important life outcomes such as health, psychological well-being, and therapeutic outcomes. The five-factor model has also been bolstered by behavioral genetic studies demonstrating substantial heritabilities of many personality traits (Rowe, 1997).

Traits are valuable descriptive features of persons, owing to their normative and nonconditional properties. But people are not reducible to their traits. To quote Ryan (1995), "Life is not lived as a trait" (p. 416). The limitations of decontextualized trait units for understanding individuality have been enumerated elsewhere (Block, 1995; McAdams, 1992; Pervin, 1994). Diener (1996) argued that when it comes to understanding a multiply determined phenomenon such as subjective well-being, traits are necessary but insufficient. He demonstrates that trait constructs fail to offer a complete account of people's evaluative responses to their lives. McAdams (1992, p. 329) argued that trait descriptions yield, at best, a "psychology of the stranger"; they are literally a first-stab attempt at describing a person.

The second level, Level II, is comprised of contextualized strategies, plans, and concerns that enable a person to solve various life tasks and achieve personally important life goals. In recent years, there has been an increasing delineation of constructs at this level of analysis as personologists turn their attention to self-regulatory mechanisms and structures that guide behavior purposefully to achieve desired goals. Constructs at this level, which include personal projects (Little, 1989), life tasks (Cantor & Zirkel, 1990), and personal strivings (Emmons, 1986), are characterized by intentionality and goal-directedness in comparison to the stylistic and habitual tendencies at Level I. Considerably more malleable than traits, these units are sometimes noncomparative, frequently highly contingent, and contextualized in time and space. Little et al. (1992) referred to these units using the acronym PAC (personal action constructs) and explicitly contrasted them with broad dispositions. Constructs at this level tend to be motivational and developmental in nature, as they focus explicitly on what a person is consciously trying to do during a particular period in his or her life. As McAdams (1992) and Pervin (1994) have forcefully argued, concepts at this level are fundamentally different from traits and cannot be reduced to traits. In a sense, Level I speaks to what a person "has" (Cantor & Zirkel, 1990), whereas Level II speaks to what a person "does." Goals are not traits, nor are they genetically based to any significant degree (though there is little hard data on this). Karoly (1993) picturesquely denotes the differences between goals and traits: "As something aspired to, a goal is inherently provisional, encompassing the romance of human possibilities—success, failure, frustration, disappointment, deferment, disallowance at the hands of others, and subversion by oneself" (p. 274).

The third level or domain, Level III, is identity, or the life narrative. Identity is reflected in the stories that people construct to provide them with a sense of overall meaning and purpose to their lives. It is the life story that renders the array of traits, strivings, and various other Level I and II elements into a more or less coherent and constantly evolving integrative unity. To quote Singer and Salovey (1993), "The stories individuals tell about their own lives are the life blood of personality" (p. 70). As opposed to the having and doing sides of personality, which are encapsulated in Levels I and II, respectively, Level III is concerned with the "making" of the self (McAdams, 1996).

FORGIVENESS AND THE THREE LEVELS OF PERSONALITY

Can this integrative, three-level model of personality offer a helpful framework for guiding conceptual and empirical efforts on personality and forgiveness? The three levels of personality structure may ultimately be useful in organizing knowledge and suggesting directions for research. Clearly, constructs and units of analysis at any of the three levels may inform research on forgiveness, and provide a framework for locating forgiveness within other aspects of psychological functioning. What the person brings with him- or herself, psychologically speaking, to a context in which forgiveness is a possible response is fundamental to understanding what will transpire in that situation. Chronic dispositions, personal goals and motives, and storied self-conceptions are likely to influence forgiveness processes in various ways. Similarly, it is possible to study forgiveness from the vantage point of any of these three levels. They each suggest constructs and measurement operations that have utility as strategies of inquiry. As the current literature on forgiveness and personality can be best understood from a trait orientation, and as trait perspectives dominate contemporary personality psychology, this chapter emphasizes trait-level constructs. Toward the end of the chapter, I consider what constructs at Levels II and III can offer the personological study of forgiveness.

Level I: Forgiveness as a Trait

One manner of studying forgiveness has been in terms of a generalized capacity or tendency to forgive others. As a decontextualized and non-conditional disposition, a generalized tendency to be forgiving transcends individual offenses and individual relationships (McCullough, Rachal, & Hoyt, Chapter 4, this volume). Several researchers have developed individual difference measures of forgiveness. McCullough and Worthington (in press) and McCullough, Rachal, and Hoyt (Chapter 4, this volume) provide a critical review of existing measures of forgiveness.

A general capacity or disposition to forgive might be called "forgivingness" (after Roberts, 1995). Forgivingness is contrasted with the act or process of forgiveness. Forgivingness, according to Roberts, is a virtue in that it is a disposition to "abort one's anger at persons one takes to have wronged one culpably, by seeing them in the benevolent terms provided by reasons characteristic of forgiving" (p. 290). A forgiving person is one who tends to be aware of anger-mitigating circumstances (e.g. sensitivity to a repentant spirit in the offender) and to have highly developed emotion-management skills that enable him or her to regulate anger and related forgiveness-inhibiting emotions. A forgiving person has a chronic concern to be in benevolent, harmonious relationships with others, the ability to take the viewpoint of sufferers and to detach him- or herself from the personal experience of having been harmed. It is this link with capacities and abilities that led Emmons (in press) to posit forgivingness as an element of spiritual intelligence. The rich conceptual analysis offered by Roberts provides fertile ground for developing an empirically valid profile of the forgiving personality and for linking forgivingness with the related interpersonal virtues of humility and gratitude (Roberts, 1995, pp. 298–299).

Given the increased attention that forgiveness is receiving from social and personality psychologists, assessing individual differences in forgivingness is likely to become a high priority. Researchers will need to justify the development of new measures. Piedmont (in press) demonstrated the value of the five-factor model (FFM) for advancing the scientific study of religion. He suggests that the FFM can provide an empirical reference point for evaluating the development of new measures of religiousness and for evaluating the meaning of existing measures. Given the historically central role of religion in forgiveness, Piedmont's recommendations are potentially applicable to the development and validation of trait measures of forgiveness as well. Ozer and Reise (1994) advise that personality researchers routinely correlate their particular measure with constructs in the FFM of personality. Given the proliferation of measurement instruments in the psychology of religion, researchers would do well to heed this advice.

A different tack for capitalizing on the McAdams framework might be to utilize constructs at Level I to examine their impact *on* forgiveness. Various dispositional traits may either constrain or facilitate the ability to both ask for and grant forgiveness. The next section of the chapter presents a detailed consideration of a construct with particular relevance for forgiveness: narcissism and the narcissistic personality.

The construct of narcissism has much to offer scientists and practitioners intent on a deeper understanding of dispositional influences on the process of forgiveness. Similarly, I argue that the concept of forgiveness is central to the understanding of narcissistic dynamics. The rich and multifaceted nature of this construct may contribute to its potential as an explanatory device for understanding conscious and unconscious motivations, prevailing affects, and implicit beliefs that underlie the forgiveness process. Narcissism is a rich, multifaceted construct, consisting of enduring attitudes toward the self and others, characteristic interpersonal orientations, and chronic emotional reactions. Therefore, narcissism and narcissistic processes ought to have considerable relevance for advancing knowledge of personality influences on forgiveness.

Narcissism and the Forgiveness–Personality Link

Theoretical constructs come and go in personality psychology. Some have flourished over the years, providing a deeper understanding of the nature and functioning of personality, while others have quickly faded into obscurity. The construct of narcissism has withstood this test of time. One hundred years ago, Havelock Ellis (1898) invoked the concept to describe a psychological state of male autoeroticism, and Freud (1914/1957) subsequently depicted narcissism as a normal stage of infant psychological development, described as a state of libidinal self-cathexis. The roots of contemporary psychodynamic formulations can be traced back to these initial conceptions. Kernberg (1975) used narcissism to refer to a pathological personality configuration, while Kohut (1977, 1985) used it to describe a separate line of personality development independent of and prior to psychosexual and ego development. Although the concept has been used to refer to a (1) developmental process, (2) a pathological category, and (3) a normal personality trait, it is this final meaning that is invoked here.

Definition and Measurement of Narcissism

Narcissism, of course, forever will be associated with the legend from Greek mythology depicting excessive and obsessive self-love. Although the term has often been viewed as synonymous with self-centeredness, its meaning has become elaborated, refined, and clarified over time. Perhaps the most comprehensive definition in the empirical literature was provided by Raskin and Terry (1988). They defined narcissism as "self-admiration that is characterized by tendencies toward grandiose ideas, exhibitionism, and defensiveness in response to criticism; interpersonal relationships that are characterized by feelings of entitlement, exploitativeness, and a lack of empathy" (p. 896).

Until the 1980s, little was known about the empirical basis of narcissism. Case studies and clinical descriptions from psychodynamically oriented psychiatrists and psychologists were one source of information, as were the writings of social critics, historians, novelists, and psychobiographers. The development of the Narcissistic Personality Inventory (NPI; Raskin & Hall, 1979) opened the door for the empirical study of narcissism as a normal personality trait. The NPI is based on the diagnostic criteria of the DSM (American Psychiatric Association, 1994) narcissistic personality disorder (NPD). The NPD is a pervasive pattern of grandiosity in either behavior or fantasy, as well as a lack of empathy and a hypersensitivity to others' criticism. Furthermore, the DSM specifies that this pattern is present from early adulthood and is manifested in all aspects or contexts of the person's life.

Although the NPI was based on DSM-IV criteria (originally, DSM-III), only extreme manifestations of those behaviors constitute the NPD, and when exhibited in less extreme forms, these behaviors are assumed to be reflective of narcissism as a normal personality trait. This assumption seems warranted in that historians such as Lasch (1979) have contended that narcissistic characteristics are prevalent in the general population.

Furthermore, Sperry and Ansbacher (1996) stated that "the narcissistic personality has become one of the most prominent personality types today in the Western world" (p. 349). As Freud noted, narcissistic processes are a universal component of personality development. Narcissistic dynamics are present in all individuals to varying degrees, depending upon developmental history and sensitivity to cultural pressures. A certain degree of self-focus and self-regard is vital to the fully functioning personality and to a coherent personality structure. Yet in a culture oriented toward personal gratification and self-enhancement, these normal tendencies can become magnified and assume prepotence in the overall personality structure.

The construct validity of the NPI has now been documented in both clinical and nonclinical samples (see Rhodewalt & Morf, 1995, for a review). The nomological network that has begun to be formed facilitates understanding of the role of the construct in personal and interpersonal functioning. Multivariate analyses of the NPI have revealed a complex factor structure ranging from a set of four to seven interrelated components that correspond to the DSM criteria. Emmons (1987) uncovered four factors identified as Exploitiveness/Entitlement, Leadership/Authority, Superiority/Arrogance, and Self-Absorption/Self-Admiration. Raskin and Terry (1988), employing different analytic procedures, uncovered a seven-factor solution in which the factors were labeled Authority, Superiority, Exhibitionism, Vanity, Exploitiveness, Entitlement, and Self-Sufficiency.

Not only is narcissism theoretically relevant to forgiveness and unforgiveness, but also it was selected to demonstrate personality influences on forgiveness in this chapter for another reason—its higher-order nature. Narcissism can be viewed as a superordinate organizing construct that subsumes several more specific traits, namely, those uncovered through the factor-analytic work on the NPI. In a study examining the thesis that personality disorders are hierarchically organized, Herkov and Blashfield (1995) demonstrated that NPD had "diagnostic dominance." When faced with a client who had a varied symptom presentation (e.g., met the criteria for two separate personality disorders), clinicians chose the narcissistic diagnosis most often. A dominant diagnosis has greater implications for treatment and understanding of the client. As a "master personality trait," narcissism and narcissistic tendencies can be expected to be activated in a wide variety of situations relevant to the psychology of forgiveness. Narcissism might serve as a central organizing construct that subsumes other forgiveness-related traits such as humility, empathy, and grandiosity.

Narcissism and Interpersonal Functioning

Problematic interpersonal relationships are a hallmark of narcissistic personalities. Negative, disdainful views of others and a chronic inability to get along are just two manifestations of a general negative orientation toward others. Millon (1998) characterizes the interpersonal aspects of narcissism brilliantly in the following passage:

> An interpersonal boldness, stemming from a belief in themselves and their talents, characterizes these persons. Competitive, ambitious, and self-assured, they naturally assume positions of leadership, act in a decisive and unwavering manner, and expect others to recognize their special qualities and cater to them. Beyond being self-confident, they are audacious, clever, and persuasive, having sufficient charm to win others over to their own causes and purposes. Problematic in this regard may be their lack of social reciprocity and their sense of entitlement—their assumption that what they wish for is their due. (pp. 89–90)

A sense of entitlement and a lack of empathy are two of the core features of narcissism. Narcissistic persons believe they are entitled to special rights and privileges, whether earned or not. They are demanding and selfish. They expect special favors without assuming reciprocal responsibilities and express surprise and anger when others do not do what they want. A lack of empathy is reflected in their difficulty in recognizing the desires, needs, and feelings of others. When recognized, the subjective experiences of others are viewed contemptuously as signs of the other's personal weakness. The sense of entitlement, combined with a lack of sensitivity to the needs of others, results in either a conscious or unconscious interpersonal exploitation (American Psychiatric Association, 1994). Other, associated features of narcissism include vulnerability in self-esteem, the need for admiration, and hypersensitivity to "injury" from criticism, failure, or humiliation.

McDonald and Waternaux (1989) and Thoresen and Powell (1992) noted several similarities between Type A and narcissistic personalities. Both are power-oriented, have concerns with their own adequacy, and are overreactive to minor frustrations; both lack a calm, relaxed manner, the ability to read interpersonal cues, and the ability to arouse nurturance in others. Both types of personalities are hostile and condescending to others, tend to create and exploit dependency, tend to be self-defensive, and lack the capacity for close relationships. In both clinical and nonclinical samples, a statistically significant association was observed by these authors between the Jenkins Activity Survey (measuring aspects of narcissism) and three measures of NPD. Along the same lines, Rhodewalt and Morf (1995) found that scores on the NPI (particularly the Entitlement/Exploitiveness element) were associated with cynical mistrust and with antagonism and disagreeableness. The narcissism–hostility link has been replicated by other researchers (McCann & Biaggio, 1989; Raskin & Terry, 1988).

NARCISSISM AND FORGIVENESS

Given the portrait of the narcissistic person as described here, compelling theoretical arguments can be made for expecting a rich network of associations between narcissism and forgiveness. In fact, conceivably, there is no other personality construct with greater relevance for forgiveness than narcissism. In many respects, the narcissistic personality is the antithesis of the forgiving personality. For various reasons to be discussed, narcissistic individuals may have great difficulty in both granting and seeking forgiveness.

Worthington's Model

Worthington (1998) has recently developed an empathy–humility–commitment model of forgiveness. In this three-part model, forgiveness is hypothesized to be initiated by empathy for the offender, furthered by humility in the offendee, and then strengthened through a public commitment to forgive the offender. The core of the model is empathy. It is not a major inferential leap to see narcissism as having an inhibitory effect on the forgiveness process. Difficulty in empathic functioning is a key dimension of narcissism, and empirical evidence of a negative association between empathy and narcissism has emerged (Ehrenberg, Hunter, & Elterman, 1996; Porcerelli & Sandler, 1995; Watson, Grisham, Trotter, & Biderman, 1984). Similarly, humility, the keeping of one's successes and positive qualities in perspective, would appear to lie at the opposite end of the narcissistic spectrum. Narcissists are prone to excessive self-enhancement and poor self-perception accuracy (Gabriel, Critelli, & Ee, 1994; John & Robins, 1994; Robins & John, 1997). Worthington states that "forgiveness is the natural response to empathy and humility" (p. 64). Unfortunately, narcissism is the natural enemy to empathy and humility. The hypothesized link between empathy and forgiveness has been empirically confirmed in a series of correlation and intervention studies by McCullough, Worthington, and their associates (McCullough, Worthington, & Rachal, 1997; McCullough et al., 1998).

Although humility is often equated in people's minds with meekness and low self-regard, in reality, humility is the antithesis of this caricature. Current writings have described the nature of humility. Humility is the disposition to view oneself as basically equal with any other human being even if there are objective differences in physical beauty, wealth, social skills, intelligence, or other resources. To be humble is not to have a low opinion of oneself; it is to have an opinion of oneself that is no better or worse than the opinion one holds of others. It is the ability to keep one's talents and accomplishments in perspective (Lebacqz, 1992; Richards, 1992), to have a sense of self-acceptance, an understanding of one's imperfections, and to be free from arrogance and low self-esteem (Clark, 1992). In most philosophical treatments of the concept, humility is considered a virtue—a desirable characteristic to cultivate. Humility has been tied to a number of personal and interpersonal life outcomes. In the health field, research has reported that a lack of humility—or the excessive self-focus found in the trait of narcissism—is a risk factor for coronary heart disease (Scherwitz & Canick, 1989). It is not surprising, then, that humility should play such a vital role in the process of forgiveness.

A scattering of empirical findings supports the supposition that narcissistic traits inhibit forgiveness. Research on sustaining fantasies—the thoughts and images that people have when trying to cope with stressful circumstances—is especially informative. A number of theorists have speculated that narcissistic fantasies protect, restore, and repair the person's sense of self-esteem. Millon (1998) asserts that vengeful gratification is a common response to narcissistic injuries. Fantasies of revenge can be a powerful means of salving narcissistic wounds. Raskin and Novacek (1991) found that narcissism was associated with fantasies of power, success, glory, and revenge. In particular, narcissistic individuals undergoing a high degree of daily stress were especially likely to experience power and revenge fantasies in which they "imagine themselves in a powerful position able to impose punishment on those who have wronged them" (Raskin & Novacek, p. 496). Similar to the Rhodewalt and Morf (1995) study cited earlier, the entitlement component of narcissism was most strongly related to these types of fantasies. McCullough et al. (1998) argue that revenge–rumination is one-half of a motivational system that underlies forgiving behavior. Their data indicate that revenge-seeking and ruminative tendencies are personality-level constructs that serve as powerful inhibitors of forgiveness.

Bushman and Baumeister (1998) designed a laboratory experiment in which subjects were given an opportunity to display aggression following insult. Subjects, preselected based on their levels of narcissism and self-esteem, wrote essays that were later evaluated in a critical or positive manner. The measure of aggression was the level of noise (computer-controlled by the subject) directed toward the source of the feedback. The combination of narcissism and insult led to high levels of aggression directed toward the source of the insult. The authors interpreted the findings of the study to support their hypothesis that "threatened egotism" is an important contributor to aggressive and potentially violent behavior. Aggression is a strategy for defending a favorable view of the self against ego threats (Baumeister, Smart, & Boden, 1996).

In the only direct test of the narcissism–forgiveness link, Davidson (1993) empirically examined the association between these constructs. Levels of narcissism (as assessed by the NPI) were inversely related to forgiveness. Both males and females who scored high on narcissism were significantly less likely to display forgiveness in response to both hypothetical and real-life hurtful situations. Davidson suggests that a relatively mature level of ego development is related to the ability to forgive and that forgiveness may be a much more difficult task for emotionally needy individuals or those with significant deficits in ego resources.

Narcissistic Dynamics and Forgiveness

The rich theoretical network surrounding the construct of narcissism enables the specification of likely pathways by which narcissism affects the process of forgiveness. Similarly, the concept of forgiveness is central to understanding narcissistic dynamics. A narcissistically vulnerable individual, hypersensitive to being offended, is likely to respond to real or perceived violations in a manner that is likely to create and/or prolong maladaptive emotional reactions and interpersonal behaviors. Brandsma (1982) outlines the general context in which forgiveness occurs, particularly for the narcissistic individual. A person is wronged—he or she experiences a violation to his or her sense of fairness. The offended person experiences a loss of esteem, followed by anger in an attempt to protect him- or herself from the offender and subsequent ego threat. Three possible responses to the offender are retribution, neutrality, or forgiveness. In order to forgive, one must reexperience the hurt of the violator, which allows less threat and greater capacity for empathy. According to Brandsma, this requires a humbling of the self and a relinquishment (at least temporarily) of grandiosity. Forgiveness also requires abandoning the egocentric position of seeing others in light of one's own needs and developing insight into the offender's own motives, needs, and reasons for acting as he or she did. In other words, the person takes a more empathic view of the other's behavior. The third and final step of the forgiveness process involves a commitment not to engage in "retributive opportunities" (i.e., taking vengeance). All three of these steps may be close to insurmountable tasks for narcissistic individuals.

Narcissistic persons may be especially forgiveness-challenged because of the psychological dynamics underlying the forgiveness process. A relatively mature level of ego development is a prerequisite to the ability to forgive. Narcissistic individuals appear to be lacking the very capacities that are required for forgiveness. Because of early childhood experiences, the inner skills needed to regulate impulses and affects, to develop strategies for effective conflict resolution and a sense of competence from successfully handling problematic interpersonal encounters are unavailable (Millon, 1998). Deep hurts may paralyze these individuals with anger and pain that inhibits any movement toward forgiveness (Davidson, 1993). To forgive, one must have the capacity to identify with others and view them as more than simply extensions of oneself. One must be able to feel a mo-

dicum of social interest, a willingness to admit a personal role in relationship dysfunctions, and genuine concern and empathy for others to be
motivated for reconciliation.

The process of reparation, in which a relationship is restored, is facilitated when a transgressor admits culpability and offers an apology. Narcissists are unlikely to acknowledge guilt (Gramzow & Tangney, 1992); they
are therefore unlikely to offer an apology. The reparation process takes
on a unique tone when narcissistic processes are operating. McWilliams
and Lependorf (1990) explore at some length the denial of remorse in
narcissistic individuals. In the words of these authors, "The organizing,
overriding issue for people with narcissistic preoccupations is the preservation of their internal sense of self-cohesiveness or self-approval, not the
quality of their relations with other people" (p. 441). Because of their desire to maintain the illusion of perfection, narcissists may be incapable of
genuine expressions of remorse. Inherent in an apology is the admission
that one is not only less than perfect, but also is in fact at fault. When an
apology is forthcoming, it is offered not in the spirit of restoring the relationship, but rather in restoring the person's illusion of perfection. Oft-
times, apologies may be little more than self-justifications or other
defensive maneuvers to deflect blame. At the other extreme, narcissists
may engage in self-recrimination ("I can't believe that I did that," "You
must think I'm a terrible person," "I don't blame you if you never forgive
me"), all of which appear to genuine, if somewhat exaggerated, forms of
apologizing. However, these, too, are intended to evoke from others reassurance that despite the transgression, the narcissist is really perfect. Ex-
posing wrongdoing from the point of view of shame rather than guilt may
be a more effective strategy to elicit strivings for forgiveness from narcissistic individuals (Pembroke, 1998). It should be evident from these illus-
trations that incorporating a psychodynamic construct such as narcissism
into theory and research on forgiveness is a reminder that behavior is not
always what it appears to be on the surface and that behavioral accounts
cannot always be taken at face value.

Clinical Implications

Awareness of narcissistic characteristics may be critical in therapeutic contexts or those that involve forgiveness interventions. Narcissistically motivated behaviors may pose significant challenges for forgiveness,
particularly in a marital relationship. Two recent studies suggest that narcissism may predispose individuals to engage in hurtful, destructive interpersonal behaviors in two marital spheres: extramarital relationships and
postdivorce parenting.

There may be no offense more challenging to forgive than adultery.
Buss and Shackelford (1997) examined a number of predictors of the sus-

ceptibility to infidelity in the first year of marriage. Although they did not examine actual infidelity, their proxy measure consisted of several specific, self-reported infidelity behaviors, including flirting with someone else, kissing someone else, having a one-night stand, and having a serious affair. Participants rated the probability of engaging in these extramarital behaviors, and then the probability that their partners would also engage in each of these activities. High scores on narcissism were strongly linked to anticipated infidelity, both in the self and in the partner. The pattern was especially strong for women. Women who scored high on narcissism estimated that they were more likely than their less narcissistic counterparts to engage in all forms of extramarital activity. The husbands of women who scored high on narcissism also predicted that their wives would engage in extramarital activity. Given that women tend to be more forgiving of affairs than men (Lawson, 1988), one would predict that narcissistic men would be the least likely to forgive indiscretions of their partners.

Marital dissolution and the custody and child access arrangements in its wake provide a real-world laboratory for the study of forgiveness processes. Ehrenberg et al. (1996) found that narcissism in ex-spouses was a strong predictor of continued conflict between them, with predictable destructive consequences for their children. Couples who disagreed about postdivorce parenting arrangements were more narcissistic, less empathic, more self-focused, and less child-oriented then were parents who were able to maintain a cooperative parenting plan after separation. This fascinating study demonstrated that a single personality trait has profound implications for one of the most pressing social issues of our time—the welfare of children following divorce.

FORGIVENESS AND OTHER LEVELS OF PERSONALITY

Traits such as narcissism (and, for that matter, forgivingness) are essential for describing the most general and observable aspects of a person's typical behavioral patterns. Vital as they are for understanding forgiveness, the limitations of decontextualized trait units for understanding individuality in its totality have been spelled out (Block, 1995; McAdams, 1992; Pervin, 1994). From a methodological standpoint, the limitations of relying exclusively on the questionnaire measurement paradigm have been noted (Diener, 1996; Gorsuch, 1984). Thus, there exists a need to identify and rigorously measure contextualized and conditional units of analysis. Level II (contextualized personal concerns and goals) and Level III (identity or the life story) in McAdams's framework remain largely unexplored and have much to offer the psychologist interested in the place of forgiveness within personality structure and functioning. By articulating concepts and mechanisms that are sensitive to interactional and situational variation, constructs at these levels can enhance the study of forgiveness beyond the previously articulated dispositional strategy.

Forgiveness Goals and Strivings

Personal strivings, as one type of middle-level unit representing personal concerns, might prove enlightening in the study of forgiveness. Personal strivings represent the typical or characteristic objectives that a person is trying to accomplish in everyday life. Emmons (1989) examined the personal strivings of individuals high and low in the trait of narcissism. One especially narcissistic individual in the study was committed to the following goals: "Be strong against people who might use me," "Reject authority—church leaders, police, my boss," and "Manipulate people to see things from my point of view." A similar strategy could be employed to identify the strivings of individuals high and low in trait measures of forgiveness, or in dispositions that enable or, conversely, inhibit forgiveness, such as humility. This would provide valuable information on how global dispositions are contextualized in concrete life situations and may also provide important leads for clinical assessment and intervention (Karoly, 1993).

In addition to considering what a person is trying to do, Level II strategies for forgiveness might entail examining mechanisms and processes that underlie the effective regulation of goal-directed behavioral sequences. How is an intention to forgive enacted and interwoven in the ongoing tapestry of a close relationship? How is the intention protected from competing goal intentions, including the desire to maintain a grudge and to hold the offender accountable for his or her actions? A cognitive–motivational approach to forgiveness can elucidate the mechanisms by which forgiveness is translated into concrete behavioral sequences across situational and temporal contexts. A number of cognitive mechanisms such as strategies, schemas, and personal scripts might be invoked to account for the translation of an abstract "forgiveness trait" into effective action to attain personally relevant goals. The cognitive–motivational approach to personality views people as intentional, usually (but not always) rational beings, who are engaged in a constant effort to shape their social worlds to pursue agendas and move toward valued life outcomes. Motivational units, such as goals, motives, and values, form a hierarchical system in which various levels could be activated depending upon environmental stimuli. Moreover, goals can be activated and subsequently guide cognitive and behavioral processing outside conscious awareness of the person (Bargh & Gollwitzer, 1994). For instance, the striving "to be more forgiving" can be removed from conscious control and still be activated by situational cues sensitizing the person to opportunities for forgiveness quite outside of his or her awareness. This dynamic approach to personality thus accommodates unconscious motivation and points to how the unconscious can be a source of goals independent of conscious intents and plans. Conflict that is experienced between strivings for forgiveness and competing tendencies might be explained through the override of conscious intentions by conflicting unconscious goals. Gollwitzer's (1993) theory of goal achievement proposes that implementation intentions are critical determiners of successful goal pursuit. Effective self-regulation proceeds through a series of stages, or "action phases," in which a person moves from an abstract goal state "to be more forgiving" to a concrete action ("Tell Jill over coffee that I understand why she treated me as she did").

The goal or personal-concerns approach to forgiveness represents a dynamic perspective and a departure from the structural approaches described earlier. Rather than being seen as competing with a dispositional level of analysis, it is an approach that leads to asking and answering questions such as "How well am I doing?" "How might I be more successful?" These applied concerns are more likely to have direct clinical relevance than a focus on more static entities such as decontextualized traits.

Forgiveness in the Life Narrative

Level III in McAdams's framework concerns how persons make sense of who they are in the world and how they create life stories that provide their lives with overall unity, meaning, and purpose. The study of narrative, both as a methodology and as a theoretical construct, has played an influential role in personality psychology in the past decade (e.g., Rosenwald & Ochberg, 1992). Nor have narrative approaches been limited to the field of personality. Sarbin (1986) has suggested that the organization of life experiences into a narrative can serve as a root metaphor for general psychology. According to Sarbin, narrative modes of explanation provide a more satisfactory account of human action than do formistic or mechanistic models. Since identity is a story, it must be understood in story terms. McAdams (1993, 1996) outlines several component features of life stories: narrative emotional tone, symbolic and metaphoric use of imagery, motivational themes, ideological setting, nuclear episodes (e.g., turning points in life), imagoes (idealized characters), and the ending provided by the generativity script. An appraisal of these features enables life stories to be systematically quantified, classified, and analyzed, much like any other data source for personologists. Concrete guidelines for the analysis of life stories are provided by McAdams (1993) and Atkinson (1998). Combining life narratives with dispositional and contextual data at Levels I and II, respectively, provides the richest possible picture of the forgiving personality.

Life stories teem with images, symbols, and metaphors that may indirectly enable forgiveness. For instance, the richness of metaphor that religious systems provide (e.g., viewing major life changes as involving the death and burial of an old life and a resurrection to a new one) may be a potent means of activating forgiving tendencies or incorporating forgiveness into one's identity. The use of religious stories or parables can serve as a powerful source of inspiration and guidance for those desiring to seek or to grant forgiveness, even under the most trying circumstances. Consider, for example, the parable of the prodigal son (Luke 15: 11–32, New Revised Standard Version). A profligate, narcissistic son squanders away his inheritance and, broken and humbled, returns, repentant, to his compassionate, loving, accepting father. The son asks for and is granted forgiveness. A number of contemporary writers have drawn out the implications of this parable for how we are to relate to one another in circumstances of offense, wrongdoing, and suffering (Nouwen, 1992; Volf, 1996). This classic story of separation followed by reconciliation serves as a paragon of forgiveness and a standard by which we might be able to judge our own ability to forgive in close relationships.

While constructs at Levels I and II can lead to a healthy understanding of forgiveness, it may be only through incorporation of constructs at Level III that a complete account of forgiveness within personality can be constructed. It has been suggested that much of the transformative power of forgiveness stems from its ability to produce a state of wholeness or integration of personality (McCullough, Sandage, & Worthington, 1997; Pargament, 1997). Forgiveness can activate integrative tendencies in the person, rescuing the psyche from inner conflict and turmoil, transforming the person from a state of fragmentation to a state of integration, from separation to reconciliation. Forgiveness is the integrated state of a person who is in a right relationship with God, with others, and within him- or herself (Bonar, 1989).

Identity is concerned with achieving unity and purpose in life. In recent years, the psychological sciences have become increasingly concerned with what constitutes "the good life." For example, the scientific study of happiness has flourished in recent years (Myers & Diener, 1995). A shift from a concern with personal happiness and satisfaction to a restoration of integration and wholeness in personality can complement the current prevailing concern with personal well-being as the sine qua non of healthy psychological development and optimal psychological functioning. Forgiveness research can demonstrate that the healing effects of forgiveness extend beyond personal happiness, health, and well-being, to a deeper sense of coherence, wholeness, and integration of the self.

CONCLUSIONS

The multiple-level approach to forgiveness and personality argued for in this chapter presents researchers with a framework of strategies for studying forgiveness. If we want to know about a generalized tendency to forgive, then we should include some trait measures. If we want to learn more about context-specific forgiveness strivings and behaviors, then we need to employ measures of personal concerns. Finally, in order to understand the role of forgiveness in self-understanding and the construction of meaning in the broader context of a person's entire life, we would be wise to collect life stories and detailed personal narratives. The collection of all three types of information provides the richest possible portrait of the forgiving personality. At the very least, the consideration of these three levels makes it clear that there are risks to a decontextualized approach to forgiveness.

Although personality psychologists generally prefer to see the person as the locus of important individual differences, a growing number emphasize the need to attend to sociohistorical and other macrolevel contexts to fully appreciate the origins of individual differences (McAdams, 1996; Singer, 1995; de St. Aubin, 1996). One's individuality is forged through the conscious and unconscious ideologies that are conveyed to the developing person by the local and global institutions within which the person is embedded. These transmitters of culture include family, school, neighborhood, church, television, theater, books, and the Internet. How might these social forces impact upon forgiveness? A number of commentators have depicted the late 20th century as "the age of narcissism" (Lasch, 1979, Mazlish, 1982; Vitz, 1994). A culture that emphasizes individual rights and entitlements is not going to be hospitable to the concept of forgiveness. Thus, societal as well as individual barriers must be confronted. This dilemma raises an intriguing question: How should society foster forgiveness in its members? It has already done a good job of fostering narcissism. What would it take to replace the age of narcissism with the age of forgivingness? While answers to this question are beyond the scope of this chapter, the study of forgiveness offers researchers the opportunity to make considerable strides toward the original goal of personality psychology: understanding the individual person in cultural context.

ACKNOWLEDGMENT

Preparation of this chapter was supported by a grant from the John M. Templeton Foundation. I am grateful to each of the three editors of this volume for their constructive comments on an earlier draft of the chapter.

REFERENCES

American Psychiatric Association. (1994). *Diagnostic and statistical manual of mental disorders* (4th ed.). Washington, DC: Author.

Atkinson, R. (1998). *The life story interview.* Thousand Oaks, CA: Sage.

Bargh, J. A., & Gollwitzer, P. M. (1994). Environmental control of goal-directed action: Automatic and strategic contingencies between situations and behavior. In W. D. Spaulding (Ed.), *Nebraska Symposium on Motivation* (Vol. 41, pp. 71–124). Lincoln: University of Nebraska Press.

Baumeister, R. F., Smart, L., & Boden, J. M. (1996). Relation of threatened egotism to violence and aggression: The dark side of high self-esteem. *Psychological Review, 103,* 5–33.

Block, J. (1995). A contrarian view of the five-factor approach to personality description. *Psychological Bulletin, 117,* 187–215.

Bonar, C. A. (1989). Personality theories and asking for forgiveness. *Journal of Psychology and Christianity, 8,* 45–51.

Bradlee, P. M., & Emmons, R. A. (1992). Locating narcissism within the interpersonal circumplex and the five-factor model. *Personality and Individual Differences, 13,* 821–830.

Brandsma, J. M. (1982). Forgiveness: A dynamic, theological, and therapeutic analysis. *Pastoral Psychology, 31,* 40–50.

Bushman, B. J., & Baumeister, R. F. (1998). Threatened egotism, narcissism, self-esteem, and direct and displaced aggression: Does self-love or self-hate lead to violence? *Journal of Personality and Social Psychology, 75,* 219–229.

Buss, D. M., & Shackelford, T. K. (1997). Susceptibility to infidelity in the first year of marriage. *Journal of Research in Personality, 31,* 193–221.

Cantore, N., & Zirkel, S. (1990). Personality, cognition, and purposive behavior. In L. A. Pervin (Ed.), *Handbook of personality: Theory and research* (pp. 135–164). New York: Guilford Press.

Clark, A. T. (1992). Humility. In D. H. Ludlow (Ed.), *Encyclopedia of Mormonism* (pp. 663–664). New York: Macmillan.

Davidson, D. L. (1993). Forgiveness and narcissism: Consistency in experience across real and hypothetical hurt situations. *Dissertation Abstracts International, 54,* 2746.

de St. Aubin, E. (1996). Personal ideology polarity: Its emotional foundation and its manifestation in individual value systems, religiosity, political orientation, and assumptions concerning human nature. *Journal of Personality and Social Psychology, 71,* 152–165.

Diener, E. (1996). Traits can be powerful, but are not enough: Lessons from subjective well-being. *Journal of Research in Personality, 30,* 389–399.

Ehrenberg, M. F., Hunter, M. A., & Elterman, M. F. (1996). Shared parenting agreements after marital separation: The roles of empathy and narcissism. *Journal of Consulting and Clinical Psychology, 64,* 808–818.

Ellis, H. (1898). *Sexual inversion.* London: Wilson & MacMillan.

Emmons, R. A. (1987). Narcissism: Theory and measurement. *Journal of Personality and Social Psychology, 52,* 11–17.

Emmons, R. A. (1989). Exploring the relations between motives and traits: The case of narcissism. In D. M. Buss & N. Cantor (Eds.), *Personality psychology: Recent trends and emerging directions* (pp. 32–44). New York: Springer-Verlag.

Emmons, R. A. (in press). Is spirituality an intelligence? Motivation, cognition, and the psychology of ultimate concerns. *International Journal for the Psychology of Religion.*

Freud, S. (1957). On narcissism: An introduction. In J. Strachey (Ed. and Trans.), *The standard edition of the complete psychological works of Sigmund Freud* (Vol. 14, pp. 67–102). London: Hogarth Press. (Original work published 1914)

Gabriel, M. T., Critelli, J. W., & Ee, J. S. (1994). Narcissistic illusions in self-evaluations of intelligence and attractiveness. *Journal of Personality, 62,* 143–155.

Gollwitzer, P. M. (1993). Goal achievement: The role of intention. In W. Strobe & M. Hewstone (Eds.), *European review of social psychology* (Vol. 4, pp. 141–185). London: Wiley.

Gorsuch, R. L. (1984). Measurement: The boon and bane of investigating religion. *American Psychologist, 39,* 228–236.

Gramzow, R., & Tangney, J. P. (1992). Proneness to shame and the narcissistic personality. *Personality and Social Psychology Bulletin, 18,* 369–376.

Herkov, M. J., & Blashfield, R. K. (1995). Clinician diagnoses of personality disorders: Evidence of a hierarchical structure. *Journal of Personality Assessment, 65,* 313–321.

John, O. P., & Robins, R. W. (1994). Accuracy and bias in self-perception: Individual differences in self-enhancement and the role of narcissism. *Journal of Personality and Social Psychology, 66,* 206-219.

Karoly, P. (1993). Goal systems: An organizational framework for clinical assessment and treatment planning. *Psychological Assessment, 3,* 273-280.

Kernberg, O. (1975). *Borderline conditions and pathological narcissism.* New York: Jason Aronson.

Kohut, H. (1977). *The restoration of the self.* New York: International Universities Press.

Kohut, H. (1985). *Self psychology and the humanities: Reflections on a new psychoanalytic approach.* New York: W. W. Norton.

Lasch, C. (1979). *The culture of narcissism.* New York: Warner Books.

Lawson, A. (1988). *Adultery.* New York: Basic Books.

Lebacqz, K. (1992). Humility in health care. *Journal of Medicine and Philosophy, 17,* 291-307.

Little, B. R. (1989). Personal projects analysis: Trivial pursuits, magnificent obsessions, and the search for coherence. In D. M. Buss & N. Cantor (Ed.), *Personality psychology: Recent trends and emerging directions* (pp. 15-31). New York: Springer-Verlag.

Mazlish, B. (1982). American narcissism. *Psychohistory Review, 10,* 185-202.

McAdams, D. P. (1992). The five-factor model in personality: A critical appraisal. *Journal of Personality, 60,* 329-361.

McAdams, D. P. (1993). *The stories we live by: Personal myths and the making of the self.* New York: William Morrow.

McAdams, D. P. (1995). What do we know when we know a person? *Journal of Personality, 63,* 365-396.

McAdams, D. P. (1996). Personality, modernity, and the storied self: A contemporary framework for studying persons. *Psychological Inquiry, 7,* 295-321.

McCann, J. T., & Biaggio, M. K. (1989). Narcissistic personality features of self-reported anger. *Psychological Reports, 64,* 55-58.

McCullough, M. E., Rachal, K. C., Sandage, S. J., Worthington, E. L., Jr., Brown, S. W., & Hight, T. L. (1998). Interpersonal forgiving in close relationships: II. Theoretical elaboration and measurement. *Journal of Personality and Social Psychology, 75,* 1586-1603.

McCullough, M. E., Sandage, S. J., & Worthington, E. L., Jr. (1997). *To forgive is human: How to put your past in the past.* Downers Grove, IL: Intervarsity Press.

McCullough, M. E., & Worthington, E. L., Jr. (in press). Religion and the forgiving personality. *Journal of Personality.*

McCullough, M. E., Worthington, E. L., Jr., & Rachal, K. C. (1997). Interpersonal forgiving in close relationships. *Journal of Personality and Social Psychology, 73,* 321-336.

McDonald, C. D., & Waternaux, C. M. (1989, August). *Narcissism and Type A personality: Associations in expert, clinical, and non-clinical studies.* Paper presented at the Annual Meeting of the American Psychological Association, New Orleans, LA.

McWilliams, N., & Lependorf, S. (1990). Narcissistic pathology of everyday life: The denial of remorse and gratitude. *Contemporary Psychoanalysis, 26,* 430-451.

Millon, T. M. (1998). DSM narcissistic personality disorder. In E. F. Ronningstam (Ed.), *Disorders of narcissism: Diagnostic, clinical, and empirical implications* (pp. 75-101). Washington, DC: American Psychiatric Association Press.

Myers, D. G., & Diener, E. (1995). Who is happy? *Psychological Science, 6,* 10-19.

Nouwen, H. J. M. (1992). *The return of the prodigal son.* New York: Doubleday.

Ozer, D. J., & Reise, S. P. (1994). Personality assessment. *Annual Review of Psychology, 45,* 357-388.

Pargament, K. I. (1997). *The psychology of religion and coping.* New York: Guilford Press.

Pembroke, N. F. (1998). Toward a shame-based theology of evangelism. *Journal of Psychology and Christianity, 17,* 15-24.

Pervin, L. A. (1994). A critical analysis of current trait theory. *Psychological Inquiry, 5,* 103-113.

Porcerelli, J. H., & Sandler, B. A. (1995). Narcissism and empathy in steroid users. *American Journal of Psychiatry, 152,* 1672-1674.

Raskin, R., & Hall, C. S. (1979). A narcissistic personality inventory. *Psychological Reports, 45,* 590.

Raskin, R., & Novacek, J. (1991). Narcissism and the use of fantasy. *Journal of Clinical Psychology, 47,* 490–499.

Raskin, R., & Terry, H. (1988). A principal components analysis of the Narcissistic Personality Inventory and further evidence of its construct validity. *Journal of Personality and Social Psychology, 54,* 890–902.

Rhodewalt, F., & Morf, C. C. (1995). Self and interpersonal correlates of the Narcissistic Personality Inventory: A review and new findings. *Journal of Research in Personality, 29,* 1–23.

Richards, N. (1992). *Humility.* Philadelphia, PA: Temple University Press.

Roberts, R. C. (1995). Forgivingness. *American Philosophical Quarterly, 32,* 289–306.

Robins, R. W., & John, O. P. (1997). The quest for self-insight: Theory and research on accuracy and bias in self-perception. In R. Hogan, J. Johnson, & S. Briggs (Eds.), *Handbook of personality psychology* (pp. 649–679). San Diego: Academic Press.

Rosenwald, G. C., & Ochberg, R. C. (Eds.). (1992). *Storied lives.* New Haven, CT: Yale University Press.

Rowe, D. C. (1997). Genetics, temperament, and personality. In R. Hogan, J. Johnson, & S. Briggs (Eds.), *Handbook of personality psychology* (pp. 367–386). San Diego: Academic Press.

Ryan, R. M. (1995). Psychological needs and the facilitation of integrative processes. *Journal of Personality, 63,* 397–427.

Scherwitz, L., & Canick, J. C. (1989). Self-reference and coronary heart disease risk. In B. K. Houston & C. R. Snyder (Eds.), *Type A behavior pattern: Research, theory, and intervention* (pp. 146–167). New York: Wiley.

Singer, J. A. (1995). Seeing one's self: Locating narrative memory in a framework of personality. *Journal of Personality, 63,* 429–457.

Singer, J. A., & Salovey, P. (1993). *The remembered self: Emotion and memory in personality.* New York: Free Press.

Sperry, L., & Ansbacher, H. L. (1996). The concept of narcissism and the narcissistic personality disorder. In L. Sperry & J. Carlson (Eds.), *Psychopathology and psychotherapy: From DSM-IV diagnosis to treatment* (pp. 337–351). Washington, DC: Accelerated Development.

Thoresen, C. E., & Powell, L. H. (1992). Type A behavior pattern: New perspectives on theory, assessment, and intervention. *Journal of Consulting and Clinical Psychology, 60,* 595–604.

Vitz, P. C. (1994). *Psychology as religion: The cult of self-worship* (2nd ed.). Grand Rapids, MI: Eerdmans.

Volf, M. (1996). *Exclusion and embrace: The theological exploration of identity, otherness, and reconciliation.* Nashville, TN: Abington Press.

Watson, P. J., Grisham, S. O., Trotter, M. V., & Biderman, M. D. (1984). Narcissism and empathy: Validity evidence for the narcissistic personality inventory. *Journal of Personality Assessment, 48,* 301–305.

Worthington, E. L., Jr. (1998). An empathy–humility–commitment model of forgiveness applied within family dyads. *Journal of Family Therapy, 20,* 59–76.

PART III

Applications in Counseling, Psychotherapy, and Health

CHAPTER 9

Forgiveness as a Process of Change in Individual Psychotherapy

Wanda M. Malcolm and Leslie S. Greenberg

There is considerable philosophical debate over how best to define forgiveness. In this chapter, we look at those aspects of forgiveness discussed in the literature that appear most relevant to forgiveness as a process of change in individual psychotherapy. In this way, we arrive at a description of what we mean when we use the term "forgiveness." This is followed by a discussion of research relevant to forgiveness in individual psychotherapy.

THE PROCESS OF FORGIVENESS

Based on our review of the literature, the following five components appear to be necessary to the process of forgiveness: (1) the acceptance into awareness of strong emotions such as anger and sadness; (2) letting go of previously unmet interpersonal needs; (3) a shift in the forgiving person's view of the offender; (4) the development of empathy for the offender; and (5) the construction of a new narrative of self and other.

Without exception, everyone who writes about forgiveness in the face of deep interpersonal hurt acknowledges that strong emotions such as anger and sadness are endemic to the forgiveness process. Acknowledgment of resentment and self-protecting anger in the face of personal injury is an appropriate response to a situation of feeling unfairly treated or violated. Anger conveys self-respect and self-worth (Haber, 1991), while experiences of grief "may concern both the loss of what was and/or could have been, and, on a deeper level, the loss of a particular way of viewing oneself and the world" (Rowe et al., 1989, p. 241). Expressions of core emotions such as these are viewed by emotion theorists and therapists as biologically adaptive (Frijda, 1986; Greenberg & Paivio, 1997; Lazarus, 1991).

In individual psychotherapy, forgiveness issues are typically set within the context of relationships with an extensive history, where individuals have struggled long and hard to make sense of the offense(s). Bass and Davis (1988) counsel survivors of sexual abuse that at some point they will need to give up trying to get anything back from their abusers. In letting go of previously unmet interpersonal needs, the forgiver is released from the traps of (1) trying to make the offender understand the magnitude of harm done, and (2) trying to get the offender to take responsibility. In letting go of unmet interpersonal needs, what was missed or lost has to be acknowledged, grieved, and relinquished.

Initially, the injured person blames the offender and wants that person to make restitution or be punished for the offense. The injured person is also likely to see the offender in wholly negative terms. In the process of forgiving, however, the injured person often experiences a shift in his or her view of the offender. As Rowe et al. (1989, p. 242) point out, this involves seeing the other "as distinct and separate from one's own needs and desires." Similarly, Al-Mabuk, Enright, and Cardis (1995) address this aspect of the process when they suggest that when an individual forgives, negative cognitions about the other often become more positive (or, at least, less negative).

A number of theorists (Brandsma, 1982; Cunningham, 1985; Fitzgibbons, 1986; Hope, 1987; Human Development Study Group, 1991; McCullough, 1997) have identified the capacity for empathy as a crucial element in successful forgiveness. McCullough, Worthington, and Rachal (1997) have proposed and investigated an empathy model of forgiveness, and McCullough, Rachal, Sandage, and Worthington (1997) have concluded that empathy and forgiveness are intimately, maybe even causally, linked. Empathy can be defined as an active effort to understand another person's perception of an interpersonal event as if one were that other person, rather than judging the other person's behavior from the perspective of one's own experience of that event.

What does the forgiving person have to show for his or her efforts once he or she has made the arduous journey in pursuit of forgiveness? The forgiveness process involves the construction of a new narrative of self and other, which entails "a shift in one's understanding of, and relationship to, the other person, oneself, and the world. The implications of the original situation are cast in a new light" (Rowe et al., 1989, p. 242). The experience of violation and its impact on the forgiving person's life is different at the end of the process than it was at the beginning. Often, the forgiving person is able to see the offender in a more complex way, as possessing both strengths and weaknesses, and is enabled to see him or herself as having been made stronger, possibly better, by the struggle to forgive.

METHODS OF STUDYING FORGIVENESS

Three distinct approaches have been used to study forgiveness as a process of change: (1) descriptions based on clinical experience; (2) phenomenological studies; and (3) research aimed at providing empirical support for specific theories and hypotheses related to forgiveness. Taking each of these in turn, we consider the contributions they have made to our understanding of forgiveness as it pertains to individual psychotherapy.

Knowledge Derived from Clinical Experience

Information about the process of forgiveness based on clinical experience offers anecdotal insights into the nature and effects of forgiveness as they unfold in the therapeutic setting. Davenport's (1991) and Fitzgibbons's (1986) attention to the need for acknowledgment and expression of the anger associated with a deep hurt is a good example of the kinds of useful insights we can glean from these accounts.

The primary difficulty with models based exclusively on clinical experience, however, is that these theoretical models have not been tested empirically. While the clinician may be convinced that the process has been correctly understood and conceptualized, there is no empirical support for the proposed models.

Phenomenological Studies

Phenomenological studies represent careful attempts to generate a model of the process of forgiveness as it is understood by those who themselves have forgiven deep interpersonal hurts. People who recount their own forgiveness experiences describe them in much the same way that clinicians describe the process of forgiveness. Curtis (1989), Rowe et al. (1989), and Truong (1991) all found evidence in their participants' forgiveness narratives of the kinds of strong emotions psychotherapists encounter in their work with clients.

In constructing his model, Truong (1991) includes the stage of "letting go" of various aspects of the hurtful experience. One of the subcategories of this stage, "letting go of expectations," corresponds well to the concept of letting go of unmet interpersonal needs.

An acquired ability to empathize with the offender was also apparent in the stories of people who participated in these studies. In perceiving the offender with empathy, "one sees the other as having acted in a way human beings do, out of his or her own needs and perceptions; there may even be the recognition that what he or she did is something one has done or could well do" (Rowe et al., 1989, p. 242).

Curtis (1989) and Rowe et al. (1989) note that the participants in their studies experienced a change in their view of self, and of the offender, as they struggled to forgive. Similarly, the final stage in Truong's (1991) model is entitled Change and Growth, and is comparable to the idea of constructing a new narrative of self and others.

The retrospective and subjective nature of phenomenological studies is their major limitation, raising the question of how reliable such accounts are, especially if the forgiveness event took place some years previously. The other difficulty with the phenomenological studies reviewed here is that the investigators solicited participants who had successfully forgiven and wanted to describe that experience, guaranteeing a positive picture of forgiveness, which might lead to the mistaken conclusion that forgiveness is good for everyone in every instance. This is a significant shortcoming in light of Trainer's (1981) study, which demonstrates that people forgive for a variety of reasons (intrinsic, role-expected, and expedient), and that these different forms of forgiveness have different consequences in terms of the forgiving person's blaming behavior, feelings, and attitudes toward themselves and the offender, and their sense of control over self, other, and life events. McCullough et al. (1997) warn that forgiving could in fact be harmful in some instances (e.g., in forgiving an unrepentant abuser in order to stay in the relationship). What is needed is a set of complementary studies that investigate the phenomenology of people who have felt justified in withholding forgiveness. Such comparative data would help clarify the experiential differences between those who forgive and those who do not.

Empirical Evidence in Support of Models of Forgiveness

Despite a large body of anecdotal and case study reports, Mauger et al. (1992) and Hebl and Enright (1993) were unable to locate any *published* empirical research on forgiveness prior to the time of their publications. McCullough, Rachal, et al. (1997, p. 5) have concluded that the literature published about forgiveness has historically been "a literature of theories without data."

What we do have prior to 1993 is a set of unpublished doctoral dissertations containing reports of empirical studies that have attempted a taxonomy of types of forgiveness (Nelson, 1992; Trainer, 1981), examined the conditions under which forgiveness is most likely to take place (Droll, 1984), investigated the efficacy of promoting forgiveness in adolescents (Gassin, 1995), and developed a measure of forgiveness (Wade, 1989).

Research findings published since 1993 have begun to provide empirical evidence in support of specific theories and/or hypotheses about forgiveness. Such investigations draw attention to many of the salient features of forgiveness and contribute substantially to a comprehensive view of the overall process. One of the more robust findings has been that forgiveness can be promoted through psychoeducational interventions (Al-Mabuk et al., 1995; Hebl & Enright, 1993; McCullough & Worthington, 1995; Worthington, Sandage, & Berry, Chapter 11, this volume).

A shortcoming of most of these studies is that participants have been self-selected and are not usually from a clinical population. McCullough and Worthington (1995) point out that while the self-selection process may not differ from the self-selection that goes on in real life in regard to seeking professional counseling, we have no way of knowing whether the levels of commitment and motivation of participants in these studies are comparable to those of actual clients. This is particularly problematic when the intervention involves a single session or very brief set of sessions, as such conditions are not analogous to the potentially drawn out nature of typical psychotherapy aimed at promoting recovery. As a result, most empirical investigations of forgiveness to date are limited in their ability to improve our understanding of how forgiveness unfolds as a process of change within individual psychotherapy.

Freedman and Enright's (1996) report on forgiveness therapy carried out with incest survivors, and Coyle and Enright's (1997) report on forgiveness therapy carried out with men postabortion are notable exceptions. The purpose of the Freedman and Enright study was to investigate the effectiveness of an intervention program for incest survivors in which forgiveness was the end goal of treatment. Coyle and Enright investigated the psychological benefits of promoting forgiveness with a set of men who identified themselves as having been hurt by a partner's choice to terminate a pregnancy. The results of these studies provide initial support for the hypothesis that forgiveness has both short- and long-term psychological benefits.

BUILDING MODELS OF FORGIVENESS

McCullough and Worthington (1994) enumerate several approaches to generating models of forgiveness, one of which is to describe the tasks involved in the process. The interventions carried out by Freedman and Enright (1996) and Coyle and Enright (1997) are based on this approach to model building and make important contributions to our knowledge about the potential benefits of promoting forgiveness in individual psychotherapy.

Unfortunately, builders of forgiveness models have tended to skip over the step of validating their models and go straight to intervention efforts, without demonstrating empirically that forgiveness in fact unfolds in the hypothesized manner. Greenberg and Foerster (1996) suggest that one of the major problems with current clinical trials is that there is a hidden, intervening variable that is not accounted for: the change processes induced by the treatment. A therapist may deliver the treatment, but does it take? Does it set the anticipated change processes in motion? If a treatment group contains some clients who become engaged in the process, others who do so only intellectually, and still others who refuse, then a true test of the active ingredients of the treatment will not be obtained. As a consequence, it is not possible to determine what portion of the positive outcome is accounted for by the forgiveness process itself compared to the portion accounted for by other factors (such as the therapeutic relationship and a good working alliance) that are known to contribute to positive therapeutic outcomes (Horvath & Greenberg, 1989; Greenberg & Newman, 1996). If, in a specified treatment, however, those clients who go through the process of change in the anticipated manner are studied to see if they change more than those who do not engage in the process, the effects of the change processes are truly being tested. Then, we can assert with some confidence that we have measured the portion of positive outcome that is accounted for by the model under investigation.

A Rational–Empirical Approach to Building Models of Change

Greenberg and his colleagues (Greenberg, 1991; Greenberg & Foerster, 1996; Rice & Greenberg, 1984) point out that a combined rational–empirical methodology is helpful in building models of change in psychotherapy. The proposed task-analytic approach to the study of specific change processes is a research method that focuses on understanding complex, ongoing change processes and has been shown to aid in understanding how people change within therapy.

Task analysis involves a close scrutiny of in-session events that have been selected as representative of clients' efforts to resolve a specific class of problem. The investigator first describes the in-session performances that "mark" the presence of the problem, along with the therapist interventions thought to facilitate the resolution of the problem. Measures of the markers and therapist interventions are then constructed, after which a rationally derived set of possible problem-solving strategies are set forth, which help the researcher conceptualize ways in which the affective problem-solving task could be carried out. This is followed by the empirical task analysis of clients' actual in-therapy problem-solving efforts. A refined model of the strategies used to solve the problem is arrived at by successive rational and empirical analyses that build on one another. The end product is a detailed description of the specific processes and possible relations among processes. The resulting description sets the stage for studies that test the model by comparing successful and unsuccessful resolutions of the problem, relating specific types of task performances to therapeutic outcomes. An example of this approach to model building that is highly relevant to forgiveness follows.

The Resolution of Unfinished Business

Unfinished business can be defined as a currently felt, lingering, unresolved, negative feeling one person holds toward another (Greenberg, Rice, & Elliott, 1993; Perls, Hefferline, & Goodman, 1951). As a concept, it derives from Gestalt therapy (Perls et al., 1951) and represents the subset of client problems that have developed as a result of repeated frustrating or traumatic situations with a significant other (Greenberg et al., 1993). It is often manifested when clients are attempting to deal with past relationship difficulties involving experiences of separation, abandonment, trauma, and abuse (Greenberg & Foerster, 1996).

Greenberg and his colleagues have found the resolution of unfinished business to be a psychotherapeutic task that may include forgiveness in significant ways, in that unfinished business can be resolved in one of two ways: (1) via self-validation, self-assertion, and holding the significant other accountable; or (2) by gaining a new view of the other, understanding the other's position, and forgiving him or her (Greenberg & Foerster, 1996).

The research carried out by Greenberg and his colleagues has been done in the context of process–experiential psychotherapy, an approach that employs Gestalt interventions embedded in Rogerian client-centered conditions. Client-centered psychotherapy offers an emphasis on the therapist qualities (i.e., empathic attunement, nonpossessive warmth, and genuineness) that are necessary to the creation of a safe environment most likely to foster productive self-awareness and change in meaning construction (Greenberg et al., 1993). Gestalt therapy provides a set of interventions that aid in facilitating emotional arousal and deeper experiencing. Empty-chair dialogue is one of the interventions drawn from Gestalt therapy (Perls et al., 1951; elaborated by Greenberg et al., 1993), and it can be used to help the client confront the significant other in imagination, in order to find new ways to come to terms with the unresolved interpersonal situation.

Building a Model of the Resolution of Unfinished Business

Over the past 15 years, a task-analytic approach has been used to study the resolution of unfinished business within process–experiential psychotherapy. The research program began by constructing a simple rational model (Greenberg & Foerster, 1996; McMain, Goldman, & Greenberg, 1996). Therapy sessions containing resolutions of unfinished business were then inspected to determine how the actual performances fit, failed to fit, or otherwise enriched the rational model. At the same time, the following methods of measuring the different components were considered.

The Experiencing Scale (EXP) is a 7-point annotated and anchored rating scale developed by Klein, Mathieu, Kiesler, and Gendlin (1969). A comprehensive review of the scale's reliability and validity is provided by Klein, Matthieu-Coughlan, and Kiesler (1986). It has been widely used to evaluate the extent and quality of clients' explorations of their inner experience to achieve self-understanding and problem resolution. At lower levels of the scale, an individual gives no indication of his or her own inner processes. Moving up the scale, the individual's personal perspective becomes clearer until, at the highest levels, the individual is actively processing his or her experience in a goal-directed manner.

The Structural Analysis of Social Behavior Scale (SASB; Benjamin, 1974) is based on a circumplex model of interaction with affiliation and interdependence axes, and provides a way to evaluate moment-by-moment transactions in the psychotherapy process. The scale's psychometric properties are reviewed in Benjamin, Foster, Giat-Roberto, and Estroff (1986). The coding of interpersonal behavior involves classifying behavior according to the focus of the transaction (e.g., self or other) and the degree of affiliation and interdependence. Segments of therapy dialogue are broken into thought units (normally including a noun, a verb and an object) and assigned a code that describes the unit. For example, the statement "I forgive you" would be coded as "disclose and express" (SASB = 2-2). The SASB coding system was used to measure the changing quality of interactions between the client and imagined significant other in the empty-chair dialogue.

The Client's Emotional Arousal Scale (EAS; Daldrup, Beutler, Engle, & Greenberg, 1988) is used to rate the verbal and nonverbal expression of primary emotions. It has demonstrated reliability (Machado, Beutler, & Greenberg, 1999). At the lowest level, the individual's expression does not disclose any emotional arousal. Midway through the scale, the client expresses feelings at a moderate level of arousal. At the highest end of the scale, there is an intense state of arousal, such that the client is expressing his or her feelings freely with voice, words, and/or physical movement.

The Needs Scale (NEED; Foerster, 1990) was constructed specifically for the research being carried out by Greenberg and his colleagues, and is based on Murray's (1938) work. It has demonstrated reliability (Pedersen, 1996). The scale involves categorical judgments of the presence in the client's dialogue of specific types of interpersonal needs based on a set of semantic criteria. For example, the words "I want you to understand how much you hurt me" would be categorized as a need for validation.

Clinical judges were trained to use these scales reliably to evaluate portions of therapy sessions identified as critical to the process of resolving unfinished business. With these rating scales, the investigators were able to evaluate the therapy sessions using measures that are independent of the necessarily subjective judgments of the therapists and clients involved in the psychotherapeutic enterprise.

The next step was to construct performance diagrams of actual dialogues in order to refine the observations derived in the rational segment of the discovery phase. Client behaviors were diagrammed to depict the experiential and interactional states in the dialogue as measured by the aforementioned rating scales. This type of fine-grained process analysis revealed more closely what the process of change involved and how the different states could be measured.

After a number of cycles of observations and model building had been undertaken, a refined model was constructed that captured the essential components of the resolution process. Figure 9.1 represents that model.

The presence of important unfinished business is typically "marked" by the inhibited expression of a currently felt, lingering, negative feeling the client holds toward a significant other.

The process of resolution can be understood to unfold as follows: Given a marker of unfinished business, the client is asked to imagine the significant person in the empty chair and make contact in imagination. The client is then encouraged to express to the imagined other the emerging feelings he or she has just been describing to the therapist. As the client engages in the process, his or her first comments to the other tend to be expressed in the form of blaming the other for the client's problems, complaining about the other's behavior, or as a sense of hurt over injury done.

There is an assumption that the client's internal representation of self and other will emerge as he or she works back and forth between the chairs, so the next step is to direct the client to enact the other as he or she imagines the other to be (i.e., rejecting, hostile, critical, uncaring, etc.). The purpose of enacting the negatively construed other is to create a sense of lively contact between the client and imagined other. It also acts as a baseline against which any shifts in the client's representation of the significant other can be checked.

Successful, lively contact between the client and imagined other will evoke specific episodic memories that formed the context for the develop-

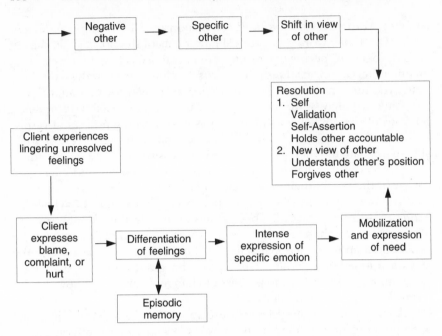

FIGURE 9.1. Refined model of the resolution of unfinished business. From Greenberg (1993). Copyright 1993 by The Guilford Press. Reprinted by permission.

ment of unfinished business. As the process unfolds, emotions are intensely aroused, and feelings are differentiated. The client shifts from a reactive, defensive stance, which is outwardly focused, to a more authentic, exploratory stance, focused on contacting and expressing core inner experience. This often comes about through the evocation and reenactment of a painful episodic memory of an earlier traumatic interpersonal event. It also often involves grieving the loss of what was missed from the other.

At this point, the wished-for aspects of the relationship are focused on in order to help the client identify his or her previously unmet interpersonal needs and express them to the imagined other. A sense of entitlement to those needs emerges as the client asserts his or her needs and examines present circumstances and personal resources in regard to the other. As the sense of entitlement and personal power emerges, the client is enabled to let go of earlier feelings of need deprivation.

Following the expression of intense emotion and unmet interpersonal needs, a schematic reorganization takes place, leading to a shift in the client's view of the significant other. In this part of the process, the client begins to view the other in a more complex, multifaceted way. The other may now be seen as separate, and as having both good and bad qualities. In effect, the client may begin to see the other from the other's point of view and as having had his or her own difficulties. This is marked by one of two outcomes. Either the client's attitude toward the other softens, and both the self and other are seen more positively (or, at least, less negatively) or, as often occurs in cases of abuse, the other is held accountable for his or her actions and is seen as deserving of the client's negative feelings. In the latter instance, the self is seen as empowered and worthwhile in relation to the other, and entitled to the negative feelings held toward the other. As the self is experienced as more powerful, the other is seen as less threatening.

When representations of both self and other undergo positive shifts, the split-off "good" aspects of the other are allowed to emerge and be experienced emotionally. The client develops a deeper understanding of the other and may forgive him or her. Instead of viewing the other from the perspective of injury, the client is able to view the other with compassion and empathy. In addition, the client typically feels a sense of resolution and completion with respect to the unfinished business with the other. This is often accompanied by a sense of optimism about the future.

The model described here, and in Figure 9.1, represents an empirically grounded discovery that forgiveness is a central ingredient in some forms of resolution of unfinished business. It also suggests a number of processes critical to therapeutic change and can be used to investigate the relationships between process and outcome (Greenberg, 1991; Greenberg & Newman, 1996).

Two studies (Foerster, 1990; Pedersen, 1996) have demonstrated that four components of the model (intense expression of emotion, expression of need, shift in view of the other, and resolution) are significantly more likely to occur in events that clients and therapists report having been resolved, than in those reported unresolved. The components of blame/complaint/hurt and enactment of negative other do not discriminate between the two kinds of events, as these elements are usually present at the beginning of all empty-chair dialogues.

Using data from a study of the effects of empty-chair dialogue on unfinished business (Paivio & Greenberg, 1995), Malcolm (1999) carried out a detailed study of the components of resolution in an effort to relate process to outcome. Audio- and videotapes of therapy sessions for 32 clients were reviewed and, for each client, segments of empty-chair dialogue thought to be the best representative of each component of the model were transcribed and submitted to clinical judges, trained to make process ratings using the rating scales previously described. These process ratings were the method used to establish the presence or absence of the components of resolution. Thirteen clients were judged to have resolved their unfinished business according to the model, and were compared to 13 clients randomly selected from the remaining pool of unresolved clients. An analysis of covariance (using the pretherapy scores as covariates of the posttherapy outcome scores) showed significant differences at termination between the resolved and unresolved groups on a number of outcome measures. These findings lend support to the hypothesis that the model of resolution of unfinished business developed and tested by Greenberg and his colleagues relates to significant improvements in psychological well-being.

Applying the Task-Analytic Process to the Study of Forgiveness

Given the discovery that the resolution of unfinished business may involve understanding and forgiving the significant other, we propose that it would be profitable to build a task-analytic model of the forgiveness process itself. We conclude this chapter with a report of the initial steps of a rational–empirical task analysis of the forgiveness process.

Our current rational model of the therapeutic steps a client will go through to forgive a significant other for a deep interpersonal hurt is outlined in Figure 9.2. The model is based on the literature and our clinical understanding of the process.

It is important to note that progress through this process is not neces-

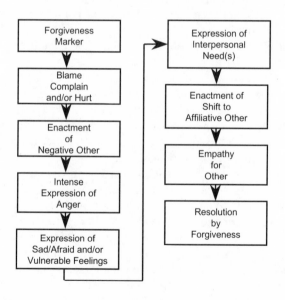

FIGURE 9.2. Initial model of the forgiveness process.

sarily linear. Rather, client and therapist are apt to revisit different aspects of the process, encountering and working on different seminal episodic memories and critical unmet needs over the course of therapy, with the result that therapist and client may loop back through parts of the model more than once. Rather than being a psychoeducational tool presented to clients as a way of understanding and thinking about forgiveness, the model is most helpful when used by the therapist as an empirically grounded map of the process of forgiveness. As such, it serves to guide the therapist to where the client is in the process of forgiving another, and it reveals how the therapist might facilitate the next processing moments (Greenberg et al., 1993).

We hypothesized that the in-session performance of a client who wishes to forgive would be marked by statements that share all the features of a marker of unfinished business (i.e., a lingering negative feeling toward a significant other) and also specifically indicate either a desire to forgive or that the inability to forgive is perceived as problematic by the client. Engaging in marker-guided therapy involves identifying such markers for intervention and allows the practitioner to facilitate forgiveness when a client indicates that this is his or her personal desire. The therapist refrains from efforts to promote forgiveness when a forgiveness marker does not appear, thereby avoiding the problem of promoting forgiveness when the client has not identified it as a desirable goal.

We expect the dialogues of clients who successfully forgive initially to contain intense expressions of anger against the offender. In addition, given the harm done to a meaningful relationship with a significant other, we expect these clients to move from intense expressions of anger to intense expressions of sadness, fear, and/or vulnerability, possibly including expressions of grief over the loss if the rupture to the relationship has been that severe.

An expression of interpersonal need(s) is expected to follow the acknowledgment and expression of these two types of strong emotion: anger directed toward the other and vulnerability in reference to the self. In successful events, a specific type of shift in view of the other is also expected. This shift should be characterized by an enactment of the other as having "softened" his or her stance and become more affiliative in response to the intense expressions of sadness, fear, and/or vulnerability on the part of the client. The change in the way the client sees the other should then lead to empathy for the offender. We predict that the process will conclude with the client expressing a new narrative of self and other, characterized by in-session performances that convey understanding and forgiveness of the other.

Having formulated this preliminary model, we moved to a consideration of the process ratings that would differentiate one component from another. Table 9.1 summarizes the expected process ratings. As in

192 APPLICATIONS IN COUNSELING, PSYCHOTHERAPY, AND HEALTH

TABLE 9.1. Summary of Expected Process Ratings

Components	Scales used	Expected process ratings
Forgiveness marker		To be rated as present
Blame, complaint, and/or hurt	EXP	Peak of 3 or less
	SASB	1-6, 2-2, and/or 2-6
	CVQ	External or limited
	EAS	Peak of 4 or less
Negative other	EXP	Peak of 3 or less
	SASB	1-5, 1-6, 1-7, 1-8, 2-5, 2-6, 2-7, and/or 2-8
	CVQ	External or limited
Intense expression of anger	EXP	Peak of 4 or more
	SASB	1-7, 2-1, 2-2, 2-7
	CVQ	Emotional or focused
	EAS	Peak of 5 or more
Intense expression of sad/afraid and/ or vulnerable feelings	EXP	Peak of 4 or more
	SASB	2-2
	CVQ	Emotional or focused
	EAS	Peak of 5 or more
Expression of interpersonal need(s)	EXP	Peak of 4 or more
	SASB	2-1 and/or 2-2
	CVQ	Emotional or focused
	NEED	Judged present; categorized by type
Shift in view of other	EXP	Peak of 4 or more
	SASB	1-2, 1-3, 1-4, and/or 2-2
	CVQ	Emotional or focused
Empathy	EXP	Peak of 4 or more
	SASB	1-1, and/or 1-2
	CVQ	Focused
	TES	5 or more
Resolution	EXP	Peak of 6
	SASB	1-2, 2-2, and/or 1-3
	CVQ	Focused

Note. EXP refers to the Experiencing Scale, on which 3 = reaction to external events; 4 = an inward focus; and 6 = synthesis leading to personally meaningful structures or resolution of issues. SASB refers to the Structural Analysis of Social Behavior Codes, on which 1-1 = freeing; 1-2 = affirm and understand; 1-3 = loving; 1-4 = trust; 1-5 = control; 1-6 = blame; 1-7 = attack; 1-8 = ignore; 2-1 = assert; 2-2 = disclose; 2-5 = submit; 2-6 = sulk; 2-7 = recoil; and 2-8 = wall off. CVQ refers to the Client Vocal Quality Scale, on which External = an outer-directed, lecturing voice; Limited = a tense, wary, low-energy voice; Focused = an inner-directed, exploratory voice; and Emotional = a voice that breaks from its normal platform in expressing emotion. EAS refers to the Emotional Arousal Scale, on which 3 = a low level of emotional arousal; and 4 = a moderate level of arousal. TES refers to the Truax Empathy Scale, on which 5 = an understanding of all the more readily discernible feelings, and many of the less evident ones.

earlier research, we used the following scales: EXP (Klein et al., 1969), SASB (Benjamin, 1974), EAS (Daldrup et al., 1988), and NEED (Foerster, 1990).

The Client Vocal Quality Scale (CVQ; Rice & Kerr, 1986) and Truax Empathy Scale (TES; Kiesler, 1973) were also used. The CVQ is a reliable classification system developed by Rice and Kerr to provide a way of assessing the quality of a client's involvement in the moment-by-moment therapy process. Client expressions can be classified as one of four types: (1) focused, an inner-directed exploratory voice; (2) emotional, a voice that breaks from its natural platform in expressing emotion; (3) external, an outer-directed lecturing voice; or (4) limited, a tense, wary, low-energy voice.

The TES (Kiesler, 1973) is a 9-point anchored and annotated scale used to rate one individual's understanding of another's internal experience and feelings. It has shown interrater reliability and predictive validity in client-centered therapy (cf. Kiesler, 1973) and was modified to fit empty-chair dialogue. The scale's range extends from a virtual lack of empathic understanding of the other person's feelings, to accurately understanding the other person's more readily discernible feelings, to an accurate understanding of the other's full range of expressed and implicit feelings.

Taking the component of sad/afraid and/or vulnerable feelings as an example, we expect intense sadness to be expressed with an inward focus, or as a proposition about the self (EXP = 4–5); in an inner-directed exploratory voice, or a voice that breaks from its normal platform in expressing emotion (CVQ = Fo or Em); at a moderate to very high level of emotional arousal (EAS = 5–7). In addition, we expect over 50% of the units of expression in such a component to be categorized on the SASB as statements that "disclose and express" (SASB = 2-2).

With our hypothesized model and ratings in hand, from a set of clients who successfully resolved their unfinished business (Malcolm, 1999), we identified one client who chose to forgive and another who resolved without forgiving. The forgiving client came into therapy with unfinished business around her mother's abandonment of the family by suicide when the client was a child. The other client had unresolved issues with a teacher who seduced and sexually abused him when he was a child. These two cases are different in a number of critical ways (particularly in terms of gender, relationship of offender to client, and type of offense). Nonetheless, they successfully demonstrate the kinds of similarities and differences we can expect to find in comparing the two types of resolution.

Table 9.2 contains brief excerpts from the therapy dialogues of these two clients that represent (or fail to represent) the critical components of the hypothesized forgiveness process. It also contains the process ratings assigned to each component.

TABLE 9.2. Comparing Resolutions with and without Forgiveness

Components and scales	Understanding and forgiving the other	Holding the other accountable without forgiveness
Forgiveness marker	*Original marker* [referring to mother's suicide] I should be able to just get on with it. . . . It's water under the bridge. Just forget it and get on with it. . . . But it's not easy to forget it. I *can't* forget it. *Forgiveness marker* As self: I've been thinking about this in the last couple of weeks and, when we ended the last time I said that I would like to forgive you and . . . I still can't bring myself to forgive you.	*Original marker* I was a very different person [before the sexual abuse]. . . . There were negative changes in me regarding trusting other people; [I was] open and invited people into my life before. . . . Later I was closed off and wanted to distance myself from others. . . . I like the person I was before more than I like the person I am now. I think I would enjoy being that person . . . but there are things I have to work through to get to that person. *Forgiveness marker* Not found
Blame/ complaint/ hurt	As self: You broke up our family; we've had so many problems that really didn't need to be there if you had dealt with whatever your problems were at the time. Whatever drove you to commit this atrocity? I just don't know what was that bad . . .	As self: You don't feel anything at a deep level for me. You feel things for yourself. . . . You have little or no regret, except for the fact that this has trashed your career in some ways . . . and has raised the ire of other people in your [work organization] . . .
EXP SASB CVQ EAS	(3) Reaction to events (1–6) Blame and belittle (Ex) External voice (4) Moderate arousal	(3) Reaction to events (1–6) Blame and belittle (Ex) External voice (2) No overt arousal
Enactment of negative other	As mother: You know how difficult it was for me when I grew up . . . and I always carried around this incredible resentment. . . . And your father, well . . . it was all his fault. He would get drunk and we would come home and get into an argument and he would slap me around, and I just couldn't live with him anymore . . .	As perpetrator: Oh, I really feel bad about this, but . . . what can I do now? Uh, I was confused then but I've really changed my ways and I'd really like to make this up to you. Uh, is there anything I can do for you or your family? Uh, I mean what do you want from me *now*? What do you want me to do?
EXP SASB CVQ	(3) Reaction to events (2–6) Sulk and appease (Ex) External voice	(3) Reaction to events (2–5) Submit and defer (Ex) External voice

(continued)

TABLE 9.2. (*continued*)

Components and scales	Understanding and forgiving the other	Holding the other accountable without forgiveness
Intense expression of anger toward the other	As self: I've got a lot of resentment and . . . I know the resentment is hurting me, because you don't care. I mean how dare you take these things away? How dare you! . . . [Therapist: What would you like to do?] What I would like to do is just wring your god-damn neck. . . . I swear to god, it's so unfair. I would like to physically lash out at you and I'm not even a physical person. . . . I'm really angry at you and I'm angry at the things that you've left me with.	As self: You physically lorded it over me for [a long time]. Now I get a chance to do it back . . . [an aside to therapist: but I'll probably feel like shit afterwards, because then it'll be me being the abuser. But . . . You know, deep down, to be honest, I'd still like to do that . . . Definitely] [Therapist: Right. So describe it.] Knocking you down. Stomping on you. Keeping you down . . . pushing your face in dog piss. . . . And of course, the final act of kicking you right in the groin.
EXP SASB CVQ EAS	(4) Inward focus (2–2) Disclose and express (1–7) Attack and reject (2–7) Protest and withdraw (Em) Emotional voice (6) High emotional arousal	(4) Inward focus (1–7) Attack and reject (Fo) Focused voice (6) High emotional arousal
Intense expression of sad/afraid and/or vulnerable feelings	As self: I've missed having you all of my life. . . . It's very difficult for me to describe how much I miss you. The sense of loss inside is . . . [Therapist: This is incredibly painful—the loss. Yes. Tell her about your tears.] I cry very often for no apparent reason. . . . I cry and I'm very emotional even at happy times . . . I cry because I miss you . . .	None found
EXP SASB CVQ EAS	(5) Proposition about self (2–2) Disclose and express (Em) Emotional voice (6) High emotional arousal	
Expression of interpersonal need(s)	As self: I've needed you very much. I would have liked to have had your approval. Your saying, "That's good," "That's bad," "That's indifferent." Even if I'd fought with you. I feel like I missed so much. . . . And the thought that I'll never be able to speak to you, never be able to tell you any of this, just tears me apart.	As self: I would demand that [you] never molest children again. I would demand that you stay out of my life.

(*continued*)

TABLE 9.2. (*continued*)

Components and scales	Understanding and forgiving the other	Holding the other accountable without forgiveness
EXP	(4) Inward focus	(4) Inward focus
SASB	(2-2) Disclose and express	(2-1) Assert and separate
CVQ	(Em) Emotional voice	(Fo) Focused
NEED	Need for affiliation	Need for inviolacy
Enactment of shift in view of the other	*To more affiliative*	*To less dominant*
	As mother: I wish there was something that I could do to change what I did. You're making me understand the devastation that I caused and the aftermath. It wasn't just about me, it was about a lot of other people. I really wish that you could forgive me. I know that you've struggled. . . . I need you to forgive me because . . . I realize this has burdened you all of your life. By forgiving me you will release yourself from the pain . . .	As perpetrator: I feel remorse. I feel like I wasted a lot of my [career] years—not just wasted, ruined that. . . . It has been ruined by the way I have behaved. . . . Yes, I coerced children but that was just a sexual release. It wasn't what I was looking for ultimately. I never found what I was really looking for.
EXP	(4) Inward focus	(4) Inward focus
SASB	(2-2) Disclose and express	(2-2) Disclose and express
	(1-2) Affirm and understand	
	(1-4) Trust and rely	
CVQ	(Em) Emotional voice	(Li) Limited voice
Empathy for the other	As Mother: I want you to think of me as someone who wasn't well. . . . I felt I had no place to turn. I was full of despair. . . . I cared about you children more than anything in the whole world. . . . My suicide wasn't about you kids at all. You're the reason I stayed as long as I did. . . . It was about a life that I just thought was hopeless. . . . You have every right to feel ashamed of what I did. And I don't want you to feel guilty. You didn't cause it. . . . It's not about you. It's about my life. It's about me being out of control. I take responsibility for what I did. . . . I was out of control.	As self: Yeah, well, sure, in some ways you felt this way—you felt compelled this way—but in another way, you made choices . . . about me that were coercive and manipulative and abusive, and what do you expect when you make those kinds of choices? That your life is going to be fulfilled? I don't think so. I think you got what you deserve, and . . . I feel great inside that [you feel] like crap. . . . I'm happy that you have this empty unfulfilled life because I don't think you deserve a happy fulfilled life given your behavior . . .
EXP	(4) Inward focus	(3) Reaction to events
SASB	(2-2) Disclose and express	(1-6) Blame and belittle
	(1-2) Affirm and understand	
	(2-3) Approach and enjoy	

(*continued*)

TABLE 9.2. (*continued*)

Components and scales	Understanding and forgiving the other	Holding the other accountable without forgiveness
CVQ	(Fo) Focused voice	(Ex) External voice
TES	(7) Accurate understanding of other	(2) Little understanding of other
Resolution	*By understanding and forgiving* As self: Mom, I'm going to try to work on positive images of you and positive images when I was a child. And I will try not to . . . focus on your leaving as being the turning point of everything. . . . I think I'm really starting to forgive you Mom. I'm really starting to feel okay about that inside. . . . I'm not in control of it and I can't be responsible for it. It's what you did for your own reasons. I'm trying to understand these reasons.	*By holding other accountable without forgiveness* As self: Look at the difference between us now. The tables have completely turned. . . . Your authority was a kind of sham; it was a facade. It was because of a role that you had taken on that you didn't deserve in any real way. My authority comes from myself, and everything I am I have earned and I deserve. . . . Yeah, I feel good with who I am and that I exposed you for the fraud that you are.
EXP	(6) Synthesis leading to resolution	(6) Synthesis leading to resolution
SASB	(1–2) Affirm and understand (2–2) Disclose and express	(2–1) Assert and separate
CVQ	(Fo) Focused voice	(Fo) Focused voice

The components and process ratings summarized in this table were inspected to determine (1) whether an actual forgiveness process resembles the hypothesized model, and (2) whether there are any noteworthy differences in content and process ratings between the two types of resolution.

An examination of the forgiving client's dialogue shows that the process she went through fits reasonably well with the model diagrammed in Figure 9.2. The process ratings assigned were also much as we expected. For example, as predicted, her sadness and vulnerability are expressed to the imagined other in the empty chair as a proposition about the self (EXP = 5), at a high level of emotional arousal (EAS = 6), and in a voice that breaks from its normal platform in expressing emotion (CVQ = Em). Most of the client's words are characterized as statements that "disclose and express" (SASB = 2-2).

Nonetheless, there were a few interesting discoveries. First of all, we had not anticipated that a desire to forgive might not be part of the original marker of unfinished business. In this client's case, the actual forgiveness marker came relatively late in therapy (during the ninth of 12 sessions), with the rest of the process unfolding fairly rapidly thereafter. Further investigation will be needed to determine whether this is unique to this particular client or apt to be true of most forgiveness events.

The second unanticipated finding was that the empathy component was enacted from the empty chair, while the client was enacting the imagined other. The client literally put herself in the mother's place and "saw" the relationship from the offender's point of view. Since it makes sense that the empathy component could be expressed from either chair, we will need to adjust the rating criteria on the SASB to reflect this possibility (i.e., add codes 2-2 = disclose and express, 2-3 = approach and enjoy, and 2-4 = trust and rely).

The third discovery also came out of an examination of the empathy component. We were intrigued by the presence of statements from the other chair indicating that the offender was imagined as taking responsibility for the offense and explicitly freeing the client from guilt and blame. Enacting the mother, the client says: "You have every right to feel ashamed of what I did. And I don't want you to feel guilty. You didn't cause it. . . . This is not about you. It's about my life. It's about me being out of control. I take responsibility for what I did. . . . I was out of control." Given that victims often question their own role in the events surrounding a deep hurt, we are left to consider the possibility that this taking of responsibility from the other chair and absolving the self of responsibility for the offense might be another necessary step in the forgiveness process. Should it be found that most successful forgiveness processes include this step, future refinements of the model will need to include a component of "taking responsibility" on the part of the imagined significant other.

An inspection of the empty-chair dialogues of the client who did not forgive showed no evidence that the client ever considered forgiving the man who had sexually abused him. It is interesting to note that when forgiveness is not offered, anger is not followed by an expression of sadness, fear, or vulnerability (which are highly attachment-related emotions that indicate an action tendency toward comfort and/or moving closer). In addition, we found that the shift in view of the other in this dialogue was to a less dominant rather than more affiliative other, with no evidence of softening toward, or empathy for, the perpetrator. The resolution components of the two dialogues also show marked differences: The client who did not forgive described himself, not as understanding the other or seeing the past situation in a new way, but as stronger in relation to the other, and as experiencing satisfaction with how he now saw himself. Resolution here comes about by dismissing the other as a source of threat and harm, and by focusing on the self in terms of self-strengthening and self-affirmation.

These differences show up in the process ratings assigned and summarized in Table 9.2. For example, there are important differences between clients in the empathy component, with the dialogue of the client who did not forgive failing to meet criteria on all four process measures. Clearly, this component is highly salient in discriminating between the two types of resolution.

These differences in content, and their attendant ratings, lend initial support to the hypothesis that there are two distinct paths possible within the resolution of unfinished business model, one that leads to a focus on understanding and forgiving the other, and another that focuses on self-strengthening and self-affirmation. This first task-analytic inspection of forgiveness is encouraging, but it will have to be followed up with further investigations of additional resolution events. Each successful replication of findings will allow us to refine the model and increase our confidence in it as a map of the way forgiveness unfolds in the therapy process.

As successive comparisons are made and evidence accumulates in support of the proposed psychotherapeutic model, we will be able to proceed to an investigation of the relationship between process and outcome. Such studies will allow us to investigate differences in outcome between those who resolve their unfinished business by forgiving their significant other and those who resolve without forgiving. We may find that clients who forgive in certain contexts for specific types of transgression enjoy increases in psychological well-being significantly different from the improvements experienced by clients who resolve their unfinished business without forgiveness.

CONCLUSION

The relative merits of forgiveness have been debated in the philosophical and religious literature for decades. In contrast, until the early 1990s, the concept of forgiveness was essentially overlooked within the field of psychology. This is an especially peculiar oversight within the field of psychotherapy research, since it is not at all uncommon for clients to struggle with the dilemma of whether to forgive in the face of deep personal hurt.

Earlier in the chapter, we noted that there have been three different approaches to the recent study of forgiveness as a process of change: case study reports, phenomenological investigations, and outcome studies. Each approach has made significant contributions to our knowledge, and they all add credibility to the hypothesis that facilitating forgiveness can be an effective way of helping people recover from the effects of deep personal hurt.

We are now at the stage where we can articulate some of the critical components of the process. Fine grained process–outcome research programs such as the one described in this chapter are now needed to move the field forward and help forgiveness gain a legitimate place in the field of research based scientific knowledge. Without this kind of research, we will be hampered in our efforts to identify (1) when it is appropriate to facilitate forgiveness in psychotherapy; (2) what the key therapeutic tasks of forgiveness are; and (3) whether it is the process of forgiveness itself, as opposed to the benefits of satisfactory psychotherapy in general, that accounts for the improvements in psychological well being that have been documented in the forgiveness literature to date.

REFERENCES

Al-Mabuk, R. H., Enright, R. D., & Cardis, P. A. (1995). Forgiveness education with parentally love-deprived late adolescents. *Journal of Moral Education, 24*(4), 427–444.

Bass, E., & Davis, L. (1988). *The courage to heal: A guide for women survivors of child sexual abuse.* New York: Harper & Row.

Benjamin, L. S. (1974). Structural analysis of social behavior. *Psychological Review, 81,* 392–425.

Benjamin, L. S., Foster, S. W., Giat-Roberto, L., & Estroff, S. (1986). Coding videotapes of family interactions by structural analysis of social behavior (SASB). In L. S. Greenberg & W. Pinsoff (Eds.), *The psychotherapeutic process: A research handbook.* New York: Guilford Press.

Brandsma, J. M. (1982). Forgiveness: A dynamic theological and therapeutic analysis. *Pastoral Psychology, 31,* 40–50.

Coyle, C. T., & Enright, R. D. (1997). Forgiveness intervention with postabortion men. *Journal of Consulting and Clinical Psychology, 65,* 1042–1046.

Cunningham, B. B. (1985). The will to forgive: A pastoral theological view of forgiving. *Journal of Pastoral Care, 39,* 141–149.

Curtis, N. C. (1989). *The structure and dynamics of forgiving another.* Unpublished doctoral dissertation, U.S. International University, San Diego, CA.

Daldrup, R. J., Beutler, L. E., Engle, D., & Greenberg, L. S. (1988). *Focused expressive psychotherapy: Freeing the overcontrolled patient.* New York: Guilford Press.

Davenport, D. (1991). The functions of anger and forgiveness: Guidelines for psychotherapy with victims. *Psychotherapy, 28*(1), 140–144.

Droll, D. M. (1984). *Forgiveness: Theory and research.* Unpublished doctoral dissertation, University of Nevada, Reno.

Fitzgibbons, R. P. (1986). The cognitive and emotive uses of forgiveness in the treatment of anger. *Psychotherapy, 23*(4), 629–633.

Foerster, F. S. (1990). *Refinement and verification of a model of the resolution of unfinished business.* Unpublished master's thesis, York University, Toronto, Canada.

Freedman, S. R., & Enright, R. D. (1996). Forgiveness as an intervention goal with incest survivors. *Journal of Consulting and Clinical Psychology, 64*(5), 983–992.

Frijda, N. (1986). *The emotions.* New York: Cambridge University Press.

Gassin, E. A. (1995). *Social cognition and forgiveness in adolescent romance: An intervention study.* Unpublished doctoral dissertation, University of Wisconsin–Madison, Madison.

Greenberg, L. S. (1991). Research on the process of change. *Psychotherapy Research, 1,* 14–24.

Greenberg, L. S., & Foerster, F. S. (1996). Task analysis exemplified: The process of resolving unfinished business. *Journal of Consulting and Clinical Psychology, 64,* 439–446.

Greenberg, L. S., & Newman, F. L. (1996). An approach to psychotherapy change process research: Introduction to the special section. *Journal of Consulting and Clinical Psychology, 64*(3), 235–238.

Greenberg, L. S., & Paivio, S. C. (1997). *Working with emotions in psychotherapy*. New York: Guilford Press.

Greenberg, L. S., Rice, L. N., & Elliott, R. (1993). *Facilitating emotional change: The moment by moment process*. New York: Guilford Press.

Haber, J. G. (1991). *Forgiveness*. Savage, MD: Rowman & Littlefield Publishers.

Hebl, J. H., & Enright, R. D. (1993). Forgiveness as a psychotherapeutic goal with elderly females. *Psychotherapy, 30*(4), 658–667.

Hope, D. (1987). The healing paradox of forgiveness. *Psychotherapy, 24*(2), 240–244.

Horvath, A., & Greenberg, L. S. (1989). Development and validation of the Working Alliance Inventory. *Journal of Counselling Psychology, 36*, 223–233.

Human Development Study Group. (1991). Five points on the construct of forgiveness within psychotherapy. *Psychotherapy, 28*(3), 493–496.

Kiesler, D. (1973). *The process of psychotherapy: Empirical foundations and systems of analysis*. Chicago: Aldine.

Klein, M., Mathieu, P., Kiesler, D., & Gendlin, E. (1969). *The Experiencing Scale*. Madison: Wisconsin Psychiatric Institute.

Klein, M., Mathieu-Coughlan, P., & Keisler, D. (1986). The experiencing scale. In L. S. Greenberg & W. Pinsof (Eds.), *The psychotherapeutic process: A research handbook*. New York: Guilford Press.

Lazarus, R. S. (1991). *Emotion and adaptation*. New York: Oxford University Press.

Machado, P. P., Beutler, L. E., & Greenberg, L. S. (1999). Emotion recognition in psychotherapy: Impact of therapist level of experience and emotional awareness. *Journal of Clinical Psychology, 55*(1), 39–57.

Malcolm, W. M. (1999). *Relating process to outcome in the process-experiential resolution of unfinished business*. Unpublished doctoral dissertation, York University, Toronto, Canada.

Mauger, P. A., Escano Perry, J., Freeman, T., Grove, D. C., McBride, A. G., & McKinney, K. E. (1992). The measurement of forgiveness: Preliminary research. *Journal of Psychology and Christianity, 11*(2), 170–180.

McCullough, M. E. (1997). Marital forgiveness. *Marriage and Family: A Christian Journal, 1*(1), 77–93.

McCullough, M. E., Rachal, K. C., Sandage, S. J., & Worthington, E. L. (1997, August). *A sustainable future for the psychology of forgiveness*. Paper presented at the American Psychological Association, Chicago, Illinois.

McCullough, M. E., & Worthington, E. (1994). Models of interpersonal forgiveness and their applications to counseling: Review and critique. *Counseling and Values, 39*, 2–14.

McCullough, M. E., & Worthington, E. (1995). Promoting forgiveness: A comparison of two brief psychoeducation group interventions with a waiting-list control. *Counseling and Values, 40*, 55–68.

McCullough, M. E., Worthington, E., & Rachal, K. C. (1997). Interpersonal forgiving in close relationships. *Journal of Personality and Social Psychology, 73*(2), 321–336.

McMain, S., Goldman, R., & Greenberg, L. (1996). Resolving unfinished business: A program of study. In W. Dryden (Ed.), *Research in counselling and psychotherapy: Practical applications*. London: Sage.

Murray, H. A. (1938). *Explorations in personality*. New York: Oxford University Press.

Nelson, M. K. (1992). *A new theory of forgiveness*. Unpublished doctoral dissertation, Purdue University, West Lafayette, IN.

Paivio, S. C., & Greenberg, L. S. (1995). Resolving unfinished business: Experiential therapy using empty chair dialogue. *Journal of Consulting and Clinical Psychology, 3*, 419–425.

Pedersen, R. (1996). *Verification of a model of the resolution of unfinished business*. Unpublished master's thesis, York University, Toronto, Canada.

Perls, F., Hefferline, R., & Goodman, P. (1951). *Gestalt therapy*. New York: Delta.

Rice, L. N., & Greenberg, L. S. (1984). *Patterns of change: Intensive analysis of psychotherapy process*. New York: Guilford Press.

Rice, L., & Kerr, G. (1986). Measures of client and therapist vocal quality. In L. S. Greenberg & W. Pinsof (Eds.), *The psychotherapeutic process: A research handbook*. New York: Guilford Press.

Rowe, J. O., Halling, S., Davies, E., Leifer, M., Powers, D., & Van Bronkhorst, J. (1989). The psychology of forgiving another: A dialogal research approach. In R. S. Valle & Steen Halling (Eds.), *Existential–phenomenological perspectives in psychology: Exploring the breadth of human experience*. New York: Plenum Press.

Trainer, M. (1981). *Forgiveness: Intrinsic, role-expected, expedient, in the context of divorce*. Unpublished doctoral dissertation, Boston University, Boston, MA.

Truong, K. T. (1991). *Human forgiveness: A phenomenological study about the process of forgiveness*. Unpublished doctoral dissertation, U. S. International University, San Diego, CA.

Wade, S. H. (1989). *The development of a scale to measure forgiveness*. Unpublished dissertation, Fuller Theological Seminary, Pasadena, CA.

Worthington, E. L., Sandage, S. J., & Berry, J. W. (1999). Group interventions to promote forgiveness: What researchers and clinicians ought to know. In M. McCullough, K. Pargament, & C. Thoresen (Eds.), *Frontiers of forgiveness*. New York: Guilford Press.

The Use of Forgiveness in Marital Therapy

Kristina Coop Gordon, Donald H. Baucom, and Douglas K. Snyder

Most persons, professionals and laypersons alike, would agree that maintaining an intimate, satisfying marriage over many decades is a significant challenge, regardless of the two people involved in the marriage. A large body of empirical findings suggests that marital adjustment is particularly sensitive to the ways that couples deal with negative events (cf. Baucom & Epstein, 1990); that is, whereas gratifying relationships likely involve a wide range of positive and mutually gratifying interactions, marital distress largely involves a significant number of negative experiences that the couple does not handle satisfactorily. These experiences can range from negative communication and interaction sequences to difficulty dealing with money, to disputes regarding in-laws, and so forth. In order to understand how couples maintain quality relationships over time, it is essential to understand how they deal with negative experiences, some of which are inevitable, and some of which are created or perpetuated by the partners themselves.

Nearly all major psychological theories of marriage (e.g., cognitive-behavioral, insight-oriented, systems, emotion-focused) devote considerable discussion to the role of negative events in marriage. At the same time, there is less understanding regarding the different types of negative events that couples encounter and how these events might call for different strategies to successfully navigate their deleterious impact. For example, a wife might find her husband's loud gum chewing annoying and, thus, be uncomfortable sitting close to him. Another wife might feel humiliated when she finds out that her husband has discussed their sexual difficulties with his parents. Serious transgressions such as the latter example given here, may require engaging in a forgiveness process, whereas minor annoyances might call for different coping strategies.

In essence, major theories of marriage have dealt extensively with the role of negative events in marriage, but overall, these same theories have largely neglected the concept of forgiveness. On the other hand, there is a growing literature reflecting theory and research on forgiveness. However, there are three significant problems in the current forgiveness literature. First, these views of forgiveness generally have not been integrated into broader theories of marriage. In addition, each theory presents a different model of how forgiveness occurs; there does not appear to be a consensus as to the critical elements in the forgiveness process. Finally, although some theories describe the behaviors that occur during the forgiveness process, few have attempted to explain why these behaviors occur. In this chapter, we attempt to (1) distill what appear to be the critical elements of forgiveness across major forgiveness theories, (2) integrate these elements within two broad theories of marriage, and (3) provide a conceptual framework for the forgiveness process that not only explains what occurs in the process, but also why it needs to occur. In addition, we describe our recent empirical findings regarding a three-stage model of forgiveness that results from this integration. Finally, we propose a new intervention program to assist couples who are struggling with a relationship trauma.

MAJOR THEORIES OF RELATIONSHIP FUNCTIONING

Two major psychological theories for understanding both individual and couple functioning are cognitive-behavioral and insight-oriented approaches. Although these two approaches often have been pitted against each other in terms of their understanding of human behavior, we believe that they both have a great deal to offer in understanding relationship functioning and, when integrated, can provide a meaningful context for understanding and promoting forgiveness within marriage. Furthermore, a recent article in the *Journal of Consulting and Clinical Psychology* indicates that both theories are considered empirically valid approaches to marital dysfunction (e.g., Baucom, Shoham, Mueser, Daiuto, & Stickle, 1998). In order to understand how these theories can assist in understanding forgiveness, it is important first to provide a brief overview of each theory of relationship functioning and describe how each theoretical approach has addressed the issue of negative marital events.

Cognitive-Behavioral Approaches to Marriage

Basic Principles

Cognitive-behavioral approaches to understanding marriage have emphasized the specific behaviors, cognitions, and emotions that contribute to gratifying interpersonal relationships. As such, cognitive-behavioral formulations generally have focused on the here and now and have explored how couples interact with each other in constructive and destructive ways that can affect their relationship quality. Initial cognitive-behavioral formulations were based on the premise that behavior, cognitions, and emotions are integrally related, and that how couples think and feel toward each other largely flow from their behavioral interaction patterns. This perspective ushered in a wave of empirical investigations exploring how couples behave toward each other. The results of these investigations confirmed that the frequency of both positive and negative behaviors is central in understanding relationship adjustment (see Baucom & Epstein, 1990, for a review). However, subsequent research showed that the same behavior could have different impacts on a couple depending on the way that the behavior was interpreted. Thus, if a husband spent a large number of hours at work, his wife might view this as positive if she interpreted it as an indication of his commitment to her and the children's economic well-being. The same behavior might have a negative impact if she were to view it as a statement of his desire to avoid spending time with her. As a result, the initial behavioral model of marriage was significantly expanded to a cognitive-behavioral model that incorporates how spouses think about and interpret each other's behavior as important factors in understanding marriage.

In order to clarify whether a spouse was likely to experience a given behavior or event as positive or negative, Baucom, Epstein, Sayers, and Sher (1989) proposed a typology of cognitions in marriage: (1) selective attention, (2) attributions, (3) expectancies, (4) assumptions, and (5) standards. Selective attention involves a cognitive–perceptual process in which an individual attends to some events and ignores others. For example, if a wife compliments her husband on his increased efforts to spend time with the children but he is absorbed in his thoughts and does not process her comments, her compliments are likely to have little impact on him. Empirical findings indicate that distressed couples selectively attend to negative events from their partners and tend to be unaware of many positive behaviors from their partners (e.g., Robinson & Price, 1980).

Given that a spouse does notice some behavior from the partner or some marital event, at times the individual will provide an explanation or attribution for why the behavior occurred. A large body of empirical literature confirms that distressed couples are more likely to interpret marital events in a more negative fashion when compared to happy couples' interpretations of the same events (Bradbury & Fincham, 1990). The prior example involving the wife's interpretations for her husband spending long hours at the office clarifies how two attributions for the same behavior might have different impacts on the wife. Not only do partners interpret behaviors that have already occurred, but they also make predictions or develop expectancies for what is likely to happen in the future. Although there has been less research conducted on expectancies in marriage, the extant findings are consistent with these results, indicating that distressed partners are more likely to make negative predictions about the future of their relationship (e.g., Notarius & Vanzetti, 1983).

Whereas these cognitions often are focal to a given set of events, spouses also have broader beliefs about marriage. First, spouses have assumptions about the way that marriages actually operate. For example, partners might have a view that marriage is a place where one can feel safe, secure, and put total trust in another person. These assumptions are important because they help to guide behavior; without basic assumptions about marriage and their partner, people would have to closely scrutinize and evaluate each separate circumstance to decide how to behave. Second, spouses not only develop assumptions about how marriages actually operate, but they also have standards about how marriages *should* function (e.g., "I should put our relationship needs before my own personal needs"). These standards involve values and moral beliefs about how one should treat a partner within an intimate relationship. Standards are critical because they serve as a road map to guide appropriate behavior. They also are important because violations of one's standards often evoke strong reactions of hurt or disappointment; in such instances, a partner's behavior might be seen not only as undesirable, but also as wrong or immoral. Again, basic research on marriage has demonstrated that a couple's assumptions and standards about marriage are related to marital adjustment (e.g., Baucom, Epstein, Rankin, & Burnett, 1996; Epstein & Eidelson, 1981).

Treatment Strategies

Based on these views of marital relationships, cognitive-behavioral interventions for relationship discord have been developed. These treatment interventions have focused primarily on the couple's current relationship. Couples are taught to pinpoint behaviors that they find rewarding and undesirable, and they are helped to negotiate changes to maximize the likelihood of the positive, gratifying behaviors while minimizing the negative, undesirable behaviors. Given that a major class of behaviors for most couples is their communication with each other, considerable effort is directed at helping couples communicate effectively. Both clinical observation and empirical findings have demonstrated that while discussing problem areas, distressed couples have a tendency to focus on the past and blame each other for previous negative events. Consequently, cognitive-behavioral marital therapists typically teach couples to avoid discussing the past or attempting to attribute blame and responsibility. Instead, couples are taught to focus on current concerns and problem-solve on how they can handle situations differently in the future. To the degree that distorted cognitions interfere with this process, they are dealt with directly (e.g., helping couples explore alternative attributions for why one partner behaved in a given way).

Applications of Cognitive-Behavioral Formulations to Recovery from Interpersonal Betrayals

Basic beliefs involving assumptions and standards are particularly important in understanding forgiveness. Not all negative marital behaviors call for forgiveness. We propose that those behaviors that disrupt important marital assumptions and violate relationship standards, particularly those behaviors involving betrayal of trust, are particularly important for understanding forgiveness. Major disruptions in marital standards and assumptions create such a high level of negative affect between the partners that the likelihood of negative cognitive distortions about the relationship and about the partners also increases significantly. Moreover, the extent to which a couple lacks communication skills for resolving this increased conflict will strongly influence the partners' ability to forgive the betrayal.

Weaknesses of the Cognitive-Behavioral Approach to Recovery from Interpersonal Betrayals

Whereas the future orientation of cognitive-behavioral marital therapy might be appropriate for a number of negative behaviors, this also can be a weakness of the model. Many problematic behaviors can be resolved by partners' agreeing how to handle similar situations in the future. However, there are some negative events that spouses have difficulty approaching from a direct problem-solving perspective. These negative events include those in which one spouse has been significantly hurt or wounded by the partner. In such instances, the injured partner simply cannot put the hurt aside and problem-solve on how to address the issue in the future. Instead, the injured partner often feels compelled to address personal injuries from the past before being able to move forward into the future. These are the negative events that often call for forgiveness. Although there is nothing inherent in cognitive-behavioral formulations that prevents a discussion and understanding of the past, until now, cognitive-behavioral theorists have not articulated when and how to help couples process such hurtful events and how to integrate such procedures with the present and the future. By contrast, this focus on understanding the past and using this understanding to change the future has been a focus and strength of insight-oriented approaches to conceptualizing relationship functioning.

Insight-Oriented Approaches to Marriage

Basic Principles

Insight-oriented models of couple therapy emphasize recurrent maladaptive relationship patterns that develop as a result of early interpersonal experiences, either within the family of origin or within other significant relationships from adolescence and early adulthood. Insight-oriented approaches to couple therapy vary in the extent to which they emphasize the unconscious nature of these relational patterns, the developmental period during which these maladaptive patterns are acquired, and the extent to which interpersonal anxieties derive from biological drives (Snyder, in press). However, these approaches all share an assumption that these maladaptive relationship patterns are likely to continue until they are explored and understood in a developmental context. This new understanding serves to reduce the couple's attendant anxiety in current relationships and permits partners to develop alternative, healthier relationship patterns.

Sustained maladaptive patterns of relating to others are viewed as defensive strategies aimed at minimizing expected traumatic or painful relationship experiences. Previous relationship injuries may contribute to persistent anxiety related to self (e.g., enduring feelings of inadequacy, guilt, and shame) or others (e.g., fears of disapproval or abandonment). A common strategy for containing such anxiety might include exaggerated efforts at controlling oneself or one's partner, such as the husband who interrogates his wife about how she spent every minute apart from him. Another problematic method partners may use to manage their interpersonal anxiety may take the form of excessive attachment, a strategy often aimed at protecting oneself against abandonment. For example, a wife may feel terrified of her husband's leaving her and may demand constant reassurance or displays of affection from him; unfortunately, these demands may exact such a burden on the husband that, eventually, he may be more likely to end the relationship. Still another strategy to manage interpersonal anxiety may be distancing oneself from the relationship, or not allowing oneself to need the other partner, in order to reduce personal vulnerability to anticipated rejection or loss. For example, a woman who observed her parents' frequent arguments and her mother's tearful responses to her father's abuse might feel insecure about appearing weak and vulnerable, and be conflicted about displaying strong emotions other than anger. Her anxiety about expressing tenderness and the desire to distance herself from potential emotional rejection could preclude her expressing vulnerable feelings toward her husband and prevent the couple from developing a sense of intimacy.

Treatment Strategies

In insight-oriented couple therapy, the developmental origins of interpersonal themes and their expression in the couple's relationship are explored through a process of "affective reconstruction" (Snyder, in press; Snyder & Wills, 1989). Previous relationships are reconstructed in order to identify how previous strategies for emotional gratification and anxiety containment were vital to prior relationships. In addition, these strategies also are examined in order to discover how they may represent inappropriate methods to create emotional intimacy and satisfaction in the current relationship. Each partner is encouraged to (1) work through previous relationship injuries, (2) grieve losses and unmet needs, (3) express ambivalence or anger toward previous significant others in the safety of the conjoint therapy, and (4) acquire increased ability to differentiate prior relationships from the present one. For example, in the case described earlier, in which the woman avoided expressing vulnerability in her marriage, insight-oriented approaches would focus primarily on helping the couple to (1) understand in greater detail how the wife learned these patterns, (2) develop empathy for her struggles, and (3) work through her problematic relationship with her parents. Consequently, as she began to understand her past relationships in a new light, she might be able to see her husband and her marriage in a more realistic perspective as well. These new perspectives might, in turn, promote greater awareness of, and comfort in expressing, feelings of tenderness and vulnerability essential to intimacy.

Examining their own developmental contributions to current marital distress offers couples several benefits. First, it grants them relief from their interpersonal anxieties by reducing their confusion about why they may be highly emotionally reactive to relationship conflicts. Second, it restores hope for greater emotional fulfillment in their relationships by resolving previous relationship injuries and helping them to develop new patterns of relating in their marriage. Third, it provides them with opportunities for greater empathy for each other and their struggles. Finally, it offers them a chance for resolution of persistent conflicts and cyclical, maladaptive patterns through redirected interpersonal strategies.

Moreover, as each spouse observes his or her partner's efforts to clarify and understand the origin of maladaptive relationship patterns, the spouse frequently comes to understand his or her partner's behaviors in a more accepting or benign manner. This change may come about through attributing damaging exchanges to the culmination of acquired interpersonal strategies to manage negative affect rather than to explicit motives to be hurtful. Armed with this greater understanding of each other, the couple may be more responsive to interventions designed to improve their marriage.

Application of Insight-Oriented Approaches to Relationship Betrayals

An insight-oriented approach provides several implications for a couple's recovery from a major interpersonal betrayal and the spouses' ability to forgive one another. First, this approach suggests that factors contributing to an individual's decision to engage in an interpersonal betrayal might include important intrapersonal issues of which he or she may not be aware. Furthermore, these factors may have their origins in relationship experiences much earlier in that person's life. To the extent that such issues remain unrecognized or unresolved, they place that person at risk for repeated destructive relationship behaviors. Second, an insight-oriented approach to couple therapy presumes that both spouses' responses to a betrayal reflect important contributions from previous relationship disappointments or injuries. Indeed, the heightened emotional turmoil characterizing the reactions of both partners to both explicit and implicit threats to their relationship make it particularly likely that both spouses will draw on exaggerated defensive strategies. In turn, these defensive strategies are likely to exacerbate the situation by interfering with (1) their understanding of the sources and consequences of the betrayal, and (2) their achieving an emotional resolution to this relationship injury.

Weaknesses of the Insight-Oriented Approach to Recovery from Interpersonal Betrayals

A potential weakness of this approach to marital therapy is that it often does not provide specific behavioral mechanisms, such as communication skills, to promote safety between the spouses as they address highly conflictual issues. The period following a major betrayal can be chaotic, and couples are likely to commit further damage to their relationship through uncontrolled negative interactions. Couples in this kind of crisis often benefit from negotiating clear, behavioral rules for interactions to prevent them from causing more relationship damage. In addition, whereas cognitive-behavioral strategies tend to slight or ignore the past, traditional insight-oriented approaches may focus so strongly on the past that they slight the present and the future. Although the enhanced understanding that couples gain from this type of therapy may be critical, they often need additional help and structure in negotiating changes to their current patterns and habits. This kind of negotiation is often facilitated through cognitive-behavioral strategies of communication training, problem solving, and cognitive restructuring.

Efficacy of Marital Therapy in Assisting Distressed Couples

From a theoretical perspective, there are numerous reasons to expect that both cognitive-behavioral and insight-oriented approaches to marital therapy will be helpful to many couples. Indeed, this assertion is affirmed by the empirical literature. Baucom et al. (1998) recently reviewed the efficacy of all theoretical approaches to marital therapy and concluded that there is widespread evidence supporting the efficacy of behavioral and cognitive-behavioral approaches. There are few studies investigating the efficacy of insight-oriented approaches to couple therapy, but thus far, the findings strongly support the efficacy of insight-oriented couple therapy (Baucom et al., 1998).

At present, there are more than two dozen controlled investigations from several countries demonstrating that cognitive-behavioral marital therapy (CBMT) is helpful to distressed couples. Unfortunately, there have been few attempts to clarify the kinds of presenting complaints for which CBMT is efficacious and those instances in which the interventions are less successful. Although there have not been any attempts to replicate the findings thus far, Bennun (1985a, 1985b) concluded from his research that CBMT was particularly effective in alleviating specific behavioral concerns that are clearly negotiable (e.g., household tasks, child-care issues, finances). However, CBMT seemed to be less successful in matters of jealousy, affection, and more emotionally based and less task-oriented concerns. It is likely that some of these emotionally based, less task-oriented marital concerns call for forgiveness. If this is true, then CBMT, as it has been commonly practiced, perhaps is not optimal for assisting couples for whom forgiveness is a major issue.

Despite their widespread use, insight-oriented approaches to couple therapy have received little empirical scrutiny. An exception to this trend is a study by Snyder and Wills (1989) comparing the effectiveness of insight-oriented marital therapy (IOMT) and behavioral marital therapy (BMT) relative to a wait-list control condition. At both termination and 6-month follow-up, both treatments proved equally efficacious in significantly reducing individuals' marital distress. However, the efficacy of insight-oriented and behavioral approaches diverged significantly when these couples were followed-up 4 years later (Snyder, Wills, & Grady-Fletcher, 1991a). During the 4 years following termination, BMT couples were more likely to show significant deterioration in their relationship adjustment as compared to IOMT couples. In discussing these findings, the authors posit an important distinction between acquisition of relationship skills through instruction or rehearsal versus interference with use of these skills on a motivational or affective basis. They further argue that spouses' negative views toward their partner's behavior "are modified to a greater degree and in a more persistent manner once individuals come to understand and resolve emotional conflicts they bring to the marriage from their own family and relationship histories" (Snyder, Wills, & Grady-Fletcher, 1991b, p. 148). These results suggest that the emphasis of IOMT on developmental contributions may be important in helping couples resolve the more emotionally based concerns that are not as effectively addressed by CBMT.

Overview of the Relevant Forgiveness Literature

Although the empirical literature on CBMT and IOMT suggests that these are both useful ways to help couples resolve marital difficulties, neither of these perspectives provides a clear, integrated conceptualization of the impact of betrayals on relationships; nor do they provide specific guidelines for how to help couples through the process of resolving these betrayals. Forgiveness is a concept that is commonly cited by successful couples and one that intuitively seems important for couples recovering from the impact of a betrayal (Fennell, 1993). Consequently, marital therapists should benefit from the development of a well-reasoned approach to forgiveness.

Basic Principles

In support of this claim, several studies have documented an association between marital adjustment and forgiveness (Holeman, 1994; Rackley, 1993; Woodman, 1992). Holeman (1994) identified a positive association between female incest survivors' forgiveness of their previous abusers and their current levels of marital adjustment; however, the mechanisms behind this association are unclear. More directly, both Rackley (1993) and Woodman (1992) addressed forgiveness occurring within a marital relationship and its association with that marriage's level of adjustment. Both studies found that forgiveness of one's spouse for major emotional injuries significantly predicted marital adjustment. However, because all three studies were correlational, it is not possible to determine a causal link between forgiveness and marital adjustment.

Furthermore, none of these studies offered a clear model of how forgiveness is accomplished or a clear theoretical basis for the association between forgiveness and marital adjustment. However, a recent study by Hargrave and Sells (1997) provides both a theoretical framework and empirical support for the importance of forgiveness in families. The authors place this model of forgiveness within a contextual family therapy perspective (Boszormenyi-Nagy, Grunebaum, & Ulrich, 1991), suggesting that family betrayals result from one member's sense of destructive entitlement. They suggest that the betraying member has experienced a violation of trust in a prior relationship and consequently feels justified in enacting hurtful behaviors within the current relationship. As a result, the betrayed partner faces the problem of how to forgive the betrayer. They further posit that the work of forgiveness is made up of both "exonerating" and "forgiving." Exonerating includes gaining insight into and understanding the motive behind the betrayal. They suggest that forgiving involves the injured person either engaging in an overt act of forgiving or giving the offender the opportunity for compensation, which seems to include acts such as apologies and other symbolic behaviors designed to create opportunities for restitution. Thus, exoneration appears to be cognitive in nature, whereas forgiving is more behavioral. They emphasize that these components are not stages that people progress through in succession; instead, they hypothesize that people vary between these strategies, or "stations," as they attempt to engage in the work of forgiveness. Hargrave and Sells provide some empirical support for this model through the validation of a scale designed to measure the four "stations" or components of forgiveness (i.e., insight, understanding, compensation, and overt acts of forgiving); however, it remains unclear how or *why* a person might choose to enact these different strategies.

The preceding studies focused specifically on forgiveness occurring within families or couples; however, more detailed theories of forgiveness that are not specific to familial relationships also have been proposed and offer potential insights on how forgiveness occurs in couples and families. Most theorists agree that forgiveness takes time and is more likely to be an ongoing process than a discrete event in time; thus, varying stage theories of forgiveness have been described (Enright and the Human Development Study Group, 1991; Hargrave & Sells, 1997; McCullough, Worthington, & Rachal, 1997; Rosenak & Harnden, 1992; Smedes, 1984). These theories differ on several levels; some include reconciliation in the process, others do not. Some place the decision to forgive early in the process; whereas others place it near the end. Some attempt to explain why a person decides to forgive, whereas others do not. However, despite these differences, most theories are fairly consistent in their definitions of the end state of forgiveness, and they indicate three common elements: (1) regaining a more balanced view of the offender and the event, (2) decreasing negative affect toward the offender, and (3) giving up the right to punish the offender further.

Furthermore, studies have emerged recently indicating that forgiveness-based interventions aimed at helping the individual cognitively reframe the interpersonal betrayal and gain a greater understanding of why the trauma occurred are effective in increasing participants' levels of forgiveness and in improving their levels of individual psychological functioning (e.g., Freedman & Enright, 1996; Hebl & Enright, 1993). In addition, McCullough et al. (1997) described results of an intervention specifically aimed at promoting forgiveness through building empathy with an offender. Despite some evidence supporting a link between empathy and forgiveness, several of their findings suggested that empathy might be only one of several possible pathways to forgiveness. In this study, empathy did not fully mediate the link between apology and forgiveness. The authors suggest that the cognitive changes effected in the didactic group also may be important in understanding forgiveness; that is, forgiveness may require cognitive as well as emotional changes in the person who is forgiving. The importance of a changed understanding of the offender in forgiveness is consistent with the "stations" of insight and understanding described in Hargrave and Sells's forgiveness model and with the strategy of cognitive reframing from the model described by Enright et al. (1991). Thus, the current literature suggests that forgiveness appears to be a complex, stage-like process that is mediated by both cognitive and affective changes in the forgiver.

Weaknesses of Forgiveness-Based Approaches to Interpersonal Betrayals

As described earlier and in the other chapters in this volume, there has been considerable progress in mapping out essential components involved in the forgiveness process. However, each forgiveness model has its own idiosyncrasies and structure; the field has yet to integrate essential components of forgiveness. Furthermore, the field lacks a coherent and comprehensive explanation about why the various stages are necessary and what motivates people to engage in this process. At present, it remains unclear how or why people progress through these similar stages or use similar forgiveness strategies.

There is another problem with current forgiveness theories when one applies them to couple and family therapy. These models primarily apply to betrayed individuals and do not include dynamic aspects of the other partners' reactions or the ongoing interactions in the relationship. Furthermore, current treatments do not include strategies to help contain the negative affect generated between the partners in response to the betrayal; damage caused by negative interactions between the partners at this point is likely to severely weaken the motivation for the forgiveness process and interfere with their chance of successful resolution. Thus, given the strength of the CBMT approaches at containing negative affect and examining distorted cognitions, and the strength of IOMT approaches at examining developmental contributions to current behaviors and at promoting empathy between the partners, the integration of these two marital models seems appropriate to promote the work of forgiveness in damaged interpersonal relationships.

A Three-Stage Model of Forgiveness in Marriage

Basic Principles

Based on existing theory, research, and clinical observations, Gordon and Baucom (1999; in press) have proposed a three-stage model of forgiveness within the context of marriage. In order to understand the forgiveness process, it is essential first to understand the kinds of negative events that call for forgiveness. Not all negative events require forgiveness. Instead, it appears to be those negative events that significantly disrupt spouses' basic beliefs about their relationships, their partners, and themselves that create the context for forgiveness. Interestingly, this same assertion has been made in trying to understand why some negative events are experienced as traumas and increase the likelihood of posttraumatic stress reactions; that is, the literature on traumatic responses suggests that people are most likely to become emotionally traumatized when an event violates basic assumptions about how the world and people operate (Janoff-Bulman, 1989; McCann, Sakheim, & Abrahamson, 1988). The cognitive disequilibrium resulting from an interpersonal trauma, such as an affair, may be more clearly understood when placed in this light. Several marital assumptions may be violated by an affair (e.g., the assumption that partners can be trusted, the assumption that the relationship is a safe place to be). The trauma literature also suggests that when these basic tenets are violated, the injured person loses a great deal of predictability for the future and, thus, experiences a loss of control. This loss of control can then lead to feelings of anxiety and depression (e.g., Joseph, Yule, & Williams, 1993; McCann et al., 1988).

Furthermore, within the context of marriage, the violation has been directly caused by an intimate partner, leading to greater feelings of interpersonal loss and hurt, as well as painful attributions of responsibility and intentional malice toward the participating partner. As long as the injured partners do not have a clear sense of why the trauma occurred, they cannot trust their partners not to hurt them again; instead, the partners are likely to be seen as malicious individuals whose very faces or voices serve as stimuli for floods of painful emotion. Unfortunately, the participating partner often is dealing with his or her own feelings of guilt, shame, anger, or depression, and thus is often ill-equipped to respond effectively to his or her partner's strong expressions of emotions.

Based on these observations, conceptualizing forgiveness as a response to an interpersonally traumatic event is likely to yield useful implications for planning effective therapy with these difficult cases (Abrahm-Spring, 1996; Coop, Baucom, & Daiuto, 1995; Glass & Wright, 1997). Consequently, many of the responses observed in injured partners during the forgiveness process can be viewed as resulting from disruption of basic beliefs and a strong need to reconstruct a shattered worldview, all the while protecting themselves from further harm from the participating partner. If forgiveness is conceptualized as a response to interpersonal trauma, then the forgiveness process can be understood as unfolding in three major stages that parallel the stages involved in the traumatic response. Thus, the three major stages of the forgiveness process include (1) absorbing and experiencing the impact of the interpersonal trauma; (2) a search for meaning as to why the trauma occurred, along with implications for this new understanding; and (3) moving forward with one's life within the context of a new set of relationship beliefs.

Our research to date has supported this conceptualization of forgiveness, although the cross-sectional nature of our research admittedly does not offer conclusive support for the stage model (Coop et al., 1995; Gordon, 1997). Using an inventory specifically designed to test this model, community couples were classified as being either in Stage I, Stage II, or Stage III of forgiveness. As predicted, partners in Stage I reported the least amount of global forgiveness on a separate one-item self-report measure and also reported the least amount of marital adjustment. Partners in Stage III reported the most forgiveness and highest marital adjustment, whereas the levels of forgiveness and marital adjustment for partners in Stage II fell between the Stage I and the Stage III individuals.

Furthermore, in order for this stage process to be initiated, an individual must believe that his or her partner has violated a major assumption or relationship standard. Thus, if a husband engages in an extramarital affair, it likely triggers a disruption of a number of standards and assumptions. As most married persons have made a commitment of sexual fidelity to their spouses, a violation of this commitment also violates the assumption that one can trust one's partner to honor the couple's other commitments. In the first stage of the forgiveness process, the impact stage, people are attempting to comprehend what has transpired. They have become aware of their partners' behavior, are attempting to clarify exactly what has happened, and begin to try to make some sense of why it has occurred. Consistent with these expectations, our findings indicate that partners classified in the Stage I group reported the most negative assumptions about themselves and their partners (Coop et al., 1995; Gordon, 1997). Partners classified in the Stage III group reported the most positive relationship assumptions, and the scores of spouses classified in the Stage II group fell between those of the Stage I and Stage III groups.

However, given that betrayals are unexpected and often have major implications for the injured person's well-being, the cognitive process described here usually is accompanied by an overwhelming array of emotions, such as fear, hurt, or anger. These emotions often alternate with a sense of numbness or disbelief. Additionally, people may find themselves acting in ways that are erratic or unlike their usual selves. Most frequently, well-ingrained behavior patterns occur within a context of having a clear view of the world around us. All persons have assumptions of how their world and relationships will be, and expect themselves and their partners to behave according to their standards. If one's spouse behaves in a way that disrupts these basic beliefs, then the injured partner's own behavior patterns no longer seem safe or make sense. The injured partner can no longer predict what will happen; thus, well-established daily patterns of behavior are questioned. As a result, the interactions between the partners are often chaotic, intensely negative, and likely to lead to further frustration and anger rather than feelings of resolution.

Given that the injured partner's sense of safety and trust typically has been violated, the injured person often retreats or establishes barriers and boundaries to protect him- or herself. This might involve responses such as sleeping in a different room, no longer sharing events of the day, and having little physical contact. In essence, the relationship no longer feels safe, so the injured person seeks to protect him- or herself from further hurt and pain; the withdrawal also can serve the purpose of punishing the participating partner. Our research has found that spouses classified as being in Stage I report more boundaries and less investment in their relationships than do partners classified as being in Stage II or Stage III; partners classified in Stage III report the fewest boundaries and most investment in their relationship (Coop et al., 1995; Gordon, 1997).

In addition, the injured person may perceive that the balance of power in the relationship has shifted; the participating or offending partner may now appear to have more power, particularly in his or her ability to hurt the injured partner. In an attempt to right this imbalance, the injured partner may lash out in destructive ways or demand that his or her partner perform extraordinary tasks in order to "even the score" between the partners or make up for what occurred. Our research indicates that spouses classified as being in Stage I report that their partners have more power in their relationships than do people classified as being in Stage II or Stage III, whereas partners classified in Stage III report the most equality in their relationships (Coop et al., 1995; Gordon, 1997).

Consequently, the first stage of the forgiveness process involves a variety of cognitive, emotional, and behavioral responses that result from the disruption of major relationship assumptions and standards. These responses include a strong need to know exactly what has happened and why, significant emotional dysregulation resulting from having one's beliefs about the partner and the relationship disrupted, and atypical behavior patterns that follow from a sense of confusion and the need to protect oneself.

The goal in the second stage, the "meaning" stage, is for the couple to explore more thoroughly why the event occurred and place it in a more understandable context. Major relationship assumptions and standards have been violated, and the injured partner must attempt to understand why. Therefore, the second stage of forgiveness involves seeking attributions or explanations for why the traumatic events have occurred. Thus, a husband might reach different understandings for why his wife displayed what he views as inappropriate affectionate behavior with a male coworker. If he viewed it as her attempt to be supportive to a coworker who was experiencing a major personal crisis, he might still be unhappy with her behavior but see her motives as honorable and unlikely to lead to repeated action once the couple has discussed the issue. If, however, the husband views her behavior as an overture to further contact and interest in an extramarital affair, then his response is likely to be one of anger and jealousy.

Typically, it is useful for couples to consider a number of factors and how they contributed to the context within which the trauma occurred. Many of these are proximal factors, that is, circumstances that were present at the time of, or immediately prior to, the trauma. This includes how each member of the couple was functioning individually, the status of the couple's relationship, and outside stressors. For example, after exploration, a couple might realize that the wife had an extramarital affair at a time when she experienced significant distress at work, felt emotionally disengaged within her marriage, and felt that her husband dealt with their increased distance by focusing his energies on his work. This understanding is not intended to blame the husband or justify the wife's decision to have an affair. What is important is for the wife in this instance to take responsibility for her decision to have an affair and for both partners to understand the factors that were salient at the time she made that decision.

In addition, couples often benefit from an increased understanding of how both partners have learned to respond to stressors in particular ways. This means that an understanding of distal factors, such as early developmental influences, often is important. In the course of a couple's attempts to work through the forgiveness process on their own, they likely vary widely in their ability or attempts to understand these developmental issues. That is why attempts to deal with significant relationship traumas often benefit from professional assistance. Consequently, in the previous example, the couple might come to recognize that the wife had learned from an early age that when she felt neglected and stressed, she could gain immediate attention and affirmation by gaining a sense of caring and security from a new dyadic relationship; that is, her long-term pattern of turning to other partners when she felt neglected or abandoned may have laid the groundwork for her recent affair. Similarly, they might learn that whenever the husband felt inadequate while growing up, he would turn to individual, intellectual activity as an arena where he knew he could succeed and regain his sense of esteem. Thus, his withdrawal response from his wife was part of a well-learned reaction to regain his self-esteem. Therefore, an understanding of both proximal and distal factors often can benefit a couple as they attempt to understand why one party would act in ways that seem contrary to the well-being of the couple and their commitments to each other.

The in-depth cognitive evaluation characteristic of this stage becomes more possible because of the change that takes place in the person's emotional experiences. At this time, it is unclear what may cause the partners to move into Stage II. The emotions literature suggests that people often are unable to sustain high levels of intense emotional arousal for an extended length of time (e.g., Selye, 1975), yet other studies do suggest that people can maintain a high level of arousal over a longer period of time. However, possibly as a result of a reduction in emotionality, people do become more able to search for the "meaning" of the trauma. This meaning may come from two sources: (1) seeking to understand the causes of the trauma or (2) attempting to find some positive impact the event had on their lives (e.g., greater spiritual growth, better understanding of life). Cognitively, this derived meaning helps victims to regain some sense of control over their lives. Knowing why it happened gives both members of the couple the ability to try to prevent it from happening again, and it may give them the sense of safety needed to "move on." From a cognitive perspective, developing more accurate and comprehensive attributions for the traumatic event can contribute to the development of new expectancies or predictions for the future; without understanding why an event occurred, it is difficult to predict whether it will recur in the future. Affectively, this search for a new understanding of the causes of the betrayal may allow the injured partner to experience more empathy for the betraying partner, particularly as it may become clear that he or she was acting out of his or her own past hurts. This empathy may in turn facilitate the search for understanding and increase the injured partner's desire to voluntarily give up the right to punish his or her partner.

Thus, the second stage of the forgiveness process is characterized by a strong need to understand why the traumatic event(s) occurred and to give them meaning; the disrupted beliefs about the partner and the marriage must be reconstructed in some meaningful way before the injured spouse feels that he or she can move forward in life. Our recent investigation of spouses' written descriptions of the forgiveness process provides data consistent with this hypothesis (Gordon, Pautsch, & Baucom, 1996). The participants' global self-report of forgiveness was predicted by the extent to which their descriptions of forgiveness included a significant amount of cognitive processing of the event and changes in attributions about the event.

Similar to trauma victims, the injured person in the third or "moving on" stage must move beyond the event and stop allowing it to control his or her life. In the current conceptualization, forgiveness involves moving forward by giving up the control that negative emotion can have over the injured person's thoughts and behaviors, and by giving up the right to punish the partner. The search for understanding in Stage II means that the couple, in essence, must reevaluate the relationship. At times this reevaluation may mean altering the relationship in significant ways. In more disruptive instances, the partners must make a decision regarding whether they wish to continue with the relationship; this decision often is quite important after relationship traumas such as physical abuse or extramarital affairs. From a psychological perspective, there is nothing in the forgiveness process that requires reconciliation. Furthermore, forgiveness does not require that anger disappear completely. In fact, it is expected that the emotions and thoughts associated with the event will reoccur, similar to flashbacks in posttraumatic stress disorder (PTSD); however, these thoughts and feelings are no longer as severe or as disruptive as they once were. Instead, in order to move forward, the injured partner needs to achieve three goals by the end of this third stage: (1) develop a realistic and balanced view of the relationship, (2) experience a release from being controlled by negative affect toward the participating or offending partner, and (3) relinquish voluntarily the right to punish the participating partner. Furthermore, it is important to note that this definition of forgiveness does not require that the person experience positive emotions toward the betrayer. We believe that, in some cases, these feelings may be impossible. Certainly, an ability to experience compassion and warmth toward the offender may ideally be the best outcome, yet we do not believe this is necessary. More research is clearly needed to explore this hypothesis.

This latter definition is consistent with the definition of the end state of forgiveness in most major theories of forgiveness (e.g., Enright et al., 1991; Rosenak & Harnden, 1992; Smedes, 1984). Our research program has attempted to find empirical support for this definition. People's written descriptions of how they had forgiven their partners were coded according to (1) valence of emotion (positive, neutral, or negative) toward the offending partner, (2) valence of current interactions between the partners, (3) their attributions of responsibility and intentionality for the offending partner, and (4) three different levels of cognitive processing of the event. The processing codes significantly predicted injured persons' emotions toward their partners, their interactions with their partners, and their attributions of responsibility and intentionality. In turn, the emotion, behavior, and attribution codes significantly predicted their level of forgiveness (Gordon et al., 1996). These results offer more concrete evidence that actively processing and thinking about the betrayal is associated with more positive emotion and behaviors toward one's partner, and more balanced, less blaming cognitions about the betrayal. Moreover, each of these three cognitive, affective, and behavioral components are in turn associated with forgiveness.

Treatment Strategies

Based on this model and evidence from our basic research, we are evaluating the efficacy of a treatment designed to aid couples in recovering from the impact of an affair, an event that violates major relationship standards and assumptions, and, therefore, calls for forgiveness. The treatment involves an integration of cognitive-behavioral strategies described in *Cognitive-Behavioral Marital Therapy* (Baucom & Epstein, 1990) and the insight-oriented treatment strategies described in Snyder and Wills's (1989) treatment–outcome study. Our treatment corresponds to our three-stage forgiveness model, and each phase of treatment targets issues and problems that are particular to that stage of the forgiveness process.

The model suggests that in the initial stage, the couple often is trying to assess the impact of the affair and contain the negative affect associated with it; thus, the treatment helps them to develop the skills to contain and regulate their negative emotions and effectively discuss with each other the impact that the affair has had on them and their relationship. Thus, the first several sessions use typical cognitive-behavioral strategies to deal primarily with helping the couple to (1) set appropriate boundaries around themselves individually and as a couple, (2) manage their emotions, and (3) express and identify their reactions to the impact of the affair. In addition, the conceptualization of the process as similar to a traumatic response is introduced and the concept of flashbacks is explained. Various reminders of the partner's affair may trigger exaggerated emotional responses similar to PTSD flashbacks. Once the partners understand this phenomenon, they are then encouraged to develop more effective means to deal with it.

In the second stage, the therapy shifts to a more insight-oriented approach as the partners attempt to explain to themselves why the affair happened and examine both current and developmental issues within themselves and the relationship that may have contributed to it. The developmental aspect of this treatment often is critical. The injured and participating partners often already know or have access to information about their relationship that may have influenced the participating partners' decision to have an affair; however, they are often unaware of deeper, or unacknowledged needs or motives from their partners' past history that may be impacting their current behaviors. Gaining this new understanding often results in an increase in compassion for the partner and tolerance of his or her flaws. Thus, our treatment is designed to help the couple to (1) explore these factors in a neutral, supportive, and structured environment; (2) develop empathy and understanding for each other to the extent possible; and (3) attempt to alter any negative or problematic issues that they pinpoint as contributors to the person's decision to have an affair.

Finally, in the third stage, the treatment again becomes more present and future focused, which in turn calls for more cognitive-behavioral strategies. As couples begin to understand why the affair happened, they need to evaluate the viability of their relationship, its potential for change, and their commitment to work toward change. In addition, the process of forgiveness becomes a focus of intervention. It is explained to couples how they have been progressing through the forgiveness process as they have gone through this treatment. Their misconceptions of, and resistance to, forgiveness are examined, and any blocks to this process are addressed. This treatment then helps them to evaluate important aspects of their relationship in order to come to a well-considered decision about whether they wish to continue their marriage. Depending on this decision, couples either continue to work on rebuilding their relationship, or they receive the therapist's support and guidance as they work through the necessary issues of terminating the marriage, while retaining their efforts toward increased understanding and forgiveness of traumatic events in the marriage in order to move on in their individual lives.

Implications of the Three-Stage Model of Forgiveness

Stage theories of human behavior are helpful in bringing order to what can otherwise seem like a random series of cognitive, emotional, and behavioral responses over a long time period in an individual's life. As such, they can have significant heuristic value in providing understanding of complex events and, for the clinician, in planning appropriate interventions. However, most stage theories by necessity oversimplify the rich complexity of emotional and behavioral functioning. Rather than occurring in discrete stages, human behavior more often appears gradual and continuous. Moreover, our stage theory of forgiveness is proposed for an event and a time period that are inherently chaotic and dysregulated; perhaps it is too much to ask that dysregulation be dealt with in an orderly manner. For example, within the context of response to trauma, a frequent phenomenon involves flashbacks to the traumatic event in which the traumatic event is reexperienced in intensely emotional ways. These flashbacks typically are triggered by stimuli related to the original trauma (e.g., someone hanging up the telephone when the wife answers, subsequent to her husband's extramarital affair). This flashback and concomitant reexperiencing of the trauma can be extremely confusing to a couple who appears to be making progress in proceeding through the forgiveness process. Consequently, any stage theory of forgiveness must acknowledge that not all individuals will progress through the process in an identical manner and must allow for a "recycling" through the process, often instigated by flashbacks to the original trauma. In spite of these caveats, there do appear to be some broad patterns that occur with enough regularity to suggest that the forgiveness model described here provides a useful means for intervening with painful and traumatic events in couple therapy.

CONCLUSIONS

Theory, research, and clinical applications of forgiveness have increased significantly in recent years. Even so, this progress has been rather slow in developing; in each of these domains, there remain significant barriers to using the term "forgiveness." Among marital researchers, research on forgiveness has been impeded for at least two reasons. First, forgiveness typically has been viewed as a spiritual construct, often derived or centered within a theological context. A recent study suggests that forgiveness is more likely to be used by clinicians with a personal religious viewpoint than by those who do not have any religious beliefs (DiBlasio & Benda, 1991). These results suggest that the rejection of forgiveness as a useful clinical strategy could be based, in part, upon nonreligious therapists' beliefs that forgiveness can only be understood from a religious perspective.

Second, constructs such as forgiveness are natural or "fuzzy" concepts (Prager, 1995). A natural concept is "one in which the boundaries that separate category members from nonmembers are fuzzy" (Prager, 1995, p. 14). Natural concepts are different from logical concepts. Logical concepts are those that include lists of characteristics that are necessary and sufficient for inclusion, along with differentiating characteristics (Cantor & Mischel, 1979). Most researchers rely upon logical constructs, and if a term cannot be clearly operationalized, then it often is not investigated. Natural or fuzzy constructs require a different set of assumptions. As Prager notes, natural constructs are not characterized by finite lists of necessary and sufficient conditions, but instead are more probabilistic in nature. Some characteristics seem more central to the construct and appear for most members in the category. In terms of forgiveness, for example, it seems likely that "moving on" is relatively central to the process of forgiveness. Other characteristics may still be included within a natural construct, but as they become less central, their boundaries with other constructs become "fuzzy." With regard to forgiveness, at times, one might not be certain whether forgiveness has actually occurred or if the injured spouse merely accepted what happened, and whether forgiveness and acceptance have clear boundaries. Although most theorists in the forgiveness area provide lists of stages or characteristics of the forgiveness process, it seems unlikely that a finite list of necessary and sufficient conditions will ever exist.

The current model proposes a remedy to these problems by integrating forgiveness within the context of two previous theoretical models of relationships and couple therapy. This integration provides an explanation of forgiveness using constructs that have already been validated by empirical research. Using these familiar constructs may facilitate research on the forgiveness process by mainstream investigators. Furthermore, the use of these constructs increases the specificity of the model by identifying specific thoughts, behaviors, and emotions that may be observed during the process, and when they may occur. This specificity may reduce the "fuzziness" surrounding forgiveness, clarifying for researchers and clinicians alike the important constructs underlying forgiveness and the mechanisms by which it occurs.

Just as the "fuzziness" of the forgiveness construct may have deterred researchers from empirically investigating forgiveness, confusion about what forgiveness means has caused some therapists to criticize its use in therapy. The basis of this misunderstanding may well be found in some people's simplistic understandings of traditional Biblical injunctions regarding forgiveness, such as "turn the other cheek" or "you must forgive seventy times seven." Often these statements are misinterpreted as meaning that one should forgive all acts and do so without reservation. Other, theorists assert that reconciliation is the ultimate or ideal form of forgiveness, implying that forgiveness is not complete unless one is reunited with the offender (e.g., Pattison, 1965; Smedes, 1984). These beliefs about forgiveness have particularly negative implications for therapists working with abused spouses. Katz, Street, and Arias (1995) found that abused women who reported being more forgiving toward their partners were more likely to return to an abusive situation. Not surprisingly, therapists working with this population are reluctant to encourage forgiveness.

However, our forgiveness model and other theoretical models suggest a different approach to forgiveness. When abused persons understand forgiveness as a means toward letting go of bitterness and anger in a safe and realistic way, then forgiveness may appear to be a better option for these populations as well. The crucial point in this application would be ensuring that the injured person understands that forgiveness does not mean reconciliation; the abused spouse can forgive her partner, but that does not mean that she should return to an unsafe situation.

Another common, problematic belief about forgiveness, particularly for people working with abused clients, is that forgiveness is "weak" and does not allow clients adequate acknowledgement of their pain or rights. Unfortunately, forgiveness is often seen as letting the offender "get away with something" or overlooking the problem. Clients often hold this view as well. However, Enright, Eastin, Golden, Sarinopoulos, and Freedman (1992) counter this by asserting that forgiveness, used properly, can have a healing effect. If one views forgiveness as a process and looks at the different stage models of forgiveness, it becomes apparent that appropriate expression of anger and other negative affect is a central part of the process. Furthermore, the process of forgiveness involves regaining a realistic view of the partner as having both positive and negative characteristics. Being able to examine oneself, one's partner, and one's relationship closely takes strength and gives people important information about their world. Thus, forgiveness need not be considered as weak, but rather as healthy and necessary for more effective relationships.

In summary, forgiveness is a concept that is likely to be of great use to marital researchers, therapists, and clients. Both the cognitive-behavioral and insight-oriented approaches to marital and couple therapy offer several important contributions to understanding these complex relationships but are incomplete in addressing a couple's response to a major interpersonal betrayal. Forgiveness comprises a critical concept, central to relationship trauma; however, the use of forgiveness in mainstream psychology has met with considerable resistance. It is likely that this resistance will decrease as the field develops clearer models of forgiveness that are specific enough to drive empirical investigations offering more support for this construct. In addition, as the field defines forgiveness more clearly and provides evidence that this process is healthy and desirable in a variety of contexts, it is expected that the resistance from clinicians should decrease as well. The model presented here can facilitate these goals by (1) providing a clear, specific three-stage model of forgiveness; (2) linking this model to previously validated approaches to intervention with distressed couples; and (3) providing an ongoing program of research that empirically supports a clear definition of the forgiveness process.

REFERENCES

Abrahm-Spring, J., with Spring, M. (1996). *After the affair: Healing the pain and rebuilding trust when a partner has been unfaithful.* New York: HarperCollins.

Baucom, D. H., & Epstein, N. (1990). *Cognitive-behavioral marital therapy.* New York, NY: Brunner/Mazel.

Baucom, D. H., Epstein, N., Rankin, L. A., & Burnett, C. K. (1996). Assessing relationship standards: The Inventory of Specific Relationship Standards. *Journal of Family Psychology, 10,* 72–88.

Baucom, D. H., Epstein, N., Sayers, S., & Sher, T. G. (1989). The role of cognitions in marital relationships: Definitional, methodological, and conceptual issues. *Journal of Consulting and Clinical Psychology, 57,* 31–38.

Baucom, D. H., Shoham, V., Mueser, K. T., Daiuto, A. D., & Stickle, T. R. (1998). Empirically supported couples and family therapies for adult problems. *Journal of Consulting and Clinical Psychology, 66,* 53–88.

Bennun, I. (1985a). Behavioral marital therapy: An outcome evaluation of conjoint, group and one spouse treatment. *Scandinavian Journal of Behaviour Therapy, 14,* 157–168.

Bennun, I. (1985b). Prediction and responsiveness in behavioral marital therapy. *Behavioural Psychotherapy, 13,* 186–201.

Boszormenyi-Nagy, I., Grunebaum, J., & Ulrich, D. (1991). Contextual Therapy. In A. S.

Gurman & D. P. Kniskern (Eds.), *Handbook of family therapy* (Vol. 2, pp. 200–238). New York: Brunner/Mazel.

Bradbury, T. N., & Fincham, F. D. (1990). Attributions in marriage: Review and critique. *Psychological Bulletin, 107,* 3–33.

Cantor, N., & Mischel, W. (1979). Prototypes in person perception. *Advances in Experimental Social Psychology, 12,* 3–52.

Coop, K. L., Baucom, D. H., & Daiuto, A. (1995, November). *Demystifying forgiveness: A cognitive-behavioral stage model.* In D. H. Baucom (Chair), Four FACTs of Marriage: Forgiveness, Acceptance, Commitment, and Trust, presented at the Annual Conference of the Association for the Advancement of Behavior Therapy, Washington, DC.

DiBlasio, F. A., & Benda, B. B. (1991). Practitioners, religion and the use of forgiveness in the clinical setting. *Journal of Psychology and Christianity, 10,* 166–172.

Enright, R. D., and the Human Development Study Group. (1991). The moral development of forgiveness. In W. Kurtines & J. Gewirtz (Eds.), *Handbook of moral behavior and development* (Vol. 1, pp. 123–152). Hillsdale, NJ: Erlbaum.

Enright, R. D., Eastin, D. L., Golden, S., Sarinopoulos, I., & Freedman, S. (1992). Interpersonal forgiveness within helping professions: An attempt to resolve differences of opinion. *Counseling and Values, 36,* 84–103.

Epstein, N., & Eidelson, R. J. (1981). Unrealistic beliefs of clinical couples: Their relationship to expectations, goals and satisfaction. *American Journal of Family Therapy, 9*(4), 13–22.

Fenell, D. L. (1993). Characteristics of long-term first marriages. *Journal of Mental Health Counseling, 15*(4), 446–460.

Freedman, S. R., & Enright, R. D. (1996). Forgiveness as an intervention goal with incest survivors. *Journal of Consulting and Clinical Psychology, 64,* 983–992.

Glass, S., & Wright, T. (1997). Reconstructing marriages after the trauma of infidelity. In W. K. Halford & H. J. Markman (Eds.), *Clinical handbook of marriage and couples interventions* (pp. 471–507). Chichester, UK: Wiley.

Gordon, K. C. (1997). *Demystifying forgiveness: A cognitive-behavioral stage model.* Unpublished doctoral dissertation, University of North Carolina–Chapel Hill, Chapel Hill.

Gordon, K. C., & Baucom, D. H. (1999). Understanding betrayals in marriage: A synthesized model of forgiveness. *Family Process, 37*(4), 425–450.

Gordon, K. C., & Baucom, D. H. (in press-b). A forgiveness-based intervention for addressing extramarital affairs. *Clinical Psychology: Science and Practice.*

Gordon, K. C., Pautsch, J., & Baucom, D. H. (1996, November). *Perceptions of forgiveness: A coding system.* Poster presented at the Annual Conference of Association for the Advancement of Behavior Therapy, New York, NY.

Hargrave, T. D., & Sells, J. N. (1997). The development of a forgiveness scale. *Journal of Marital and Family Therapy, 23,* 41–63.

Hebl, J. H., & Enright, R. D. (1993). Forgiveness as a psychotherapeutic goal with elderly females. *Psychotherapy, 30,* 658–667.

Holeman, V. T. (1994). *The relationship between forgiveness of a perpetrator and current marital adjustment for female survivors of childhood sexual abuse.* Unpublished doctoral dissertation, Kent State University, Graduate School of Education, Kent, OH.

Janoff-Bulman, R. (1989). Assumptive worlds and the stress of traumatic events: Applications of the schema construct. *Social Cognition, 7,* 113–136.

Joseph, S., Yule, W., & Williams, R. (1993). Post-traumatic stress: Attributional aspects. *Journal of Traumatic Stress, 6*(4), 501–513.

Katz, J., Street, A., & Arias, I. (1995, November). *Forgive and forget: Women's responses to dating violence.* Poster presented at the Annual Conference of the Association for the Advancement of Behavior Therapy, Washington, DC.

McCann, I. L., Sakheim, D. K., & Abrahamson, D. J. (1988). Trauma and victimization: A model of psychological adaptation. *Counseling Psychologist, 16,* 531–594.

McCullough, M. E., Worthington, E. L., & Rachal, K. C. (1997). Interpersonal forgiving in close relationships. *Journal of Personality and Social Psychology, 73*(2), 321–336.

Notarius, C. I., & Vanzetti, N. A. (1983). The marital agendas protocol. In E. E. Filsinger (Ed.), *Marriage and family assessment: A sourcebook for family therapy* (pp. 209–227). Beverly Hills, CA: Sage.

Pattison, E. M. (1965). On the failure to forgive or to be forgiven. *American Journal of Psychotherapy, 31,* 106–115.

Prager, K. J. (1995). *The psychology of intimacy.* New York: Guilford Press.

Rackley, J. V. (1993). The relationships of marital satisfaction, forgiveness, and religiosity. *Dissertation Abstracts International, 54*(4-A), 1556. (University Microfilms No. DA9319792)

Robinson, E. A., & Price, M. G. (1980). Pleasurable behavior in marital interaction: An observational study. *Journal of Consulting and Clinical Psychology, 48,* 117–118.

Rosenak, C. M., & Harnden, G. M. (1992). Forgiveness in the psychotherapeutic process: Clinical applications. *Journal of Psychology and Christianity, 11,* 188–197.

Selye, H. (1975). Implications of the stress concept. *New York State Journal of Medicine, 75,* 2139–2145.

Smedes, L. B. (1984). *Forgive and forget: Healing the hurts we don't deserve.* New York: Harper & Row.

Snyder, D. K. (in press). Affective reconstruction in the context of a pluralistic approach to couples therapy. *Clinical Psychology: Science and Practice.*

Snyder, D. K., & Wills, R. M. (1989). Behavioral versus insight–oriented marital therapy: Effects on individual and interspousal functioning. *Journal of Consulting and Clinical Psychology, 57,* 39–46.

Snyder, D. K., Wills, R. M., & Grady-Fletcher, A. (1991a). Long-term effectiveness of behavioral versus insight-oriented marital therapy: A four year follow-up study. *Journal of Consulting and Clinical Psychology, 59,* 138–141.

Snyder, D. K., Wills, R. M., & Grady-Fletcher, A. (1991b). Risks and challenges of long-term psychotherapy outcome research: Reply to Jacobson. *Journal of Consulting and Clinical Psychology, 59,* 146–149.

Woodman, T. A. (1992). The role of forgiveness in marriage and marital adjustment. *Dissertation Abstracts International, 53*(4–B), 2079. (University Microfilms No. DA9225999)

Group Interventions to Promote Forgiveness

What Researchers and Clinicians Ought to Know

Everett L. Worthington, Jr., Steven J. Sandage, and Jack W. Berry

Most of the outcome research in the scientific study of forgiveness has involved interventions with ad hoc groups of participants. People who might or might not have a common problem are brought together with a facilitator, therapist, or group leader, and an attempt is made to teach them how better to forgive someone who has hurt or offended them.

In our laboratory, we have conducted several such groups, most of which were psychoeducational groups with university students. We have also conducted interventions with community couples (Ripley, 1998). On the basis of our experience with these groups and through the review of published and other available studies aimed at promoting forgiveness, we offer several suggestions in this chapter. Our intended audience is both intervention researchers and clinicians who might conduct therapeutic, psychoeducational, or preventive groups aimed at promoting forgiveness. The present chapter is aimed at providing practical suggestions in designing and conducting groups in research and clinical situations. Throughout our discussion, we interweave findings from a meta-analytic review of the existing research on group interventions to promote forgiveness.

CONCEPTUAL ISSUES IN RUNNING GROUPS
TO PROMOTE FORGIVENESS

Definitions

Definitions of interpersonal forgiveness are varied and often depend on the investigator's theoretical (and often theological) presuppositions (see Enright & North, 1998; Worthington, 1998a). We have been concerned with interpersonal forgiveness as distinct from Divine forgiveness. We define interpersonal forgiveness as a motivation to reduce avoidance of and retaliation (or revenge) against a person who has harmed or offended one, and to increase conciliation between the parties if conciliation is safe, prudent, or possible. This definition is largely consistent with, but not identical to, a previous definition by McCullough, Worthington, and Rachal (1997), who defined forgiveness as a summary term representing efforts to reduce the motivation to avoid and to seek revenge, and increase the motivation to reconcile or seek conciliation. We thus see forgiveness as an internal motivation (or summary for a set of motivations). Group members might confuse forgiveness with reconciliation, which we define as the restoration of trust in a relationship through mutually trustworthy behaviors of the participants (Worthington, 1998b; Worthington & Drinkard, 1998). This definition of reconciliation is consistent with earlier definitions by Enright and the Human Development Study Group (1994) and McCullough and Worthington (1994). Thus, forgiveness is an internal, intrapsychic event or process, whereas reconciliation is an external, interpersonal event or process. Forgiveness is granted or received, whereas reconciliation is earned through trustworthy behavior.

Interpersonal forgiveness and reconciliation can be affected by transactions between individuals, which we call "forgiveness transactions" to distinguish the term from interpersonal forgiveness (i.e., forgiveness of one person by another). Baumeister, Exline, and Sommer (1998) discussed what we would call forgiveness transactions under the rubric of "interpersonal forgiveness," but we prefer to reserve the term "interpersonal forgiveness" to refer to two people forgiving each other, as distinct from Divine forgiveness. Forgiveness transactions involve discussions about forgiveness in which people make requests for accounts of behaviors, give accounts, accept or reject accounts, apologize, accept or reject apologies, seek forgiveness, express the granting or withholding of forgiveness, ask for restitution, grant or refuse restitution, and state intentions to try not to harm the other person again (similar to the offense under discussion). Forgiveness transactions can influence or be influenced by intrapersonal forgiveness. Similarly, forgiveness transactions can influence or be influenced by efforts at reconciliation. Forgiveness transactions are often part of efforts toward reconciliation (Worthington & Drinkard, 1998).

It is incumbent on leaders of groups, then, to define carefully interpersonal forgiveness at the outset of the group interaction. This can often be done by presenting terms or phrases and allowing group members to discuss what they think forgiveness is or is not. Following a group discussion, the facilitator or leader can draw common themes from the discussion and might present a summary of the definition that can be used throughout the remainder of the group interaction. It is important not to imply that this is the "correct" definition lest the group members become defensive about differences between the proposed definition and their own. Presenting definitions of forgiveness and reconciliation, and drawing distinctions between the two, can often forestall later confusion and misinterpretation.

Generally, in psychoeducational groups that we have conducted, group members might privately hold different definitions of forgiveness than those the group uses as its working definition. That has not typically presented a problem in the dynamics of the group. Social pressure in a well-facilitated group is usually high enough that participants do not overtly challenge the authority of the group's working definition. Obviously, when a participant disagrees substantively with the definition of forgiveness, he or she is less likely to benefit from the group.

Goals of Intervention

Groups function best if the goals are made clear early in the intervention. Goals can range from forgiving an individual who has harmed one a single time to forgiving a person who has harmed or offended one repeatedly. Another goal might be to become a more forgiving person across situations. If the group facilitator does not suggest a goal for the group, individual participants might adopt idiosyncratic goals and thus be disappointed because the group does not focus on their specific goals.

Making clear the expected scope of forgiveness is also important. In a group focusing on forgiving a single act of harm or offense, group members might think that the implied goal of the group is to achieve immediate forgiveness. However, the group leader or researcher might hope to achieve pervasive, lasting forgiveness. On rare occasions, a group leader might want group members to develop a more permanent capacity and willingness to forgive, reflecting the strengthening of "trait forgivingness." (That usually is a more ambitious goal than can be achieved in a brief group.) Group leaders should deliberately plan and communicate to group members the amount of explicit attention to be devoted to the maintenance of gains in forgiveness and to the transfer of forgiveness across situations and people.

Optimal Amount of Intervention

Dose–Effect Relationship

Sheer time spent thinking about forgiveness within a supportive group might be one of the most powerful factors determining the effectiveness of the group. Forgiveness is in many ways a process, though decisions to forgive might be made in a brief period of time (DiBlasio, 1998; Worthington & DiBlasio, 1990). People cognitively and emotionally elaborate on their experiences and deepen their level of forgiveness as the group meets and during intervals between group meetings. We would anticipate that in a group setting, the time spent thinking about and discussing forgiveness would be related to the amount of forgiveness promoted.

Method

To explore this hypothesis, we examined the available intervention outcome studies (Al-Mabuk, Enright, & Cardis, 1995, Studies 1 and 2; Bryant, 1998; Coyle & Enright, 1997; Freedman & Enright, 1996; Hebl & Enright, 1993; Hepp-Dax, 1996; Kurusu, 1996, 1998; Luskin & Thoresen, 1998; McCullough & Worthington, 1995; McCullough et al., 1997; Ripley, 1998; Rye, 1998, secular and religiously integrated conditions). All but two intervention studies (Coyle & Enright, 1997; Freedman & Enright, 1996) have used groups to deliver the intervention. We did not include Hepp-Dax's (1996) intervention because it was the sole intervention with children. We have examined only the groups that sought to promote forgiveness (not the control groups), tabulating data on the group interventions in Table 11.1. Two documents each contributed two forgiveness interventions to Table 11.1: Al-Mabuk et al. (1995), who reported two studies, and Rye (1998), who used two forgiveness groups, both aimed at producing forgiveness (one secular and one religiously integrated). In some cases, multiple measures of forgiveness were used, but we did not report or aggregate all measures. For example, a number of studies used several of Wade's (1989) nine subscales to measure forgiveness. We selected revenge, avoidance, and conciliation subscales (if those were used) and ignored the others to permit more comparability across studies. Altogether, the analyzed interventions represent 393 participants in forgiveness interventions delivered in group format.

To examine the relationship between the amount of time that people spend reflecting on forgiveness within a group and the outcome of forgiveness, we plotted a modified dose–effect curve in Figure 11.1. (In biological sciences, dose–effect curves typically use the logarithm of the dose; we did not use the logarithm.) The abscissa is hours of group intervention, and the ordinate is preintervention to postintervention effect size.

TABLE 11.1. Summary of Characteristics of Outcome Interventions Conducted with Groups

Study	Study N	Treat. Group n	No. of groups	Percent male	Forgiveness measures	Post-pre	SD pooled	ES	Hours	Weeks
Kurusu (1996)	100	80	8	24	Wade	6.0	20.8	0.28	1	1
McCullough & Worthington (1995)	86	30	4	24	Wade (Revenge, Avoidance pooled)	a	a	0.08	1	1
Bryant (1998)	106	28	4	30	Wade (Revenge, Avoidance pooled)	b	b	.37	2	1
Kurusu (1998)c	64	55	11	9	Wade (Revenge, Avoidance, Conciliation)	3.27	14.86	.22	2	1
Al-Mabuk, Enright, & Cardis (1995), Study 1	48	24	1	23	Psychological Profile of Forgiveness	-3.7	11.9	-0.31	4	2
Ripley (1998)c	96	28	6	50	Wade (Revenge, Avoidance, Conciliation)	1.6	5.4	0.30	6	1
Sandage (1997)	136	31	4	29	Enright Forgiveness Inventory	32.6	62.6	0.52	6	1
Luskin & Thoresen (1998)	55	28	2	23	Wade (Revenge, Avoidance, Conciliation)	d	d	.24	6	6
Al-Mabuk, Enright, & Cardis (1995), Study 2	45	24	1	25	Psychological Profile of Forgiveness	20.5	16.2	1.27	6	6
Hebi & Enright (1993)	24	13	1	0	Psychological Profile of Forgiveness	11.9	15.6	0.76	8	8
McCullough, Worthington, & Rachal (1997)	134	13	2	42	Enright Forgiveness Inventory (5 items only)	4.8	5.1	0.94	8	1
Rye (1998), religiously integrated	58	19	3	0	Rye (1998)	e	e	1.47	9	6
Rye (1998), secular	58	20	3	0	Rye (1998)	f	f	1.45	9	6

Note. Effect sizes are computed by taking pre- to posttest differences in variables measuring forgiveness and dividing by the pooled standard deviations. Whenever several dependent variables were relevant, (1) only measures of actual forgiveness were used (not hypothetical situations) and (2) effect sizes for different dependent measures were pooled. (Subscales that should decrease with increased forgiveness [e.g., Revenge, Avoidance] were reverse-scored.) Thus, all effect sizes that are positive show increased forgiveness from pre- to posttest.

[a] Revenge ES = 1.1/8.8; Avoidance ES = 0.2/8.0.

[b] Bryant (1998) reported Avoidance (reverse-scored) ES = 1.54/7.56; Revenge (reverse-scored) ES = 2.46/4.62.

[c] Kurusu (1998) and Ripley (1998) reported Wade Conciliation, Revenge (reverse-scored), and Avoidance (reverse-scored) summed.

[d] Revenge (Malice) ES =7/4.4; Avoidance (Estrangement) ES =.8/7.4; Conciliation ES = 2.4/5.3.

[e] Forgiveness, Affective, ES = 6.79/6.20; Forgiveness, Appraisal, ES = 6.81/3.73; scales created by Rye (1998).

[f] Forgiveness, Affective, ES = 6.10/5.14; Forgiveness, Appraisal, ES = 8.53/4.98; scales created by Rye (1998).

Effect size was determined by subtracting the preintervention group mean on the main forgiveness measure (or occasionally an aggregate of measures, where subscales that were expected to decrease with increasing forgiveness were reverse-scored) from the postintervention group mean and dividing by the pooled standard deviations of the pre- and post-intervention scores. In the event that no pretest was reported (i.e., Al-Mabuk et al., 1995; Luskin & Thoresen, 1998), the control group post-intervention mean was taken to be equivalent to what would have been the preintervention mean (resulting in Cohen's d). We preferred to use preintervention means when available, using the participants as their own controls (and thus minimizing differences due to sampling that are inherent in using Cohen's d).

Most studies used either a version of Enright's Psychological Profile of Forgiveness (Al-Mabuk et al., 1995; Hebl & Enright, 1993), the Enright Forgiveness Inventory (Subkoviak et al., 1995) in whole (Sandage, 1997) or in part (McCullough et al., 1997), the Avoidance, Revenge, and Conciliation subscales (or shortened versions) of Wade's (1989) forgiveness measure (Kurusu, 1996; Luskin & Thoresen, 1998; McCullough & Worthington, 1995; Ripley, 1998), or the Avoidance and Revenge subscales of Wade's measures (later shaped into the Transgression-Related Interpersonal Motivations Inventory; TRIM; McCullough, Rachal, Sandage, Worthington, Brown, & Hight, 1998). Rye (1998) used two subscales of a

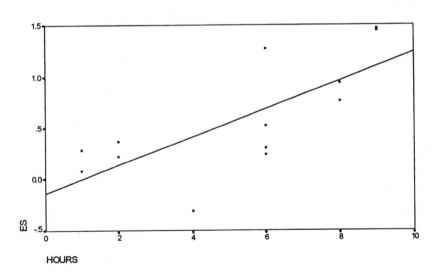

FIGURE 11.1. Dose–effect relationship for group interventions to promote forgiveness.

measure created for his study (Forgiveness Affect and Forgiveness Appraisal). McCullough et al. (1997) used a 5-item scale from the Enright Forgiveness Inventory, which is not recommended for future research.[1] Data were analyzed by considering each forgiveness group as a data point. Bivariate correlations between time (i.e., hours or weeks) of group intervention and effect size were calculated.

Results

Overall, we found a marked dose–effect curve. We fit a linear curve to the data. The beta coefficient for the weighted least squares regression between hours of intervention and effect size was $R = .70$, $p < .007$. The regression line is drawn in Figure 11.1. We calculated a weighted mean effect size ($ES_{weighted} = .43$) and 95% confidence interval (95% CI = .29/.57). (Weights were the inverse of the variance of the effect size estimates.) The 95% confidence interval around the weighted mean effect size did not contain zero, indicating that a homogenized "forgiveness intervention" that did not consider duration of the intervention can be expected (with 95% confidence) to produce an effect. However, that statistic is relatively meaningless in light of our argument that there is a dose–effect relationship. One should not care about whether homogenized "forgiveness interventions" produce an effect different from zero. One should care whether clinically relevant interventions (we defined those as interventions of 6 or more hours) are different from zero, and whether experimentally interesting but nonclinically relevant interventions (we defined those of 1 or 2 hours) are different from zero.[2] Clinically relevant forgiveness interventions ($k = 8$ studies) can be expected, with 95% confidence, to produce forgiveness ($ES_{weighted} = .76$; 95% CI = .57/.95). Nonclinically relevant forgiveness interventions ($k = 4$) can also be expected, with 95% confidence, to produce a small but measurable amount of forgiveness ($ES_{weighted} = .24$; 95% CI = .04/.44). We offer these conclusions with the caveat that our analysis is based on little power, and the conclusions are thus suspect.

Tentative Conclusions

Data suggest that amount of time thinking about forgiveness is important in the amount of forgiveness a person can experience. The 1- and 2-hour interventions are virtually inert. Al-Mabuk et al.'s (1995) Study 1 used only the first 10 (of 17) steps in Enright's process model. The group actually had a negative effect, suggesting that if people reflect on their hurts without being led toward forgiveness, the effects might be counterproductive. Study 1 might be contrasted to Al-Mabuk et al.'s Study 2, in which people were led through Enright's full process model. Confounded with changes in content are changes in (1) duration of the intervention (6 weeks rather than 2 weeks) and (2) number of sessions (six rather than four).

Based on the dose–effect curve using studies from different theoretical positions, one might initially conclude that the content of the interventions might not be as important as the sheer amount of time spent thinking about forgiveness or interacting about it within the group context (and thus experiencing other benefits of groups such as social support, seeing other examples of forgiveness and unforgiveness, spending more time experiencing empathy, expressing more affect, experiencing more group affiliation, etc.). The same trend obtains within intervention models. Within studies that tested Enright's model (Al-Mabuk et al., 1995, Study 1, Study 2; Hebl & Enright, 1993) and those that tested McCullough and Worthington's model (Bryant, 1998; Kurusu, 1996, 1998; McCullough & Worthington, 1995; McCullough et al., 1997; Ripley, 1998; Sandage, 1997), differences in time seem to account for much of the improvement (though the n is too small for a statistical test). Presumably, much of the same content could be covered within the models. Albeit, in greater amounts of time, more content could be covered. Researchers and clinicians who plan interventions should be cognizant of an effect for time and should not think that interventions can be dramatically shortened and still achieve strong effects.

We recommend that group interventions aimed solely at promoting forgiveness last at least 6 hours. Interventions that are adjuncts to therapy or occur within an ongoing group not aimed solely at producing forgiveness might be shorter, but the leader should not expect large changes in forgiveness to occur.

Spacing of Sessions

The spacing of sessions might also be a factor (see Table 11.1). For example, McCullough and Worthington's interventions have taken place on an intensive weekend, where participants met in groups on Friday nights for 2–3 hours and continued the group on Saturday from 3 (Ripley, 1998; Sandage, 1997) to 6 (McCullough et al., 1997) hours. Another model has involved weekly group meetings of 1 hour (Al-Mabuk et al., 1995, Study 2; Hebl & Enright, 1993; Luskin & Thoresen, 1998), 1½ hours (Rye, 1998), or 2 hours (Al-Mabuk et al., 1995, Study 1). We recalculated the dose–effect regression using duration in weeks (instead of hours of intervention). The R was .64, $p < .02$ ($R^2 = .35$). Of course, duration in weeks and time spent in group are confounded, so it is impossible to determine the unique effects of each with such sparse data as are currently available. Nonetheless, we would tentatively recommend (subject to more precise investigations) that, to some degree, sessions be spaced rather than massed.

Time-Limited, Closed-Membership Groups or Open-Ended, Open-Membership Groups

Psychoeducational and most therapy groups to promote forgiveness will generally be time-limited. All groups that have been investigated experimentally have been time-limited (see Table 11.1). Duration has varied from 1 to 9 hours. In contrast to group approaches, in one investigation of women who had experienced some form of sexual abuse, Freedman and Enright (1996) used individual counseling, which they continued until people had forgiven (mean of 14 months of weekly sessions). In contrast to time-limited groups, open-membership groups would add new members as they became available, and old members would drop out as they achieved their criterion of forgiveness. An open-membership, open-ended group would typically (though not necessarily always) preclude any curriculum limited to promoting forgiveness unless the curriculum was brief and repeated periodically. The group would likely be oriented toward a more general goal—such as toward improving interpersonal relationships (of which forgiveness might be an important part). This is not to say that forgiveness could not be dealt with effectively in open-ended, open-membership groups, but doing so faces substantial challenges in designing and carrying out a curriculum.

Clientele

Severity and Chronicity of Harm or Offense

Groups that have attempted to promote forgiveness have differed in the amount of specificity with which the participants were selected. Some groups have targeted people with precisely defined harms. Al-Mabuk et al. (1995) aimed groups at parentally love-deprived college students. Hebl and Enright (1993) sought to promote forgiveness in the elderly. Severe and long-lasting harms have not been addressed via group interventions. On the other hand, some groups have targeted more general populations and recruited participants who wanted to forgive a person for a particular offense or harmful act (Kurusu, 1996, 1998; McCullough & Worthington, 1995; McCullough et al., 1997; Sandage, 1997). In those groups, the harm or offense was generally perceived to be fairly severe by the participants, usually rated between severe and very severe. Still other groups (Ripley, 1998) have taught forgiveness as a general skill (for enhancing marriage and preventing future problems) without targeting a particular hurt. For example, Ripley ran groups of couples, solicited from the community, whose aim was to enhance intimacy and prevent harm from escalating in their relationship. Ripley did not select couples who had particular harms or offenses with which they wanted to deal. In fact, in that enrichment setting, many couples denied having *any* unresolved hurts.

We recommend that the boundaries within which forgiveness interventions can be helpfully applied be investigated scientifically. Severity of hurts and offenses seems to greatly influence the ease with which people are able to forgive. There might be some evidence that hurts and offenses that are extremely severe result in a revision of people's cognitive framework for understanding existence (Flanigan, 1998). Such cognitive reorganizations would undoubtedly require either a long time to repair or an extremely powerful intervention—probably beyond the capability of most interventions developed to date. Thus, we recommend that clinicians and researchers prepare longer, powerful interventions aimed at groups of people with severe or chronic unforgiveness.

Who Attends the Groups?

Because forgiveness is something one person grants another and is often intimately tied to reconciliation or a lack of reconciliation, the issue of whether participants within a group are to be individuals or whether both participants are to be present is difficult to resolve. When both partners are present in the group, forgiveness is not as simple as when only the offended or harmed person is the group member. Screening couples is, we believe, more important than screening individuals. Couples who are highly vocal and in very conflictual relationships can dominate group interactions. Couples who admit to partner violence, we believe, should be either treated individually (as a couple or as two individual partners) or treated in groups of couples who are struggling with the same issue.

Interpersonal transactions around forgiveness, such as how partners seek forgiveness (Enright & the Human Development Study Group, 1996), whether and how one apologizes for wrongdoing, how explicit the confession of wrongdoing is, how each partner accounts for wrongdoing (Sitkim & Beis, 1993), and whether one is willing to accept forgiveness once it has been offered are important components of the forgiveness process (Baumeister et al., 1998). Reconciliation becomes mixed with forgiveness (Worthington & Drinkard, 1998); that is, people who forgive a friend or partner who is present in the same group can spontaneously attempt to repair the relationship and can thus engage in reconciliation behaviors. Alternatively, partners attending the group together can rekindle conflicts and subvert the group's focus on forgiveness through having arguments or harmful and toxic interactions. Thus, conducting groups on forgiveness in which both partners are present is riskier than conducting groups of individuals who forgive an absent offender. On the other hand, if both partners are present, forgiveness can be dealt with in context. Furthermore, opportunities are available for partners to learn by watching other couples. When couples are present, the group leader should probably focus on forgiveness within a broad twofold context of (1) conflict management to handle differences and (2) reconciliation to repair any harm from attempting to resolve conflict.

Potential Target Populations

There are many potential populations for forgiveness interventions. We have grouped some of these populations into three categories according to common sources of unforgiveness (see Table 11.2). First, some potential targets for forgiveness are due to events within large social or political contexts. Second, many opportunities for forgiveness occur within families and romantic relationships. People living in close proximity and communicating intimately provide numerous opportunities for misunderstandings and for harmful interactions. Third, people's health and health care provide another category in which opportunities to forgive abound. People are highly invested in their health and in receiving good medical treatment; disappointments are legion.

Groups Tailored to Clientele

Groups designed to promote forgiveness should be tailored to the clientele. If forgiveness were addressed in communities using Alcoholics Anonymous 12-step programs, personal confession might be greatly valued; whereas, in some other communities, personal confession might not be expected nor appreciated. In religious communities, forgiveness might be embedded within a religious framework, whether that be Jewish (Dorff, 1998), Christian (Marty, 1998), or generally Judeo–Christian (Rye, 1998). Different subcultures have different norms that would be expected in the conduct of different groups. The role of guilt, apology, or confession might be high in some religious communities, whereas in other religious communities, those might be minimized.

Subgroup norms can be important to the effectiveness of the group because they may activate variables that mediate or moderate (see Baron & Kenny, 1986) the impact of intervention on forgiveness. For instance, McCullough et al. (1997) found data consistent with the hypothesis that empathy is a proximal cause of forgiveness. Thus, subcultures that value empathy might be more prone to respond to forgiveness interventions than would groups that do not value empathy. Similarly, variables such as guilt (Baumeister, Stillwell, & Heatherton, 1994), shame (Tangney, Wagner, Barlow, & Marschall, 1996), humility (Means, Wilson, Sturm, Piron, & Bach, 1990), self-esteem (Baumeister, Exline, & Sommer, 1998), apology (Weiner, Graham, Peter, & Zmuidinas, 1991), or one's status as either victim or perpetrator (Stillwell & Baumeister, 1997) might affect the outcomes and conduct of a group. For example, dealing with forgiveness in

TABLE 11.2. A Three-Category Listing of Some Pertinent Target Groups for Forgiveness

People in whom unforgiveness is stimulated by social or political issues

Victims of crime
Victims of unethical work practices
Victims of workplace aggression or discrimination
People who have been "downsized" into unemployment
People who have experienced racial, ethnic, gender, age, or religious discrimination
People who belong to ethnic groups who have a history of mutual conflict and harm

People in whom unforgiveness is stimulated by romantic or family relationships

Divorced, separated, or divorcing partners, or children in divorced or divorcing families
Victims of aggressive traumas (e.g., sexual abuse, physical abuse, domestic violence, rape, etc.)
People who are (or have been) involved in intrafamily and intergenerational conflict
People who are married or in a cohabiting relationship in which one partner has been (or is) sexually unfaithful
Children who are developing the capacity to forgive
People who have experienced romantic rejections
Those who have been harmed or rejected by a deceased parent
Caretakers who do not receive adequate support from other family members

People in whom unforgiveness is stimulated or exacerbated by medical or health issues

People facing the end of their lives through disease
HIV-infected people
Patients with cardiovascular disease or people at risk for developing it
People with mental health problems that might be related to unforgiveness
Hypertension or stroke patients
People who have problems in substance or alcohol abuse
People who are elderly and are dealing with end-of-life stress issues
Victims of failed medical treatment

offender–victim reconciliation programs provides many special challenges (see Couper, 1998; Dickey, 1998).

Alternative Treatments: Is Forgiveness the Target or a Means to an End?

When people have been hurt or offended, they do not necessarily seek treatment for forgiveness or reconciliation. Often, they seek treatment for the mental health consequences and emotional distress they feel. Consequently, practitioners and researchers might use groups aimed at promoting forgiveness as freestanding adjuncts to psychotherapy.

Alternatively, interventions to promote forgiveness could be integrated into other group treatments to deal with mental health difficulties, emotional distress, or relational problems. Several theoreticians (e.g., Fitzgibbons, 1986; Luskin & Thoresen, 1998) have developed cognitive-behavioral models of forgiveness. Others have written psychodynamic theoretical expositions of forgiveness (e.g., Gartner, 1988; Vitz & Mango, 1997), though none have been tailored to groups. Theoreticians have asserted (as yet without empirical support for their assertions) that the emotions most commonly associated with unforgiveness are either fear or anxiety (Worthington, 1998b) or anger (Fitzgibbons, 1986; Kaplan, 1992; Luskin & Thoresen, 1998). Thus, anxiety-management treatments (e.g., systematic desensitization in its variants), treatments of social anxiety (Lindemann, 1996), or anger-management treatments (e.g., Deffenbacher, 1995) might serve as bases into which elements of forgiveness are integrated. In addition, target problems, such as marital discord or sexual abuse (e.g., see Jacobson & Gurman, 1995; Madanes, 1991), or drug and alcohol addiction, might provide platforms that can launch modules on forgiveness. Preventive or enrichment programs, such as preparation for marriage, parenthood, or other life transitions, might also provide a platform to discuss forgiveness and reconciliation. Special attention must be given to whether participants are willing to accept forgiveness as a legitimate portion of the intervention to which they have subscribed.

The question of whether forgiveness is indeed a target of a group intervention should be considered prior to the onset of a group. For instance, forgiveness, reconciliation, communication training, or even support during separation, might be legitimate goals in groups of spouses dealing with marital infidelity. The target of intervention must be clearly articulated if the group is to be successful. Some consensus on the goals of the group is necessary for harmonious group process as well as achievement of goals of individual members.

RESEARCH CONSIDERATIONS

Numerous sources have described how to conduct effective intervention research. Generally, well-designed research is more likely to detect differences than is less well-designed research (see Cooper & Hedges, 1994). Wampold et al. (1997) have shown that with well-designed research, interventions that are intended to produce a therapeutic effect are usually effective and are usually no more effective than other interventions. Wampold et al.'s findings seem consistent with the dose–effect relationship we detected in the present chapter, in that theoretical perspective seemed to make less difference than did time spent in the intervention. Thoresen, Luskin, and Harris (1998) have described some of these considerations as they apply to research on forgiveness, so we will not attempt to duplicate those here. We note a few considerations arising from our review.

Participant Variables

Personality Attributes Affecting Receptivity to Forgiveness

Numerous variables might impinge on why people do or do not forgive (for a review, see McCullough, Exline, & Baumeister, 1998). One candidate for a personality or person variable that might affect people's receptivity to treatment is empathic capacity (McCullough et al., 1997). People with low empathic capacity, such as those with narcissistic, borderline, antisocial, or avoidant personality disorders or traits, are unlikely to benefit from interventions that attempt to generate empathy to stimulate forgiveness.

Gender is also potentially important. Women seem more likely to forgive and certainly are more likely to participate in forgiveness research. If extant studies are analyzed according to gender, the 13 forgiveness groups (see Table 11.1) show that 79% of the total participants have been women. No studies have investigated gender differences in actual forgiveness. To estimate the likelihood of a gender–forgiveness effect, across the 13 studies summarized in Table 11.1, we correlated effect size and percent males using weighted least-squares regression (to adjust for sample size). The correlation was $R = .34$, with the standardized beta being $-.34$, $p = .26$, $R^2 = .11$. The negative beta indicated that males tended toward being less forgiving than were females; however, the correlation was not significant. When considering these findings together—that fewer men than women volunteer for forgiveness interventions and that even among the ones who volunteer, forgiveness tends not to be achieved as often for men as for women—we can conclude (tentatively) that men are substantially more at risk for holding onto unforgiveness than are women. We very tentatively recommend that additional studies of gender effects be undertaken and that perhaps groups be designed, targeted specifically at men's issues, and that roadblocks to their forgiving be identified.

Religion is another potentially important participant variable to consider in forgiveness intervention research (McCullough & Worthington, 1999). People who are from a strongly religious, conservative Christian tradition have strong group norms that mandate forgiveness (Girard & Mullet, 1997; Rokeach, 1973), making it likely that such people will self-report forgiveness, and this might affect initial values of forgiveness because of response bias. High self-reported levels of initial forgiveness might affect the possible gains these people make because of ceiling effects. Rye (1998) found no interaction among time, secular versus religious condition, and high versus low (using a median or mean split) intrinsic religiosity. However, evidence exists that splitting a general population at the mean of religious measures is unlikely to produce many effects of religious variables (see Worthington, Kurusu, McCullough, & Sandage, 1996, for a review). Worthington has hypothesized that only people higher than one standard deviation from the mean of religious variables generally perceive the world according to religious categories. Thus, the hypothesis that forgiveness might be experienced differently for highly religious individuals relative to those of moderate and less religiosity has not yet been addressed empirically. We recommend that interventions, such as Rye's (1998) intervention aimed at Christians, be applied to groups in which people are all highly religious.

Culture

According to speculation by some writers, culture and race appear also to be important factors in forgiveness (McAleese, 1998). People from cultures such as Northern Ireland, South Africa, or Rwanda have many factors beyond the individual hurts that make extending forgiveness difficult for them. In addition, African Americans who feel that their race has been systematically discriminated against have legitimate concerns about social power that complicate dealing with an offense by an individual of a different race.[3] Those culturally loaded issues often must be addressed. Ethnicity of the group leader might be important in groups of people of color, though we could find no evidence that addressed that hypothesis directly.

Situational Variables

People who are in ongoing relationships in which offenses are continual or frequent might be unable to benefit from interventions designed to stimulate forgiveness. Ongoing conflict is so powerful that recent events tend to undo benefits of the group almost immediately.

Independent Variables

The independent variable is the nature of the forgiveness intervention. Many factors affect the effectiveness of interventions. For instance, the degree of standardization of the forgiveness intervention is important in knowing exactly what causes an intervention to succeed or fail. The content might be important. At present, treatments are complex and multifaceted. With the findings presented in this brief meta-analysis, we believe that no conclusions can be drawn about which elements of various interventions are effective, which are harmful, and which are inert (with the possible exception that the connection between forgiveness and empathic concern might be well enough supported to merit a recommendation that investigators include such considerations in designing interventions to promote forgiveness).

When we examined the content of the interventions (in a non-systematic manner), we found substantial agreement on the content across studies. All interventions (1) invited people to reflect on specific hurts or offenses; (2) emphasized empathic capacity; (3) treated forgiveness as if people must consider emotional, behavioral, and cognitive elements (rather than any single element); (4) moved people toward a conscious decision to grant forgiveness; and (5) invited participants to reframe the event (though the ways people were invited to reframe were different). Less agreement was found on whether participants were taught to modify self-statements using cognitive-behavioral methods (Luskin & Thoresen; Rye), deal explicitly with anger management (Luskin & Thoresen; Rye), adopt a perspective of humility (Bryant; Enright; Kurusu; Ripley; Rye; Sandage), or consider the fundamental attribution error (McCullough, Rye).

Treatment Manuals

One standard by which most intervention studies are judged is the presence of a detailed treatment manual (Kazdin, 1994). Controversies surround the use of treatment manuals because to the extent that interventions are prescribed and followed rigorously, creativity and responsiveness to unforeseen situations within groups or within a client's interaction with a leader are precluded. On the other hand, to the extent that a leader is flexible in responding to individual personalities and events, treatment manuals become increasingly meaningless. Nonetheless, modern psychotherapy research is built on the expectation that treatments in intervention studies will be based on a manual that will be created, followed, and made available to other researchers. Clinically wise group leaders and therapists expect to deviate at times from the manual when clinical intuition or experience dictates.

Groups per Treatment

One issue of particular importance in group research is the number of groups that are run within each treatment condition (Burlingame, Kircher, & Honts, 1994; Hoyle & Crawford, 1994). If, for example, a design had one treatment and one control condition, and one treatment group and one control group were run in each condition, a reader could not interpret the meaning of a finding that showed that the treatment condition was superior to the control condition. Groups develop unique characteristics as individuals in the groups interact with each other. Thus, the single group per condition would confound the particular people who are in each group, the leader, setting, time of day, and so on, with the content of the intervention.

It is advantageous to allow several leaders to run at least two groups in each treatment (and control) condition.[4] This combats the concerns that (1) leaders are confounded with treatment condition, and also (2) leaders are confounded with groups. It allows generalization. After groups have been run, analyses of variance should be conducted to determine whether the groups (nested within conditions) affected dependent variables equally (Burlingame et al., 1994; Hoyle & Crawford, 1994). Researchers might check leaders' preferences for each intervention to discern whether such preferences might make a difference in outcome.

Effective Leaders

The relationship between outcome and amount of leader training in conducting interventions designed to promote forgiveness has not been considered. In the studies in Table 11.1, training of leaders was reported only for McCullough and Worthington (1995; 1 hour plus use of cue sheets), McCullough et al. (1997; 4 hours, use of manual), Sandage (1997; 2 hours, use of manual), Rye (1998; 1 hour plus 1 hour per week supervision), Ripley (1998; 4 hours, use of manual), Kurusu (1996; 2 hours, use of manual), Kurusu (1998; 3 hours, use of manual), Bryant (1998; 2 hours, use of manual), and Al-Mabuk et al. (1995; "some" training). Characteristics of leaders who are more or less effective at running groups that promote forgiveness have not been determined. All groups except one (Hebl & Enright, 1993) have been conducted by graduate students. Clinical experience of leaders—and especially experience specifically with forgiveness groups—might affect outcome. No studies have conducted process research on variables affecting the delivery of the intervention. Consequently, at this point, no conclusions can be drawn about who can conduct forgiveness interventions effectively.

Setting

The setting in which a forgiveness intervention is delivered might affect the treatment. For example, a religiously oriented forgiveness intervention delivered to theologically conservative religious participants within a church setting might differ in its effectiveness from the same treatment delivered in the office of a therapist or in a university clinic setting (Pargament, 1997; Rye, 1998). Similarly, such a group leader who is a member of the clergy might be expected to achieve different results than would a psychologist or a graduate student. In short, there is an expected interaction between the characteristics of the leader or facilitator, setting, and relevant personal attributes of group members.

Control Group

Choice of a control group must be made within several boundaries. An ethical boundary must be adhered to in that treatment should be provided to patients who need treatment if it is possible to provide that treatment. Thus, no-treatment conditions in clinical settings should be avoided.

An alternative is to use a waiting-list control condition. After a suitable waiting period in which people on a waiting list complete the same assessments as do those in the treatment condition(s), the people on the waiting list would then receive the intervention. This satisfies ethical requirements in that if the clinician is not able to provide treatment during the waiting-list period but does provide treatment later, then the participants do have the opportunity to receive the treatment of interest. A waiting-list design has two problems: (1) It precludes any possibility of additional long-term follow-up; (2) in existing research in which complex interventions have usually been compared to waiting-list control groups, there is no way to discern which element within that complex intervention is actually responsible for producing forgiveness.

Analog research is needed to dismantle complex interventions or to build up interventions from their basic elements. Such research designs can allow investigators to determine the critical parts of the program that are causing the effects.

Yalom (1970) has identified curative factors that occur by virtue of participating in a group. These factors include such elements as installation of hope, universality, psychoeducation, altruism, corrective recapitulation of the primary family group, development of socialization, imitation, interpersonal learning, cohesiveness, catharsis, and existential factors. Investigators should create control-group conditions that provide nonspecific group effects without including forgiveness as an intervention. Alternatively, some process measures of the response to the curative factors might be statistically removed from the outcome in comparing group treatments with control conditions that do not involve a group.

Another possible control condition is an alternative treatment. An alternative treatment might be an intervention similar to the full treatment except for the presence of elements promoting forgiveness. For example, in studying the empathy model of forgiveness, an alternative treatment would induce empathy with the offender but make no attempt to promote forgiveness. Al-Mabuk et al. (1995) employed a variant of this methodology. In Study 1, participants received 10 of 17 steps in Enright's process model. In Study 2, participants received all steps. Due to differences between Studies 1 and 2 (e.g., time of treatment, spacing of treatment, etc.), it is not possible to conclude that the addition of steps 11–17 caused more forgiveness than occurred in Study 1. Nonetheless, Al-Mabuk et al.'s article is the only attempt at identifying active components of intervention in the available literature. An alternative treatment might also be an intervention aimed at changing a correlate of unforgiveness, such as anxiety (anxiety-management training) or anger (anger control) or relationship problems (such as communication training).

Attrition

It is not always easy to ensure that people who begin a treatment will finish it. Some participants selectively are more likely to drop out of forgiveness treatments. Such people often tend to be the people who need forgiveness the most; that is, people in ongoing and hurtful relationships who consequently cannot see the benefits of participation in the group. In addition, people who have settled into a generally unforgiving life pattern are likely to drop out of treatment because they might view forgiveness as an indication of weakness, or they might simply find forgiveness too difficult because it works in opposition to their normal behavior. An effort to become a more forgiving person might be met with cynicism and distrust within their friendship network. Their participation in a forgiveness group might thus be punished by their friends and colleagues who do not treat their efforts to forgive as serious. In addition, people who have personality problems might also selectively drop out of interventions. Group leaders might make themselves available to discuss such concerns or refer people to therapy, though each solution might compromise the integrity of the study.

Dependent Variables

Choice of Dependent Measures

The choice of dependent variables is also of crucial importance in outcome research on forgiveness. Clearly, dependent variables should be chosen that are related to the goals of the intervention. If the intervention aims to help an individual forgive one person for one hurtful event, then that should be measured as the dependent variable. Generalization should be tested to see whether effects were achieved on the person's personality, whether the person became more forgiving as a person, or on the relationship, and whether the relationship benefited.

Multiple Dependent Variables

In addition to measuring degree of forgiveness directly in terms of self-report, it is advantageous to use a multitrait, multimethod strategy to infer the effectiveness of group interventions. These multiple methods might involve the report of others as to whether a person appears more forgiving. They might include physiological measures, which might indicate whether forgiveness has taken place. For instance, it might be found that forgiveness is correlated with lower measures of stressfulness (e.g., blood cortisol level), lowered psychophysiological reactivity, reduced physical indications of fear or anger, and the like. Such physiological measures might "triangulate" with self-reports and other-reports of forgiveness to boost confidence that forgiveness has indeed occurred after an intervention.

Forgiveness has not yet been shown empirically to correlate with improved health, though hypotheses have been advanced that suggest such a connection. Potential correlates with state forgiveness or trait forgivingness might include measures of Type A behavior (Friedman et al., 1986; Kaplan, 1992), immune functioning (Herbert & Cohen, 1993; Kiecolt-Glaser et al., 1996), trust, hostility (Williams, 1989), relationship or dyadic satisfaction and commitment (Rusbult, Verette, Whitney, Slovik, & Lipkus, 1991), and others such as anxiety, anger, or other emotional states. It is likely that chronic unforgiveness (or trait unforgivingness) rather than acute unforgiveness will be found to be related to negative health indices and that trait forgivingness rather than states of forgiveness will be related to positive health indices. In spite of there being no extant evidence that directly links unforgiveness, unforgivingness, forgiveness, or forgivingness to health correlates, researchers should consider measuring health variables to establish whether there are any associations between health and unforgiveness or forgiveness.

Additionally, forgiveness is intrapersonal and has been measured by assessing individuals. However, transactions around forgiveness might affect and be affected by interpersonal forgiveness and might affect and be affected by reconciliation. Future studies need to attend to ramifications of interpersonal forgiveness on transactions around forgiveness and vice versa. In addition, forgiveness and transactions need to be considered within the context of reconciliation. Measures need to be developed and refined to measure the host of interrelated constructs associated with forgiveness.

Degree of Change

The degree of change in such measures is important. Researchers must consider not only how much forgiveness is statistically significant, but also how much is clinically significant. What degree of unforgiveness is conducive to poor health outcomes or poor relational outcomes? What degree of reconciliation is related to better or worse relational outcomes?

Timing of Taking Dependent Measures

Earlier, we mentioned that follow-up measurements had been made in a number of intervention studies that attempted to promote forgiveness. One question that the researcher must address is the appropriate amount of time after a treatment ends for a follow-up measurement to be taken. Most measurements have been made at either 3- or 4-weeks postintervention. At that time, the effects of treatment have generally been maintained, perhaps with slight decay.

The researcher must consider the reasonable amount of time for a forgiveness intervention to last. One would hope that if people forgive those who have harmed them, then that forgiveness will last forever. However, in relationships that are ongoing, other relationship events intrude between the end of treatment and the follow-up assessment. Thus, the likelihood increases that other hurtful or offensive events may take place, or alternatively, that other healing events might take place in the relationship that obscure the effects of the treatment. One technical solution to the problem would be to measure the relationship events that might have occurred since the end of treatment. Those events could serve as dependent variables as a consequence of treatment and also as variables that become new moderating variables or new independent variables for other outcomes.

In this chapter, we have suggested considerations necessary to conduct good research on groups to promote forgiveness. Clearly, the scientific study of the promotion of forgiveness is embryonic. Four groups of researchers have conducted all the studies reported to date, and most of those studies come from two groups of researchers. In the early stages of scientific study, a diversity of methods is recommended for effective study. Thus, we advocate case studies, multiple $n = 1$ studies, and other approaches that are likely to uncover findings that might be obscured by sole reliance on a single methodology (i.e., the studies reviewed in the present chapter).

CLOSING

Generally, in group interventions to promote forgiveness and reconciliation, the effects of one or two group facilitators are leveraged so that they can (we hope) help many people at once. With leverage, though, come special considerations needed to conduct effective groups and to produce meaningful research on group interventions. Consequently, group treatments deserve specific focused attention. In particular, many special considerations are necessary in designing and conducting groups in such a way that the effects can be clearly discerned and the outcomes can be attributed to the parts of the treatment that promote forgiveness.

Several research issues are of pressing concern to the field. These include the following:

- Continued research on populations to which group interventions can and cannot be applied effectively.
- Process analyses that determine the active ingredients of established group interventions.
- Creation of other effective groups by researchers who approach the topic from other (than the four established programs) theoretical frameworks, followed by intervention research to determine which elements of the new groups are effective.

In addition, an essential question must be addressed. Given the findings we have presented about the dose–effect relationship, is there benefit to addressing forgiveness briefly? For example, in an interpersonal group, if the topic of unforgiveness arose for group members, would it be worthwhile to address the topic in an hour or two, given the research indicating that such interventions will likely produce minimal effects?

This question might be extended beyond the bounds of the present chapter. The dose–effect relationship seems strong within groups. Two studies to date have investigated forgiveness in individual psychotherapy (Coyle & Enright, 1997; Freedman & Enright, 1996). Both have used long-term interventions of 18 and 60 weeks. If we had included the data, they would have fit the dose–effect curve for group interventions. Will brief interventions intended to promote forgiveness in individual psychotherapy produce meaningful effects?

The present meta-analysis on the relationship between dose and effect throws down a set of challenges. It challenges theoreticians to establish that aspects of their theory that they claim to be distinct from other theories actually model a difference in outcome. It challenges practitioners to consider whether to make a focus on forgiveness a larger or smaller emphasis than it currently is, and whether to conduct groups targeted at promoting forgiveness. It challenges researchers to attempt to partial out the effects of groups to determine the unique effects of dealing with the content of forgiveness. The field of research on interventions to promote forgiveness is wide open, and there are more than enough challenges to occupy theoreticians, clinicians, and researchers for years to come.

ACKNOWLEDGMENT

Preparation of this chapter was partially supported by a grant from the John Templeton Foundation. The Foundation's generous support is gratefully acknowledged.

NOTES

1. The 5-item measure assesses a cognitive component of forgiveness. Enright has requested that it not be used in future research because it operationalizes forgiveness inadequately. McCullough, Worthington, and Rachal concur. Instead we recommend either the full Enright Forgiveness Inventory (Subkoviak et al., 1995), portions of Wade's (1989) measure, or the TRIM (McCullough et al., 1998), Hargrave and Sells's (1997), Mauger's measure of trait forgivingness (see Mauger et al., 1992) or Rye's (1998) measure as some of the most promising measures of forgiveness.

2. We use the term "clinically relevant," but we acknowledge that legitimate clinical interventions are needed to deal with issues of forgiveness within the clinic in individual counseling and in psychotherapy groups oriented toward interpersonal group psychotherapy. We treat a group intervention as "clinically relevant" if its primary purpose is to promote forgiveness. Such interventions are likely to be effective (according to our dose–effect curve) only if they occupy a substantial amount of time.

3. For example, how can African Americans possibly forgive European Americans who have historically oppressed African Americans, even though the particular modern-day African American might not have experienced much of that oppression? Social power is certainly an issue in that situation, just as it is when a child forgives a parent, a traditional female spouse forgives her traditional husband, an abused woman forgives her spouse, or an employee forgives his or her employer. Issues of social power affect the forgiveness transactions, which affect ease of both interpersonal forgiveness and reconciliation.

4. It is by no means clear that blocking interventions within leaders is the best solution to this problem. By blocking groups within leaders, we assure that a nonhelpful leader will not contribute differentially to the effectiveness of conditions. However, this solution lacks external validity. In practice, leaders prefer only one approach and do not conduct approaches of which they might not approve. Such reasoning might argue that external validity would be improved if the researcher nested leaders within interventions. A priori, a researcher would want to ensure that leaders are matched on experience, degree, gender, ethnicity, and other variables that might reasonably be expected to influence income. After the intervention, the researcher would want to check that leaders in each condition were rated equally on relationship variables (though one might argue that such a rating could be interpreted as a dependent variable).

REFERENCES

Al-Mabuk, R. H., Enright, R. D., & Cardis, P. A. (1995). Forgiving education with parentally loved-deprived late adolescents. *Journal of Moral Education, 24,* 427–444.

Baron, R. M., & Kenny, D. A. (1986). The moderator–mediator distinction in social psychological research: Conceptual, strategic, and statistical considerations. *Journal of Personality and Social Psychology, 51,* 1173–1182.

Baumeister, R. F., Exline, J. J., & Sommer, K. L. (1998). The victim role, grudge theory, and two dimensions of forgiveness. In E. L. Worthington, Jr. (Ed.), *Dimensions of forgiveness: Psychological research and theological speculations* (pp. 9–28). Philadelphia: Templeton Foundation Press.

Baumeister, R. F., Stillwell, A. M., & Heatherton, T. F. (1994). Guilt: An interpersonal approach. *Psychological Bulletin, 115,* 243–267.

Bryant, W. (1998). *The application of cognitive dissonance theory in a forgiveness workshop: Inducing hypocrisy to create a commitment to forgive.* Unpublished doctoral dissertation, Virginia Commonwealth University, Richmond.

Burlingame, G. M., Kircher, J. C., & Honts, C. R. (1994). Analysis of variance versus bootstrap procedures for analyzing dependent observations in small group research. *Small Group Research, 25,* 486–501.

Cooper, H., & Hedges, L. V. (1994). *The handbook of research synthesis.* New York: Russell Sage Foundation.

Couper, D. (1998). Forgiveness in the community: Views from an Episcopal priest and former chief of police. In Robert D. Enright & Joanna North (Eds.), *Exploring forgiveness* (pp. 121–130). Madison: University of Wisconsin Press.

Coyle, C. T., & Enright, R. D. (1997). Forgiveness intervention with postabortion men. *Journal of Consulting and Clinical Psychology, 65,* 1042–1046.

Deffenbacher, J. L. (1995). Ideal treatment package for adults with anger disorders. In H. Kassinove (Ed.), *Anger disorders: Definition, diagnosis, and treatment* (pp. 151–172). Washington, DC: Taylor & Francis.

DiBlasio, F. A. (1998). The use of a decision-based forgiveness intervention within intergenerational family therapy. *Journal of Family Therapy, 20,* 77–94.

Dickey, W. J. (1998). Forgiveness and crime: The possibilities of restorative justice. In R. D. Enright & J. North (Eds.), *Exploring forgiveness* (pp. 106–120). Madison: University of Wisconsin Press.

Dorff, E. N. (1998). The elements of forgiveness: A Jewish perspective. In E. L. Worthington, Jr. (Ed.), *Dimensions of forgiveness: Psychological research and theological speculations* (pp. 29–55). Philadelphia: Templeton Foundation Press.

Enright, R. D., & the Human Development Study Group. (1994). Piaget on the moral development of forgiveness: Identity or reciprocity? *Human Development, 37,* 63–80.

Enright, R. D., & the Human Development Study Group. (1996). Counseling within the forgiveness triad: On forgiving, receiving forgiveness, and self-forgiveness. *Counseling and Values, 40,* 107–126.

Enright, R. D., & North, J. (Eds.). (1998). *Exploring forgiveness.* Madison: University of Wisconsin Press.

Fitzgibbons, R. P. (1986). The cognitive and emotive uses of forgiveness in the treatment of anger. *Psychotherapy, 23,* 629–633.

Flanigan, B. (1998). Forgivers and the unforgivable. In R. D. Enright & J. North (Eds.), *Exploring forgiveness* (pp. 95–105). Madison: University of Wisconsin Press.

Freedman, S. R., & Enright, R. D. (1996). Forgiveness as an intervention goal with incest survivors. *Journal of Consulting and Clinical Psychology, 64,* 983–992.

Friedman, M., Thoresen, C. E., Gill, J., Ulmer, D., Powell, L. H., Price, V. A., Brown, B., Thompson, L., Rabin, D., Breall, W. S., Bourg, W., Levy, R., & Dixon, T. (1986). Alteration of Type A behavior and its effect on cardiac recurrences on postmyocardial infarction patients: Summary results of the Recurrent Coronary Prevention Project. *American Heart Journal, 112,* 653–665.

Gartner, J. (1988). The capacity to forgive: An object relations perspective. *Journal of Religion and Health, 27,* 313–320.

Girard, M., & Mullet, E. (1997). Forgiveness in adolescents, young, middle-aged, and older adults. *Journal of Adult Development, 4,* 209–220.

Hebl, J., & Enright, R. D. (1993). Forgiveness as a psychotherapeutic goal with elderly females. *Psychotherapy, 30,* 658–667.

Hepp-Dax, S. (1996). *Forgiveness as an intervention goal with fifth grade inner city children.* Unpublished doctoral dissertation, Fordham University.

Herbert, T., & Cohen, S. (1993). Stress and immunity in humans: A meta-analytic review. *Psychosomatic Medicine, 55,* 364–379.

Hoyle, R. H., & Crawford, A. M. (1994). Use of individual-level data to investigate group phenomena. *Small Group Research, 25,* 464–485.

Jacobson, N. S., & Gurman, A. S. (Eds.). (1995). *Handbook of couple therapy.* New York: Guilford Press.

Kaplan, B. H. (1992). Social health and the forgiving heart: The Type B story. *Journal of Behavioral Medicine, 15,* 3–14.

Kazdin, A. E. (1994). Methodology, design, and evaluation in psychotherapy research. In A. E. Bergin & S. L. Garfield (Ed.), *Handbook of psychotherapy and behavior change* (4th ed., pp. 19–71). New York: Wiley.

Kiecolt-Glaser, J. K., Newton, T., Cacioppo, J. T., MacCallum, R. C., Glaser, R., & Malarkey, W. B. (1996). Marital conflict and endocrine function: Are men really more physiologically affected than women? *Journal of Consulting and Clinical Psychology, 64,* 324–332.

Kurusu, T. A. (1996). *The effectiveness of pretreatment interventions on a forgiveness-promoting psychoeducational group.* Unpublished master's thesis, Virginia Commonwealth University, Richmond.

Kurusu, T. A. (1998). *The effectiveness of pretreatment intervention on participants in forgiveness-promoting psychoeducation in various stages of change.* Unpublished dissertation, Virginia Commonwealth University, Richmond.

Lindemann, C. (Ed.). (1996). *Handbook of the treatment of anxiety disorders.* New York: Jason Aronson.

Luskin, F., & Thoresen, C. (1998). *Effects of forgiveness training on psychosocial factors in college age adults.* Unpublished manuscript, Stanford University, Northport, NY.

Mauger, P. A., Perry, J. E., Freeman, T., Grove, D. C., McBride, A. G., & McKinney, K. (1992). The measurement of forgiveness: Preliminary research. *Journal of Psychology and Christianity, 11,* 170–180.

Madanes, C. (1991). Strategic family therapy. In A. S. Gurman & D. P. Kniskern (Eds.), *Handbook of family therapy* (Vol. 2, pp. 396–416). New York: Brunner/Mazel.

Marty, M. E. (1998). The ethos of Christian forgiveness. In E. L. Worthington, Jr. (Ed.), *Dimensions of forgiveness: Psychological research and theological speculations* (pp. 9–28). Philadelphia: Templeton Foundation Press.

McAleese, M. (1998). *Love in chaos: Spiritual growth and the search for peace in Northern Ireland.* New York: Continuum.

McCullough, M. E., Exline, J. J., & Baumeister, R. F. (1998). An annotated bibliography of research on forgiveness and related concepts. In E. L. Worthington, Jr. (Ed.), *Dimensions of forgiveness: Psychological research and theological speculations* (pp. 193–317). Philadelphia: Templeton Foundation Press.

McCullough, M. E., Rachal, K. C., Sandage, S. J., Worthington, E. L., Jr., Brown, S. W., & Hight, T. L. (1998). Forgiving in close interpersonal relationships: II. Theoretical elaboration and measurement. *Journal of Personality and Social Psychology, 75,* 1586–1603.

McCullough, M. E., & Worthington, E. L., Jr. (1994). Encouraging clients to forgive people who have hurt them: Review, critique, and research prospectus. *Journal of Psychology and Theology, 22,* 3–20.

McCullough, M. E., & Worthington, E. L., Jr. (1995). Promoting forgiveness: The comparison of two brief psychoeducational interventions with a waiting-list control. *Counseling and Values, 40,* 55–68.

McCullough, M. E., & Worthington, E. L., Jr. (1999). Religion and the forgiving personality. *Journal of Personality.*

McCullough, M. E., Worthington, E. L., Jr., & Rachal, K. C. (1997). Interpersonal forgiving in close relationships. *Journal of Personality and Social Psychology, 73,* 321–336.

Means, J. R., Wilson, G. L., Sturm, C., Piron, J. E., & Bach, P. J. (1990). Humility as a psychotherapeutic formulation. *Counseling Psychology Quarterly, 3,* 211–215.

Pargament, K. I. (1997). *The psychology of religion and coping: Theory, research, practice.* New York: Guilford Press.

Ripley, J. S. (1998). *Marriage contracts and covenants: The effects of marital values on outcomes of marital-enrichment workshops.* Dissertation in progress, Virginia Commonwealth University, Richmond.

Rokeach, M. (1973). *The nature of human values.* New York: Free Press.

Rusbult, C. E., Verette, J., Whitney, G. A., Slovik, L. F., & Lipkus, I. (1991). Accommodation processes in close relationships: Theory and preliminary empirical evidence. *Journal of Personality and Social Psychology, 60,* 53–78.

Rye, M. S. (1998). *Evaluation of a secular and a religiously integrated forgiveness group therapy program for college students who have been wronged by a romantic partner.* Unpublished dissertation, Bowling Green State University, Bowling Green, OH.

Sandage, S. J. (1997). *An ego-humility model of forgiveness.* Unpublished dissertation, Virginia Commonwealth University, Richmond.

Sitkim, S. B., & Beis, R. J. (1993). Social accounts in conflict situations: Using explanations to manage conflict. *Human Relations, 46,* 349–370.

Stillwell, A. M., & Baumeister, R. F. (1997). The construction of victim and perpetrator memories: Accuracy and distortion in role-based accounts. *Personality and Social Psychology, 23,* 1157–1172.

Subkoviak, M. J., Enright, R. D., Wu, C. R., Gassin, E. A., Freedman, S., Olson, L. M., & Sarinopoulos, I. (1995). Measuring interpersonal forgiveness in late adolescence and middle adulthood. *Journal of Adolescence, 18,* 641–655.

Tangney, J. P., Wagner, P., Barlow, D. H., & Marschall, D. E. (1996). Relation of shame and guilt to constructive vs. destructive responses to anger across the lifespan. *Journal of Personality and Social Psychology, 70,* 797–809.

Thoresen, C. E., Luskin, F., & Harris, A. H. S. (1998). The science of forgiving interventions: Reflections and suggestions. In E. L. Worthington, Jr. (Ed.), *Dimensions of forgiveness: Psychological research and theological speculations* (pp. 163–190). Philadelphia: Templeton Foundation Press.

Vitz, P. C., & Mango, P. (1997). Kernbergian psychodynamics and religious aspects of the forgiveness process. *Journal of Psychology and Theology, 28,* 72–80.

Wade, S. H. (1989). *The development of a scale to measure forgiveness.* Unpublished doctoral dissertation, Fuller Graduate School of Psychology, Pasadena, CA.

Wampold, B. E., Mondin, G. W., Moody, M., Stich, F., Benson, K., & Ahn, H. (1997). A meta-analysis of outcome studies comparing bona fide psychotherapies: Empirically, "all must have prizes." *Psychological Bulletin, 122,* 203–215.

Weiner, B., Graham, S., Peter, O., & Zmuidinas, M. (1991). Public confession and forgiveness. *Journal of Personality, 59,* 281–312.

Williams, R. (1989). *The trusting heart.* New York: Times Books.

Worthington, E. L., Jr. (Ed.). (1998a). *Dimensions of forgiveness: Psychological research and theological speculations.* Philadelphia: Templeton Foundation Press.

Worthington, E. L., Jr. (1998b). The pyramid model of forgiveness: Some interdisciplinary speculations about unforgiveness and the promotion of forgiveness. In E. L. Worthington, Jr. (Ed.), *Dimensions of forgiveness: Psychological research and theological perspectives* (pp. 107–137). Philadelphia: Templeton Foundation Press.

Worthington, E. L., Jr., & DiBlasio, F. A. (1990). Promoting mutual forgiveness within the fractured relationship. *Psychotherapy, 27,* 219–223.

Worthington, E. L., Jr., & Drinkard, D. T. (1999). Promoting reconciliation through psychoeducational and therapeutic interventions. *Journal of Marital and Family Therapy.*

Worthington, E. L., Jr., Kurusu, T. A., McCullough, M. E., & Sandage, S. J. (1996). Empirical research on religion and psychotherapeutic processes and outcomes: A ten-year review and research prospectus. *Psychological Bulletin, 119,* 448–487.

Yalom, I. D. (1970). *The theory and practice of group psychotherapy.* New York: Basic Books.

Forgiveness and Health

An Unanswered Question

Carl E. Thoresen, Alex H. S. Harris, and Frederic Luskin

Exploring possible relationships among forgiveness, disease, and physical health is truly at the frontiers of forgiveness research. To date, no controlled studies have demonstrated that forgiveness affects physical health outcomes either positively or negatively. While some data suggest that a secular approach to increasing forgiveness improves some mental health measures, such as depression and anger (see Thoresen, Luskin, & Harris, 1998; Worthington, Sandage, & Berry, Chapter 11, this volume), no controlled studies have yet reported improved physical health in persons with major diseases. Forgiveness has, however, been part of several successful multifactor intervention trials for patients with serious health problems, such as cancer and heart disease, but the specific effects of forgiveness in these studies have not been assessed (e.g., Friedman et al., 1986; Ornish, Brown, Scherwitz, & Billings, 1990; Spiegel, Bloom, Kraemer, & Gottheil, 1989).

Some retrospective anecdotal evidence (e.g., Albom, 1997; Flanigan, 1992) suggests a positive relationship between forgiveness and heath outcomes, although no prospectively designed case-study research is available. A literature also exists linking physical health outcomes with factors that are conceptually related to forgiveness, such as anger, blame, and hostility (e.g., Booth-Kewley & Friedman, 1987). This research has led us to consider the possibility that a forgiveness and physical health relationship may exist. Interestingly, health professionals have at times recommended forgiveness to their patients, apparently because they believe forgiveness improves health (e.g., Caudill, 1995; Weil, 1997).

254

Historically, anecdotal religious literature spanning many centuries has also commonly cited the health benefits of forgiveness (e.g., Easwaran, 1989; Marty, 1998). Because we understand forgiveness to involve, in part, the release of chronic negative cognitions and affectivity toward the offender, and we recognize the negative health implications of these negative thoughts and feelings, we wonder if these age-old adages might be supported by empirical research. Does forgiveness, for example, yield improved physical health in those who are more spiritually or religiously active than those who are less active? Although our initial intuition is that forgiveness is salubrious, forgiveness may be found empirically to be unrelated or, in some cases, negatively related to physical health status in specific contexts. Relatedly, we believe research needs to demonstrate that observed health outcomes result from the conscious decision to forgive and the related reduction of situated anger, blame, and resentment specific to the offense rather than the nonspecific reduction of global anger, blame, and resentment. We also note that other psychosocial factors known to influence physical health need to be controlled in forgiveness studies, such as perceived social support. These are empirical questions that we hope will be explored by the kind of research we discuss later (also see Worthington, Sandage, & Berry, Chapter 11, this volume).

In this chapter, we elaborate on why we are encouraged to pursue this line of research, discuss conceptual frameworks that are potentially useful in understanding the possible link between forgiveness and physical health, and consider some conceptual and methodological issues. We do so in the spirit of trying to encourage breadth as well as depth of research in this empirically deprived area. We first comment briefly on the term "forgiveness" as used in this chapter.

THE DECISION TO LET GO

Currently, no "gold standard" definition of forgiveness exists (see McCullough, Pargament, & Thoresen, Chapter 1, this volume). We offer a working definition of forgiveness here and refer the reader to McCullough and Worthington (1994) for a discussion of the various process models of forgiveness that have been proposed. Interpersonal forgiveness can be seen as the decision to reduce negative thoughts, affect, and behavior, such as blame and anger, toward an offender or hurtful situation, and to begin to gain better understanding of the offense and the offender. The choice to let go of the negative affect, cognitions, and behaviors may commonly occur in the beginning phases of the forgiveness process, yet the various outcomes of forgiveness, such as reduced anger and blame, may not occur for weeks, months, or perhaps years. Furthermore, the offender is not required in this perspective of forgiveness to acknowledge the offense, seek forgiveness, or make restitution (see Rye et al., Chapter 2, this volume; Worthington, 1998). Forgiveness can be viewed as part of the "life cycle of an offense" involving many steps or processes, depending on one's model. We hypothesize that the ability and willingness to forgive may be one of the characteristics of positive overall health and well-being.

SPIRITUAL OR SECULAR?

Forgiveness may be seen as closely connected to various religious beliefs and formal practices or as a purely secular, psychosocial factor, without any explicit or implied belief or concern with a transcendent relationship with God or any other universal power or force. In other words, we believe forgiveness can be conceived of as a spiritual or religious principle with often-specified practices or as a secular, individualized psychosocial construct. We suspect either perspective (or a blend of perspectives) may be beneficial when it comes to physical health, depending upon various situational factors (e.g., cultural factors or spiritual backgrounds of those involved).

Forgiveness may be undertaken with various motivations and experienced with various levels of enthusiasm. Although interpersonal forgiveness has received by far the most empirical attention, other types of forgiveness may be found that influence health outcomes. Self-forgiveness may turn out, for example, to be linked to interpersonal forgiveness, perhaps in a moderating or mediating role, and may be a major factor in the reduction of guilt, anger, and depression, as well as the enhancement of health. People also refer at times to the need to receive forgiveness as a means to release the negative affect associated with some traumatic events. Very little is known empirically about this type of forgiveness (see Exline & Baumeister, Chapter 7, this volume). Other empirically unexplored but potentially fruitful areas involves asking for forgiveness or accepting the request from others to forgive. Only a few empirical studies of seeking forgiveness have been reported in the social-psychological literature (e.g., Weiner, Graham, Peter, & Zmuidinas, 1991), but no clinical investigations have been undertaken using this type of intervention, nor have the health-related correlates been explored.

HOW MIGHT INTERPERSONAL FORGIVENESS INFLUENCE PHYSICAL HEALTH?

How might forgiveness-related processes influence physical health and disease outcomes? We will only have reliable answers after controlled studies have been completed. We can, however, begin to examine the evidence that some components related to the forgiveness processes, such as blame, anger, and hostility, influence health. Although there is currently no evidence available that forgiveness is associated with positive health outcomes, there are studies documenting the fact that blaming others and chronic hostility are associated with negative health outcomes. For example, Affleck, Tennen, Croog, and Levine (1987) demonstrated that cardiac patients who blamed their initial heart attack on other people were more likely to have reinfarctions, even when several other biological and psychosocial variables were controlled. Tennen and Affleck (1990) reviewed 25 published studies reporting the health impact of blaming others for threatening events. Blaming others for one's misfortune (e.g., heart attacks, failure to conceive) was associated with impairments in emotional well-being and physical health. In multivariate analyses, anger and hostility over many years have both been predictive of all-cause mortality in several but not all studies (Miller, Smith, Turner, Guijarro, & Hallet, 1996). Future research may reveal that forgiveness is salubrious to the extent that it is helpful in reducing chronic blaming, anger, and hostility.

In a series of studies, McCraty, Atkinson, Tiller, Rein, and Watkins (1995) demonstrated that increasing positive emotional states, compared to negative emotions (e.g., depression, anger, fear), produces improved immune competence and reduced heart rate, blood pressure, and respiratory variability. For example, strong positive emotionality led to greater synchronization of immunological and cardiovascular functioning. Forgiveness may be one factor that fosters such synchronization via reducing negative emotionality and enhancing cognitive processes associated with more compassion and understanding of others.

Hopelessness, the belief that there is nothing that one can do to make changes or influence the future positively, is conceivably involved with those people whose guilt and resentment prevent them from forgiving themselves for their felt inadequacies and perceived past failures. Hopelessness has been shown to predict all-cause mortality spanning several years, controlling for several other possible explanatory factors (e.g., Everson, Goldberg, Kaplan, & Cohen, 1996).

Although these studies have demonstrated relationships between anger, hostility, and hopelessness, with various physical health outcomes, the connection with forgiveness remains unexamined. What we suggest is examination of forgiveness in ways that will allow researchers to assess the possible unique or shared contributions of forgiveness to physical health. In other words, we recommend that research examine the mechanisms by which forgiveness reduces "pathogenic" factors (e.g., chronic anger), resulting in beneficial physical changes. Next, we discuss briefly some possible mechanisms through which forgiveness may mediate or moderate positive health outcomes.

Possible Physiological Mechanisms

The underlying pathways, both psychosocial and physiological, remain quite complex and a great deal of work remains to be done. As to possible physiological mechanisms that might explain how forgiveness processes could influence physical health, Scheidt's (1996) perspective on psychosocial factors and coronary heart disease seems most promising. Scheidt offered over 12 possible physiological and psychosocial mechanisms. Of these, he rated chronic sympathetic nervous system (SNS) hyperarousal influencing endocrine production (e.g., norepinephrine) as the most empirically supported mechanism. By decreasing chronic SNS arousal, demands upon the cardiovascular system are reduced (e.g., lowered blood pressure, endogenous production of low density lipoproteins, heart rate variability, atherosclerosis).

Jiang et al. (1996) demonstrated that patients with elevated levels of silent ischemia (short-term contractions of coronary arteries) during stressful tasks associated with SNS arousal were almost three times more likely to suffer a major coronary event over 5 years than those with less reaction to emotional stress. These results were not explained by several physiological variables. In addition, immune competence (e.g., increased natural killer [NK] and t-cells [CD4]) can be enhanced when SNS arousal is diminished. Anderson et al. (1998) recently demonstrated that in women with breast cancer, psychological stress reduces NK cell and CD4 activity, as well as lowering immune response to cytokine proteins. Several biological and demographic factors were controlled, but psychosocial stress still mediated diminished immune competence over several months (see also Pennebaker, Kiecolt-Glaser, & Glaser, 1988; Petrie, Booth, & Pennebaker, 1998).

Perhaps one of the most promising explanations concerns the notion of allostasis, the ability of several physiological systems to achieve and maintain stability when trying to adapt to stress (McEwen & Stellar, 1993). By means of allostasis, the autonomic nervous system, the hypothalamic–pituitary–adrenal (HPA) axis, and the cardiovascular, metabolic, and immune systems all make needed changes to adapt and stabilize in the face of internal and external stress (perceived demands). Major life events, trauma, and abuse, for example, represent stressful experiences taking place at home, at work, or in the neighborhood. Both chronic and acute stress (e.g., hostility and public speaking, respectively) present challenges requiring physiological systems to adapt. These changes involve different physiological response patterns. The long-term physiological price of chronic over- or underactivity of allostatic systems is called "allostatic load" (McEwen, 1998). Normally, a stressor results in arousal and then recovery in, for example, blood pressure or heart rate variability. However, high allostatic load can result in maladaptive changes such as extended length of arousal, with some or no recovery, or failure to adapt (no arousal) at all.

For example, excessive and prolonged activation of the SNS and HPA pathways can alter brain functioning (hippocampal cell damage) that accelerates aging. McEwen (1998) describes several diseases that might be due to inadequate or inappropriate physical changes. Overall, the concept of allostasis, adaptive physiological changes to stressful experiences over time, suggests that forgiveness experiences might enhance health by reducing excessive physiological burden that comes with unresolved stressful experiences, such as the hurt and offense attributed to others (see McEwen, 1998, for further discussion).

Conceivably, increased frequency of forgiving others, oneself, and of asking for and accepting forgiveness, might function to reduce the chronicity of distress (e.g., anger, blame, and vengeful thoughts and feelings) that has prospectively been shown to alter brain, coronary, and immune functioning. Such reductions could encourage diminished SNS arousal in frequency, magnitude, and duration; resulting over time in less physical disease risk.

Possible Psychosocial Mechanisms

Besides the possible physiological mechanisms of reduced sympathetic tone and reactivity, possible psychosocial mechanisms may also be at work in how forgiveness might alter physical status. Some possibilities include the following:

1. Forgiveness may foster more perceived security and/or greater positive self-evaluative and optimistic thoughts that strengthen "host resistance" to taking offense. Doing so might reduce the probability of fear, anxiety, anger, hostility, depression and/or hopelessness, all of which have been shown in varying degrees to increase physical disease risk (e.g., Segerstrom, Taylor, Kemeny, & Fahey, 1998; Everson, Goldberg, Kaplan, Julkunen, & Salonen, 1998; Everson, Kauhanen, & Kaplan, 1997).

2. Forgiveness may foster stronger perceived competence or self-efficacy to take needed steps to reduce disease-enhancing or pathogenics "agents" (e.g., take action to alter chronic hostile feelings, helpless beliefs, stable and global attributions), which, in turn, may increase positive stimulus–outcome expectations (e.g., "In potentially hurtful situations, I can manage my anger well enough and not be offended") (Bandura, 1997; Thoresen et al., 1998).

3. Forgiveness may provide higher levels of perceived social and emotional support, especially from more intimate close friendships. This includes the experience of a greater sense of community, often from be-

ing of service to others, and of feeling more belonging and connectedness to others, all of which may promote physical health (House, Landis, & Umberson, 1988; Oman, Thoresen, & McMahon, 1999).

4. Forgiveness may encourage a greater sense of a transcendent consciousness (or moving "beyond the ego") and more inner experiences of communion with God, a Higher Power or an Infinite/Universal Energy, especially among more spiritually or religiously oriented persons (Albom, 1997; Richards & Bergin, 1997; Walsh & Vaughn, 1993).

Note that these possibilities are clearly tentative but seem promising enough to consider exploring empirically. Also, note that possible psychosocial explanations for specific chronic diseases, such as coronary heart disease and cancer, may share these same possible psychosocial explanations for improved health (see Thoresen & Hoffman Goldberg, 1998; Allan & Scheidt, 1996).

For those who doubt the plausibility of a forgiveness relationship with physical health, we are reminded of how implausible the role of psychosocial factors in the body's immune system was considered just two decades ago. Since then, the field now known as psychoneuroimmunology (PNI) has emerged (Coe, 1997). Because of PNI, we now know, for example, that chronic psychosocial distress in humans (and nonhuman primates) lowers immune competence, thus lowering a person's host resistance to cope with biological and psychosocial pathogens or agents (e.g., Stone, Cox, Valdimarsdottir, & Jandorf, 1987; Cohen, Tyrrell, & Smith, 1991).

CONCEPTUAL FRAMEWORKS TO CONSIDER

At the beginning stages of inquiry in any health-related area, it is important to examine the psychosocial and health literature for conceptual frameworks that have proved useful in explaining and predicting health outcomes. Such frameworks can be useful in designing assessment instruments and interventions. In this case, we have searched for conceptual frameworks that have been useful in understanding the effects of psychosocial, cognitive, and emotional factors on physical health, particularly those factors that may be conceptually related to forgiveness (i.e., anger, Type A behavior, narcissism, depression, and self-efficacy). Others, of course, are possible, but we will limit discussion to these five factors. Note that how we conceptualize forgiveness and its possible link to physical health outcomes will strongly influence what we choose to measure, how we choose to measure it, and what we focus on in forgiveness interventions.

Constructive Anger

Understandably, anger commonly is experienced when someone feels hurt, offended, or abused. Surprisingly, however, anger has not received the major attention it deserves in terms of what forgiveness is and how forgiveness processes work (Thoresen et al., 1998). Given the demonstrated role of anger and hostility in altering physiological processes (e.g., Williams & Williams, 1993) and anecdotal data implicating anger and hostility (e.g., hostile cognitions) in hurtful, offensive, or abusive situations, we believe this topic deserves primary attention. Here, only introductory comments are possible, with references offered for further reading (e.g., Williams & Williams, 1993; Deffenbacher, 1994; Smith, 1992; Spielberger, Reheiser, & Sydeman, 1995).

Few studies in forgiveness have assessed anger or hostility, either in correlational or experimentally designed interventions (Luskin & Thoresen, 1998). Worthington, Sandage and Berry (Chapter 11, this volume) note that anger remains a promising yet unexamined construct in the forgiveness literature, especially with respect to intervention studies.

An intriguing model of anger in relation to health has been recently offered by Davidson and her colleagues (Davidson, Stuhr, & Chambers, in press). She proposes a distinction between the experience of anger and the expression of anger. Arguing that anger is a multidimensional construct that cannot be adequately captured in any single measure (or mode of assessment), Davidson et al. focus on anger expression for two major reasons: Very few existing measures assess anger expression, focusing instead primarily on dispositional anger. However, it is the expression of anger over time, not its immediate reactive experience, that may influence health and disease status more dramatically. From this perspective, getting angry per se is less of a problem than how long one remains angry and how it is expressed during that time (Tavris, 1989; Pickering & Gerin, 1990).

Based on the existing anger literature, Davidson et al. (in press) describe two major features of anger expression: constructive and destructive anger. The former involves such things as engaging in instrumental thoughts and actions to rectify the situation, cognitive restructuring, and interpersonal problem solving. Destructive anger involves harm, rage, revenge, retaliation, as well as hostile ruminations and imagery. Finally, constructive and destructive anger expression is divided into verbal, nonverbal (e.g., facial or physical expression), and cognitive categories. Changes in systolic and diastolic blood pressure were used as the major physical health variables.

Some initial data offer support for the "recovery conjecture"; that is, the health risk due to anger may lie in how long the arousal persists rather than the immediate physiological reactivity (e.g., Hall, Davidson, Mac-

Gregor, & MacLean, 1998). Assessing systolic and diastolic blood pressure as the outcome, several existing self-report anger questionnaires were compared in three studies, one with a 2-year follow-up. Using multiple regression analyses, popular anger questionnaires were compared with behavioral ratings from a brief, videotaped structured interview, the Constructive Anger Behavior–Verbal Interview (CAB-V). In addition, a self-rated questionnaire version of the CAB-V was also developed.

Results indicated significant negative relationships for all popularly used anger questionnaires with the CAB-V interview ratings (e.g., Spielberger Trait Anger Scale, $-.18$, $p < .05$), indicating that self-reports from questionnaires tapped different facets of anger than observed interview behavior. In addition, only the CAB-V interview ratings predicted recovery rate of diastolic blood pressure from stress. Note that diastolic, or resting blood pressure, is more stable and difficult to alter than systolic pressure. Interestingly, these findings support the findings of Shedler, Mayman, and Manis (1993), who found that commonly used questionnaires of depression, anxiety, and other emotions often fail to relate to physiological measures and clinical interview assessments of the same emotions (e.g., roughly 30% of those clinically disturbed missed by questionnaires).

Application to Health-Related Forgiveness Research

If forgiveness interventions seek to help participants reduce their anger, then anger should be assessed as an outcome variable. Also, the multidimensional concept of anger presented earlier can help to distinguish types of anger expression that are hazardous to health from the more benign or constructive anger that may in fact facilitate physical health. Health-related forgiveness researchers could benefit from assessing constructive and destructive anger expression in participants, and using these categories as variables in comparing responsiveness to forgiveness interventions. Theoretically, persons with more destructive anger expression stand to benefit more from the advantages of forgiveness, such as the reduction of rage and hostile ruminations, than those who express anger more constructively. Conversely, those with greater destructive anger expression may need more extensive anger interventions. Finally, the anger research discussed earlier should remind those in health-related forgiveness research of the importance of multiple methods and modes of assessment, especially the need to complement self-report questionnaires with various combinations of interviews, and behavioral and physiological measures.

Type A Behavior and Narcissism

Type A behavior has been closely linked conceptually to the narcissistic personality (Thoresen & Powell, 1992). Empirically, narcissism has been positively related to hostility, a major Type A component (Rhodewalt & Morf, 1995). Emmons (Chapter 8, this volume) and others have suggested that both commonly involve an exaggerated sense of entitlement, superiority, and arrogance, as well as extreme sensitivity to criticism and a quickness to anger and vengeful ideation. In addition, narcissistic persons often present as decisive, persuasive, and ambitious, if not slick and audacious.

Noteworthy for forgiveness-related health research are the shared Type A and narcissistic characteristics of being easily aggravated and angered by others, readily blaming others, taking offense quickly, and manifesting cynical hostility (i.e., viewing others as untrustworthy and uncaring). These characteristics may readily set the stage for these persons to experience the actions of others as offensive, if not deliberately disrespectful. For example, Dodge and Frame (1982) found that aggressive boys ("bullies") routinely interpreted neutral or accidental events as intentionally hostile, in a fashion similar to the narcissist's negative attributional style about others.

Although none of the Type A-related interventions independently assessed narcissism using the Narcissistic Personality Inventory (NPI; Raskin & Hall, 1979), reductions in Type A behavior have been associated with reduced physical disease (e.g., fatal and nonfatal myocardial infarctions) in controlled interventions (see Linden, Stossel, & Maurice, 1996). Interestingly, the Type B behavior pattern (Price, 1988) closely resembles a personality profile compatible with the characteristics associated with forgiveness (e.g., high empathic understanding, high threshold for taking offense). Unknown at present, however, is the proportion of the variance in improved physical health that might be attributed to forgiveness.

Application to Health-Related Forgiveness Research

The marked prevalence of narcissism and Type A behavior in the United States needs, we believe, to be considered by those designing assessment and forgiveness intervention studies (Thoresen & Powell, 1992). Using Type A and narcissistic personality measures in research designs as possible moderators may help explain differential effects of programs designed to foster interpersonal forgiveness. Researchers should also be aware that efforts at promoting self-forgiveness or interpersonal forgiveness, in which partners are actively involved (e.g., married couples) in the intervention, may prove much less effective if one or both persons evidence elevated levels of Type A behavior and/or narcissism. The research on Type A personalities also reminds and encourages us that changes in behaviors and psychosocial factors, such as learning to forgive and take offense less easily, might have significant physical health consequences.

Depression

Research on depression over the last decade has increasingly focused on using an information-processing model that seeks to clarify how and why some persons become clinically depressed and frequently relapse (Gotlib, Gilboa, & Kaplan, in press). For example, persons have been found prospectively to experience more clinical depression if they characteristically recall negative life events (termed "depressive schema") compared to those with less negative recall bias. Depression is currently viewed as a multidimensional psychosocial construct, predictive of physical health outcomes, with several components, such as cognitive bias and problems in attention, memory, and judgment (Gotlib et al., in press).

Some prospective research in depression (e.g., Roberts, Gilboa, & Gotlib, in press) suggests that these chronic negative ruminations predict higher and more substantial levels of negative mood and behavior. Another study (Hammen & Goodman-Brown, 1990) found that a young person's negative self-schema and overall self-concept were highly associated with the onset of clinical depression as well as negative life events over several years. Other studies speak to the value of helping persons learn how better to manage their attention to internal and external responses, as well as to select goals, and use behavioral strategies (see Gotlib et al., in press).

Application to Health-Related Forgiveness Research

We believe that this research literature offers some exciting perspectives on how researchers can clarify the various processes in forgiveness. Problems of what the offended person focuses on, how that focus or attention permeates negative or positive emotions, and what factors influence judgments and evaluations about the offender appear to be potentially relevant. Attending to hostile or helpless ruminations about the offender may elicit angry and/or depressive emotions that in turn may fuel harsh or hostile judgments, as well as avoidance or anger. Research can help clarify whether processes similar to those at work in depression are present and active in those who find it difficult to forgive, to ask for forgiveness, or to accept forgiveness. Perhaps those strategies found to be efficacious in the treatment of depression could be adapted to foster forgiveness. Conceivably, those offended, for example, may find a spiritually oriented form of cognitive-behavioral therapy to be more effective than a secular version (Propst, Ostrom, Watkins, & Dean, 1992).

Importantly, over time, researchers in this area of depression have also learned the value of combining standardized self-report measures with other modes of outcome and process assessments, such as interviews, physiological monitoring, and behavioral ratings by others. Earlier research in depression, relying exclusively on questionnaire methodology, proved inadequate in clarifying what cognitive and social–emotional processing variables might be involved. Researchers, we believe, can greatly benefit from the experience of depression researchers, especially in clarifying how cognitive and behavioral factors may influence forgiveness and health variables over time.

Self-Efficacy and Forgiveness

The concept of self-efficacy, the level of perceived confidence to take action (perform a task), seems especially relevant in designing forgiveness assessments and interventions. The importance of self-efficacy has been successfully demonstrated in literally hundreds of empirical studies (Bandura, 1997). The accumulated evidence demonstrates that efficacy beliefs strongly influence a person's efforts to change. If a person has fairly high levels of perceived efficacy to engage successfully in certain tasks (in the 70% range or higher), such as taking steps to reduce anger toward someone who has been offensive, then that person is much more likely to engage in that action. In addition, a person with higher offense-related self-efficacy, faced with a problem, will exert more energy, persist longer at the task, and acquire more knowledge and skills compared to someone with a lower sense of efficacy. In addition, the level of self-efficacy beliefs has been found to powerfully influence the chances that people will attain their desired outcomes (Bandura, 1997).

Use of self-efficacy theory in studying health and disease processes and outcomes has been extensive (e.g., biochemical effects, autonomic activity, catecholamine and opioid changes, pain regulation, and immune functioning). Behavioral effects have also been observed (e.g., changing personal behaviors, such as smoking, eating, and exercising; reducing tension headaches, bulimic behavior, and adherence to medical regimens). Such changes include increasing or decreasing activities as well as relapse prevention and the maintenance of health-related behaviors. Especially notable is the role that self-efficacy beliefs play in self-regulation and perceived control. Gordon, Baucom, and Synder (Chapter 10, this volume) have discussed loss of control by the person offended and how important building greater perceived control may be for forgiveness to occur.

Applications of Self-Efficacy

Two successful examples of using self-efficacy as a major conceptual model in health research stand out. DeBusk et al. (1994) developed a self-efficacy-based computer-managed program to encourage coronary patients to engage in regular exercise, improve nutrition, manage body weight, and quit smoking permanently. Each participant used individualized self-efficacy belief ratings for engaging in several specific, health-related activities. Result to date have been very impressive, including the cost–benefit evidence of this program. An area to consider, based on this successful program, is developing a computer-mediated intervention program for a specific major disease category, in which a forgiveness program could be included along with other health topics. Applications in health behavior programs without computers deserve consideration as well.

The second example involves a behavioral self-management group program for osteoarthritis patients (Lorig & Holman, 1989). Similar to the aforementioned program, each major intervention activity uses self-efficacy ratings (e.g., efficacy to practice relaxation or walk for 30 minutes). If a task is perceived by the patient as being less likely to be completed successfully (e.g., rating below 30%), the task is altered to one that yields a higher efficacy rating by the participant. A unique feature of this program is that it is peer-managed, in that groups are led by patients who have completed highly structured training in how to use a very detailed manual of operations. Furthermore, this approach has been successfully replicated in several different countries with impressive results. Currently, this efficacy-based model is being used to demonstrate that mixed groups of patients with several different diseases can also be effectively treated together (Lorig, 1999).

Example of Using Self-Efficacy in Forgiveness Research

To date, only one study (Luskin & Thoresen, 1998) has explored the use of self-efficacy in a forgiveness intervention for young adults. Randomized participants in the intervention or control groups were assessed using self-efficacy items designed to highlight major intervention targets. Using a scale from 0 to 100, participants were asked to rate how confident they were about doing certain tasks, such as "I can think about the offense and remain calm and peaceful," or "I can take responsibility for the angry thoughts that arise toward the offender."

Given the exploratory nature of this intervention, results were encouraging. Compared to wait-list control participants, those treated substantially increased their overall efficacy beliefs to forgive (ES = 0.6, $p <$ .001), which was maintained at 10-week follow-up (ES = 0.5, $p <$ .01). The emphasis of this intervention on primary prevention, that is, on learning how to use forgiveness in future hurtful episodes rather than only focusing on the offending person and the particular situation, was revealed in the relative improvement in efficacy ratings. While both improved significantly, greater increases were found in efficacy to forgive others across a variety of situations than efficacy to forgive the identified offender ($p <$ .05). At follow-up, a major interpersonal hurt not covered in the intervention was used as a forgiveness simulation task. Compared to controls, significantly higher self-efficacy was found in those receiving the intervention (ES = 0.7, p < .05).

Applications to Health-Related Forgiveness Research

The value of efficacy-based forgiveness research seems particularly promising in serving to align the focus of interventions with clearly identified tasks that are designed to produce outcomes. In this way, a close and ongoing connection is created between participants' initial efficacy beliefs about how well they can perform certain tasks and the specific steps in the intervention process, whether individually or group based.

Optimally, as in the DeBusk et al. (1994) and Lorig and Holman (1989) programs, efficacy belief ratings would be used repeatedly during the intervention, as well as serving as outcome variables. One of the benefits of repeated efficacy assessments is the motivational consequences that come from participants observing their growth in confidence and improved performance. Fortunately, there are many examples of self-efficacy-based studies, including guidelines for how to construct self-efficacy scales tailored to the problem area, and how to link assessments more directly with the sequence of intervention (Bandura, 1995).

QUESTIONS FOR FUTURE RESEARCH

Having cited some promising conceptual frameworks, we now turn to some questions and issues we believe are important to address in future research. Many of the questions have been raised by others as well (see Thoresen et al., 1998; Worthington, Sandage, & Berry, Chapter 11, this volume).

1. Does some form of self-forgiveness play a consistent role in the effects of forgiveness on physical health? Little, if anything, is known from controlled studies about forgiving oneself. Perhaps the process of forgiving someone for a serious offense almost invariably involves some degree of self-reflection about one's present and past action toward others. If so, assessing self-forgiveness could prove informative, as it may be a moderating variable in the interpersonal forgiveness process and influence health. Conceivably, the long-term influence of forgiveness on general health may lie in reframing basic beliefs (along with selected attributions, expectations, and "rules to live by") about oneself. Such reframing may need to be transformational in the sense of persons becoming much less self-involved and egocentric, as well as much more caring and serving those in need (Markus, Reaff, Conner, Pudberry, & Barnett, in press; Oman et al., 1999).

2. What differences a person's spiritual and religious background, beliefs, attitudes, and practices, including ways of coping, make in terms of forgiveness as it relates to health? It may be that people who are more intrinsically religious or spiritual (Gorsuch & Miller, 1999) forgive others more readily and more often than those less religiously affiliated or spiritually involved (Pargament, 1997). Perhaps for some people who are highly active in a religion in an extrinsic sense, forgiveness may be more difficult or may create a greater challenge in general or for specific types of offenses. With rare exception, published forgiveness interventions to date have been secularized, not even assessing spiritual and religious factors or incorporating these factors directly into the intervention. Rye and Pargament (1997) describe the only comparative evaluation of religiously integrated and secular forgiveness intervention which was for women wronged by a romantic partner. Both interventions were effective, with no significant differences between them. More research would help clarify the conditions under which either approach (or a blend of both approaches) might increase forgiveness and positive health outcomes.

3. What roles do significant others (e.g., spouse, parent, and sibling) play for a person in forgiving others or oneself? Gordon, Baucom, and Synder (Chapter 10, this volume) raise this issue, noting the lack of evidence regarding couples faced with an offense between partners. We suspect that such influences may parallel findings about spouses in the physical health literature (e.g., recovery process from myocardial infarction). Active participation by spouses, for example, in cardiac rehabilitation and in weight management programs, often improved patient's physical health and sometimes the spouse's health as well (e.g., Ewart, Taylor, Reese, & DeBusk, 1983; Brownell & Wadden, 1992). Would couples or partners participating together in forgiveness interventions prove more effective, even when the offense involved a third party? Would the partner not directly offended experience improved physical health and increased forgiveness by participating in the forgiveness intervention (also see Malcolm & Greenberg, Chapter 9, this volume)?

4. Is it possible to develop simulated forgiveness situations linked to serious physical health problems for which persons at high risk could be helped to practice the forgiveness process? Or would forgiveness simulations not related directly to health problems prove more effective because they would be less threatening and easier to practice? Simulations could be used in disease-related primary prevention programs with a focus on raising the threshold for taking offense at others' actions. Simulated practice in forgiveness could be based on the participant modeling strategy (Bandura, 1986) in which persons practice specific steps in the forgiveness process immediately after observing others engaging in these forgiveness behaviors. Immediately following this, they would receive corrective feedback and support, and try again if needed. Goldfried (1980) identified

such opportunities to observe and practice the target actions, with immediate feedback as essential ingredients for all successful psychotherapeutic interventions across different theoretical orientations.

5. Does a person need to empathize in some way with the offender in order for forgiveness to take place? Some retrospective anecdotal data have suggested that not everyone who presumably forgives evidences any change in empathy and understanding for the offender (Flanigan, 1992). Does the magnitude and/or the duration of the offense make a difference in the need for empathetic understanding to occur? We believe that empathy, gaining some understanding and insight into the offender's situation, operates in all genuine forgiveness (see McCullough, Worthington, & Rachal, 1997). However, the need for empathy in forgiveness still remains an open question, especially with respect to demonstrating a relationship to physical health outcomes.

TOWARD A PLURALISTIC METHODOLOGY

In the very early stages of scientific inquiry, such as the empirical study of forgiveness-related factors and physical health, a variety of research-design and data-analytic methods seem essential to provide an empirically grounded foundation for research (Cook, 1985; Mahoney, 1995; Suppe, 1977). Clearly, one methodological size does not fit all questions and issues. Worthington, Sandage, and Berry (Chapter 11, this volume) and McCullough, Rachal, and Hoyt (Chapter 4, this volume) note the paucity of different research methods and designs used in forgiveness studies. They raise many issues that deserve attention, such as the lack of studies using methods other than brief questionnaire self-reports, the lack of studies involving the offender along with the offended party in assessment and intervention studies, and the lack of studies of persons of different cultural and ethnic backgrounds. They also note the preponderance of female college students participating in studies. Malcolm and Greenberg (Chapter 9, this volume) lament the lack of empirically based process studies that are essential in validating theoretical models of forgiveness. They advocate the use of carefully analyzed interview data to capture more fully forgiveness processes and to evaluate whether conceptions of forgiveness fit the data.

We briefly mention some measurement and research design issues involved in forgiveness that may help address some of the experiences and processes not adequately assessed by questionnaires used in cross-sectional designs. We focus here on measurement strategies using structured interviews and daily self-monitoring methods, as well as the design strategies of randomized controlled trials (RCTs) and single-subject ($N = 1$) experimental designs.

Each of these strategies can help researchers address what cognitive scientists often refer to as "situated" cognitions and actions (e.g., Greeno,

1998), that is, the need to assess interactions between what the person is thinking and doing in a particular situation when faced with a specific task. Each of these methods bridge the now popular, if controversial, concern with qualitative and quantitative inquiry. We cannot deal with all the features of this "postmodern versus positivist" controversy other than to argue that both perspectives offer useful methods, each suited to certain issues and questions. Since the questions we face in the forgiveness/physical health arena are truly impressive, we favor an open-minded, pluralistic perspective, one that often combines various methods depending upon the problem. As a noted philosopher of science (Kaplan, 1964) once complained, scientists are too often like the little boy given a hammer, in that once given a hammer, everything seems to need hammering (e.g., everything needs questionnaires or t-tests).

We strongly recommend that readers examine carefully Denzin and Lincoln's *Handbook of Qualitative Research* (1994). This comprehensive resource includes 36 chapters covering a broad range of design and analysis methods. Particularly recommended are chapters comparing paradigms within qualitative research, case studies, grounded theory, interviewing, data management, and data-analysis methods.

We now offer more detailed comments on the use of two measurement strategies, structured interviews and daily self-rating methods, and two research design issues, $N = 1$ experimental designs and RCTs.

Structured Interviews

Using interviews for assessment offers a rich array of approaches, from asking a prepared list of questions orally (often for those who are limited in reading comprehension abilities) to opened-ended questions or comments (e.g., "How do you feel about forgiveness?"). Malcolm and Greenberg (Chapter 9, this volume) describe the use of therapy interviews to study the verbal processes of clients who forgive others. Semistructured interviews were used by Kleinman and Becker (1998), as well as other researchers, in exploring societal and cultural features of experience, especially differences, that may influence physical health and disease ("sociomatics"). Such differences can influence the quality and quantity of information available about symptoms, treatments, compliance, and relapse, as well as emphasize certain values, attitudes (such as the role of forgiveness), and concepts of health and disease (Kleinman, Eisenberg, & Good, 1978).

Discovering Spiritual Factors

Folkman (1997) and Richards and Folkman (1997) used semistructured interviews to explore the cognitive and emotional coping experiences of surviving caretakers of deceased AIDS patients. In analyzing the narrative transcripts of answers to such questions as "What have you learned from this period in your life?" and "What's important to you now?", these researchers discovered an unanticipated factor: spiritually related themes of coping. Roughly 50% ($N = 120$) of participants spontaneously cited spiritual topics, such as concerns with personal meaning and purpose in life or use of prayer or meditation. When the interview sample was then divided into spiritual versus nonspiritual theme groups, these researchers found that the groups differed significantly on standardized measures of coping as well as depression and anxiety questionnaire measures. Interestingly, while those citing spiritual or religious themes reported significantly higher levels of anxiety and depression, along with more physical symptoms (but not differences on medical HIV status) immediately after the death of the patient, than the nonspiritual group, they also demonstrated significantly more use of adaptive coping, such as positive reappraisal and planful problem solving. Follow-up several months later, again using interviews and questionnaires, demonstrated a noteworthy outcome: Participants in the spiritual theme group had significantly less anxiety and depression, while the nonspiritual participants had become substantially more anxious and depressed.

Here we have an example of the value of combining methods, with each providing partial information but the two together offering a more complete portrayal of coping over time. Note that without the interview, the results of the questionnaire data would have presented a much less accurate picture, since the crossover effect of emotional and coping data would have been obscured.

Note also the unanticipated discovery of spiritual factors that emerged from using the interview method. First, open-ended questions facilitated comments concerning coping processes that were unanticipated yet relevant to the study's objectives. Second, a rigorous and systematic narrative-analysis method revealed these themes in the data. Just using interviews without rigorous data analysis might not have revealed the spirituality variable and its role in emotional states and coping.

We have also already noted the use of a structured interview to assess types of anger and hostility, such as constructive anger (Davidson et al., in press). Also see Barefoot (1992) for another example of how behavior rated from a structured interview significantly improves the predictive validity of health outcomes when compared to questionnaires dealing with a sensitive psychosocial topic such as hostility. Forgiveness may also be a sensitive topic, one that some find difficult to describe or discuss.

Assessing Nonverbals

Often missed in psychosocial research concerned with physical health and not yet examined in forgiveness research is nonverbal behavior, such as facial expression or gestures. Note that the aforementioned Davidson et al. (1998) model of constructive anger contains three components: verbal, nonverbal, and behavioral activities. It remains to be seen if nonverbal elements of forgiveness play any significant role in health outcomes. However, given the often-cited proportion of nonverbal factors involved in effective interpersonal communication, it seems reasonable to believe that giving and receiving forgiveness may involve an important nonverbal component . Use of structured interview and behavioral ratings of verbal and nonverbal affect and behavior during interventions could provide valuable information in forgiveness research and health.

Daily Monitoring/Self-Rating Methods

The previous discussion has already introduced the idea of repeated measures rather than assessment on one or a few occasions. A single example can illustrate a methodology already found to be useful (and publishable) in the psychosocial health area.

Pain, Self-Efficacy, and Emotions: Exploring Processes over Time

Keefe and others (e.g., Keefe et al., 1997; Affleck, Tennen, Urrows, & Higgins, 1991) have studied pain in persons suffering from different chronic diseases, such as rheumatoid and osteoarthritis patients. Pain, particularly chronic pain, confronts researchers with a host of methodological problems, including the marked variability of pain within and between persons as to severity, duration, and frequency. The challenge of understanding pain has moved researchers toward gathering the kind of data that will better inform theory as well as clinical practice. Given the effectiveness of self-efficacy in pain management, as noted earlier in Lorig and Holman (1989), pain researchers have begun to explore how self-efficacy works in helping patients reduce negative moods, increase physical functioning, and alter pain-related symptoms.

Acknowledging the serious limitations of cross-sectional and pre–post group designs, Keefe and colleagues (Lefebvre et al., in press) explored how daily ratings of joint pain, pain coping strategies, and positive and negative moods related to self-efficacy and medical states over 30 days. Using a time interval, within-person design, separate self-efficacy ratings for pain and physical function were found to predict mean joint pain reduction far more substantially than disease status measures or demographic factors. In addition, self-efficacy beliefs were also significantly more predictive of specific coping strategies, such as relaxation, seeking emotional support, and expressing emotions. Self-efficacy measures were negatively related to all disease status measures as well as negative mood. Interestingly, seeking spiritual support, which was rated daily as one of the main coping strategies, was found to be highly predictive of reduced joint pain the next day.

Impressively, Keefe and his colleagues have developed a strategy for assessing 30 consecutive daily ratings of efficacy, pain, function, and mood, with over a 90% compliance rate. We believe that forgiveness researchers could use this methodology to examine several theoretical process variables, especially how particular factors, such as anger or empathy for the offender, vary with other forgiveness-related variables.

Currently, in a pilot study, we are exploring ways to adapt the daily monitoring/self-rating procedure described earlier with structured interviews in a forgiveness intervention study. We hope others will use this methodology as a complement to standardized questionnaires and other procedures, such as interviews.

Uniformity Myths, RCTs, and Single-Case ($N = 1$) Experimental Designs

Clearly, a need exists for randomized clinical trials (RCTs) to answer some major questions about the efficacy of forgiveness interventions and health outcomes. Often, the designation of an intervention approach as "empirically validated" requires data from RCTs. Such designs offer a great deal of experimental control within a study, increasing confidence that the reported outcomes (e.g., morbidity and mortality) are more likely related to the treatment. Recently, researchers have discussed the pros and cons of RCTs, especially problems of relying solely on RCTs to evaluate interventions, in special issues of the *Journal of Consulting and Clinical Psychology* (e.g., Compas, Haaga, Keefe, Leitenberg, & Williams, 1998) and *American Psychologist* (e.g., Barlow, 1996), devoted to empirically validated treatments in psychotherapy.

We mention RCTs and psychotherapy intervention research because this topic has received by far the most critical and sustained attention over the years. Furthermore, many of the issues that have been considered are directly germane to ways to improve forgiveness and health research. Thoresen et al. (1998) provide a more extended discussion of lessons learned from empirical research in counseling and psychotherapy and how they may apply to improving forgiveness research (also see Worthington, Sandage, & Berry, Chapter 11, this volume).

All the Same?

Two issues, however, deserve brief mention here. First is the need to recognize the role of individual differences in forgiveness research. These include differences in gender, ethnicity, educational level, religion, spirituality, age, and basic value systems, as well as the type of offense and its frequency, severity, and duration. Kiesler (1966) long ago highlighted the problem in ignoring these differences, terming them "uniformity myths" among researchers, that is, the tendency to consider all participants with a particular problem as essentially the same (patient uniformity myth) and thus needing the same treatment (treatment uniformity myth).

One of the major criticisms of RCT designs is that they uniformly assume that the same intervention will work for all participants. While participants may have the same general health problem (e.g., recovering from acute myocardial infarction or chronic lower back pain), they commonly differ in ways related to the validity of an assessment method or in responsiveness to a particular intervention (Barlow, 1996). We recognize the need for standardization of intervention regimens and the value of manualized treatments, but such standardization should not be prematurely emphasized, nor should participants who fail to benefit from a treatment be ignored or labeled simply as outliers. Rather, these differences are not necessarily random or noisy fluctuations. Instead, they can provide opportunities to learn more about what works with whom and why. Examining person and contextual variables early on with smaller N designs can help reduce premature use of RCTs that assume uniformity among participants.

$N = 1$ Experiments: Feasible and Functional

Second, of experimental, single-case research designs ($N = 1$), while typically ignored, remain a valuable research tool (Hillard, 1993). $N = 1$ designs will not provide convincing confirmatory evidence that an intervention or assessment works well with most persons concerning forgiveness or a host of other problem areas (Thoresen & Powell, 1992). But $N = 1$ experimental designs can offer very effective, low cost ways to assess and evaluate a particular forgiveness intervention approach or assessment procedure. Multiple measures can be gathered before, during, and after an intervention, or different treatment components can be tried in sequence, in time-lagged, overlapping designs.

One of the distinguishing features of $N = 1$ is the process-related nature of the design. Instead of gathering, for example, baseline data on one occasion (pretest), $N = 1$ designs involve collecting data repeatedly over many hours, days, or weeks, depending on the type of information being gathered. Doing so can establish a more reliable baseline and also reveal fluctuations in data related to particular times and situations. For example, participants in a forgiveness intervention could complete daily ratings of anger and blame as well as empathy for an offender. This could be done with simple, inexpensive daily diary protocols or with electronic ambulatory monitors that can be programmed to prompt self-reports of particular moods or cognitions at selected or random times during the day.

Such devices can also monitor heart rate and blood pressure repeatedly during the day (Taylor, Fried, & Kenardy, 1990).

Typically, intervention data are collected before, after, and at one or more follow-up occasions. By contrast, using $N = 1$ designs, one or more dependent variables can be gathered throughout the intervention, allowing for analysis of patterns of change during the intervention rather than simply point estimates. To control for possible assessment effects, some participants can engage only in assessment while others receive the intervention. See Kazdin (1982) for a comprehensive presentation of $N = 1$ design options, such as multiple baseline, alternating treatment, and time-lagged multiple interventions designs. Also discussed are different data-analysis techniques, such as distribution-free methods and autoregressive integrated moving average analyses that control for the nonindependence of often-repeated measures.

Finally, rather than again relying on only one occasion to collect posttreatment or follow-up data, $N = 1$ methodology offers a time-series perspective on patterns of change, if any, over time. Such data can be mined for systematic fluctuations associated with different features of the intervention, such as the introduction of a new intervention procedure. For example, did any discernible change occur in selected physiological indicators during the days surrounding the participant's stated decision to begin the forgiveness process, to begin "letting go?" If the same participant is also collecting data concerning an offense by another person who is not the direct focus of the intervention, analyses of generalization effects are possible.

The variations of $N = 1$ experimental designs are almost limitless, yet they are feasible, since so few participants are involved. Some may consider this type of research too painstaking and laborious, without ample enough reward. Yet as part of an overall research program or as early steps in a clearly innovative study area, $N = 1$ designs offer well-controlled data, especially in the discovery phases of empirical research (Suppe, 1977).

CLOSING COMMENTS

Evidence that forgiveness influences physical health does not yet exist. Still, we have reason to suspect that physical health status may indeed be related, probably indirectly, to forgiveness. Some of the major components believed to be involved in forgiveness, such as anger, hostility, and blame, have been implicated in physical disease risk. While scores of retrospective accounts ("stories") have attributed improvement in physical health to forgiveness, these narratives at best only hint at possibilities.

Some of these conceptual frameworks and research methods could be used to explore possible connections between forgiveness and physical health. Such examination will be well served if a pluralistic perspective can be adopted theoretically and methodologically. We are mindful of several noted philosophers of science (e.g., Whitehead, 1967) who recognized the inevitable tension in science between faith and doubt; that is, the scientist must believe in what he or she is doing yet balance that faith with a healthy and rigorous skepticism of their beliefs. Popper (1965) expressed this well in his demand that scientists use disconfirmatory logic, in effect seeking to disconfirm their theoretically favored hypotheses. For example, researchers need to consider other explanations for data that seem to support the notion that forgiveness benefits health. By using a variety of research methods, and by recognizing that no single methodology by itself can adequately examine and document the phenomena of forgiveness and physical health, researchers are more likely to produce meaningful evidence and sound theory.

We suspect that the potential physical health benefits of forgiveness not only exist but also that forgiveness may promote optimal health and well-being (Diener, 1996), what Emmons (Chapter 8, this volume) calls "the good life." Forgiveness as a major coping style for dealing with life's inevitable hurts, frustrations, and offenses, often yields a calmer and more caring way of living (Kushner, 1996). Learning about forgiveness and how to use forgiveness skills conceivably might enhance health status not only through reduced sympathetic hyperarousal and risky health behaviors but also through a more optimistic and hopeful outlook on life, or what Antonovsky (1979) termed a greater "sense of coherence." Such a perspective has long been advanced by various religiously inspired "wisdom traditions" as the path to living with greater meaning, direction, and health (e.g., Smith, 1989). The question raised here, however, is whether empirically based research can begin to demonstrate that forgiveness does promote better physical health. It is a question well worth answering.

REFERENCES

Affleck, G., Tennen, H., Croog, S., & Levine, S. (1987). Causal attributions, perceived benefits and morbidity after heart attack: An 8 year study. *Journal of Consulting and Clinical Psychology, 55,* 29–35.

Affleck, G., Tennen, H., Urrows, S., & Higgins, P. (1991). Neuroticism and the pain–mood relation in rheumatoid arthritis: Insights from a prospective daily study. *Journal of Consulting and Clinical Psychology, 60,* 119–126.

Albom, M. (1997). *Tuesdays with Morrie.* New York: Doubleday.

Allan, R., & Scheidt, S. (1996). Empirical basis for cardiac psychology. In R. Allan & S. Scheidt (Eds.), *Heart and mind: The practice of cardiac psychology* (pp. 63–123). Washington, DC: American Psychological Association.

Anderson, B. L., Farrar, W. B., Golden-Kreutz, D., Kutz, L. A., MacCallum, R., Courtney, M. E., & Glaser, R. (1998). Stress and immune responses following surgical treatment of regional breast cancer. *Journal of the National Cancer Institute, 90,* 30–36.

Antonovsky, A. (1979). *Health, stress, and coping.* San Francisco: Jossey-Bass.

Bandura, A. (1986). *Social foundations of thought and action: A social cognitive theory.* Inglewood Cliffs, NJ: Prentice-Hall.

Bandura, A. (1995). *Manual for the construction of self-efficacy scales.* Department of Psychology, Stanford University, Stanford, CA 94305-2130.

Bandura, A. (1997). *Self-efficacy: The practice of control.* San Francisco: Freeman.

Barefoot, J. C. (1992). Developments in the measurement of hostility. In A. W. Siegman & T. W. Smith (Eds.), *Anger, hostility and the heart* (pp. 43–66). Hillsdale, NJ: Erlbaum.

Barlow, D. (1996). Health care policy, psychotherapy research, and the future of psychotherapy. *American Psychologist, 51,* 1050–1058.

Booth-Kewley, S., & Friedman, H. S. (1987). Psychological predictors of heart disease: A quantitative review. *Psychological Bulletin, 101,* 343–362.

Brownell, K. D., & Wadden, T. A. (1992). Etiology and treatment of obesity. *Journal of Consulting and Clinical Psychology, 60,* 505–517.

Caudill, M. A. (1995). *Managing pain before it manages you.* New York: Guilford Press.

Coe, C. (1997). Sociality and immunological health revisited. *Psychosomatic Medicine, 59,* 222–223.

Cohen, S., Tyrell, D. A. J., & Smith, A. P. (1991). Psychological stress in humans and susceptibility to the common cold. *New England Journal of Medicine, 325,* 606–612.

Compas, B. E., Haaga, D. A. F., Keefe, F. J., Leitenberg, H., & Williams, D. A. (1998). Sampling and empirically supported psychological treatments from health psychology. *Journal of Consulting and Clinical Psychology, 66,* 89–112.

Cook, T. D. (1985). Postpositivist critical multiplism. In R. L. Shotland & M. M. Mark (Eds.), *Social science and social policy* (pp. 21–62). Beverly Hills, CA: Sage.

Davidson, K., Stuhr, J., & Chambers, L. (in press). Constructive anger behavior as a stress buffer. In K. D. Craig & K. S. Dobson (Eds.), *Stress, vulnerability and reactivity.* Thousand Oaks, CA: Sage.

DeBusk, R. F., Miller, N. H., Superko, H. R., Dennis, C. A., Thomas, R. J., Lew, H. T., Berger, W. E., Heller, R. S., Rompf, J., & Gee, D. (1994). A case-management system for coronary risk factor modification after acute myocardial infarction. *Annals of Internal Medicine, 120,* 721–729.

Deffenbacher, J. L. (1994). Anger reduction: Issues, assessment and intervention strategies. In A. W. Siegman & T. W. Smith (Eds.), *Anger, hostility and the heart* (pp. 239–269). Hillsdale, NJ: Erlbaum.

Denzin, N. K., & Lincoln, Y. S. (Eds.). (1994). *Handbook of qualitative research.* Thousand Oaks, CA: Sage.

Diener, E. (1996). Traits can be powerful, but are not enough: Lessons from subjective well-being. *Journal of Research in Personality, 30,* 389–399.

Dodge, K. A., & Frame, C. L. (1982). Social cognitive biases and deficits in aggressive boys. *Child Development, 53,* 620–635.

Easwaran, E. (1989). *Meditation.* Tomales, CA: Nilgiri Press.

Everson, S. A., Goldberg, D. E., Kaplan, G. A., & Cohen, R. D. (1996). Hopelessness and risk of mortality and incidence of myocardial infarction and cancer. *Psychosomatic Medicine, 58,* 113–121.

Everson, S. A., Goldberg, D. E., Kaplan, G. A., Julkunen, J., & Salonen, J. T. (1998). Anger expressed and incident hypertension. *Psychosomatic Medicine, 60,* 730–735.

Everson, S. A., Kauhanen, J., & Kaplan, G. A. (1997). Hostility and increased risk of mortality and acute myocardial infarction: The mediating role of behavioral risk factors. *American Journal of Epidemiology, 146,* 142–152.

Ewart, C. T., Taylor, C. B., Reese, L. B., & DeBusk, R. F. (1983). Effects of early post-myocardial infarction exercise testing on self-perception and subsequent physical activity. *American Heart Journal, 51,* 1076–1080.

Flanigan, B. (1992). *Forgiving the unforgivable.* New York: Macmillan.

Folkman, S. (1997). Positive psychological states and coping with severe stress. *Social Science and Medicine, 45,* 1207–1221.

Friedman, M., Thoresen, C., Gill, J., Ulmer, D., Powell, L. H., Price, V. A., Brown, B., Thompson, L., Rabin, D., Breall, W. S., Bourg, W., Levy, R., & Dixon, T. (1986). Alterations of Type A behavior and its effects on cardiac recurrence in post-myocardial infarction patients: Summary results of the coronary prevention recurrence project. *American Heart Journal, 112,* 653–665.

Goldfried, M. R. (1980). Toward the delineation of therapeutic change principles. *American Psychologist, 35,* 991–999.

Gorsuch, R. L., & Miller, W. R. (1999). Measuring spirituality. In W. R. Miller (Ed.), *Integrating spirituality into practice: A practitioner's guide.* Washington, DC: American Psychological Association.

Gotlib, I. H., Gilboa, E., & Kaplan, R. (in press). Cognitive functioning in depression: Nature and origins. In R. J. Davidson (Ed.), *Wisconsin Symposium on Emotion* (Vol. 1). New York: Oxford University Press.

Greeno, J. G. (1998). The situativity of knowing, learning and research. *American Psychologist, 53,* 5–26.

Hall, P., Davidson, K., MacGregor, M., & MacLean, D. (1998). *Expanded Structured Interview: Assessment manual.* Halifax, Nova Scotia: Heart Health of Nova Scotia.

Hammen, C., & Goodman-Brown, T. (1990). Self-schemas and vulnerability to specific life stresses in children at risk for depression [Special Issue: Selfhood processes and emotional disorders]. *Cognitive Therapy and Research, 14,* 215–227.

Hilliard, R. B. (1993). Single-case methodology in psychotherapy process and outcome research. *Journal of Consulting and Clinical Psychology, 61,* 373–380.

House, J. S., Landis, K. R., & Umberson, D. (1988). Social relationships and health. *Science, 241,* 540–545.

Jiang, W., Babyak, M., Krantz, D. S., Waugh, R. A., Coleman, R. E., Hanson, M. M., Frid, D. J., McNulty, S., Morris, J. J., & O'Connor, C. M. (1996). Mental stress—induced myocardial ischemia and cardiac events. *Journal of the American Medical Association, 275,* 1651–1656.

Kaplan, A. (1964). *The conduct of inquiry.* San Francisco: Chandler.

Kazdin, A. E. (1982). Single-case experimental designs in clinical research and practice. *New Directions for Methodology of Social and Behavioral Science, 13,* 33–47.

Keefe, F. J., Affleck, G., Lefebvre, J. C., Starr, K., Caldwell, D. S., & Tennen, H. (1997). Pain coping strategies and coping efficacy in rheumatoid arthritis: A daily process analysis. *Pain, 69,* 35–42.

Kiesler, D. J. (1966). Some myths of psychotherapy research and the search for a paradigm. *Psychological Bulletin, 65,* 110–130.

Kleinman, A., & Becker, A. E. (1998). "Sociosomatics": The contributions of anthropology to psychosomatic medicine. *Psychosomatic Medicine, 60,* 389–393.

Kleinman, A., Eisenberg, L., & Good, B. (1978). Culture, illness, and cure: Clinical lessons from anthropologic and cross-cultural research. *Archives of Internal Medicine, 88,* 251–258.

Kushner, H. (1996). *How good do we have to be?* New York: Little, Brown.

Lefebvre, J. C., Keefe, F. J., Affleck, G., Raezer, L. B., Starr, K., Caldwell, D. S., & Tennen, H. (in press). The relationship of arthritis self-efficacy to daily pain, daily mood, and daily pain coping in rheumatoid arthritis patients. *Pain.*

Linden, W., Stossel, C., & Maurice, J. (1996). Psychosocial interventions for patients with coronary artery disease: A meta-analysis. *Archives of Internal Medicine, 156,* 745–752.

Lorig, K. (1999, March). *Self-management groups for chronic disease patients: Invited address.* Paper presented at the Society of Behavioral Medicine, San Diego, CA.

Lorig, K., & Holman, H. R. (1989). Long-term outcomes of an arthritis self-management study: Effects of reinforcement efforts [Special Issue: Health self-care]. *Social Science and Medicine, 29,* 221–224.

Luskin, F. M., & Thoresen, C. E. (1999). *The psychosocial effects of forgiveness training in young adults.* Unpublished manuscript, Stanford University, Stanford, CA.

Mahoney, M. J. (Ed.). (1995). *Cognitive and constructivist psychotherapies: Theory, research, and practice.* New York: Springer.

Markus, H. R., Reaff, C. D., Conner, A., Pudberry, E. K., & Barnett, K. L. (in press). "I am responsible": Themes and variations in American understandings of Responsibility. In A. S. Rossi (Ed.), *Caring and doing for others: Social responsibility in the domains of family, work, and community.* Chicago: University of Chicago Press.

Marty, M. (1998). The ethos of Christian forgiveness. In E. L. Worthington (Ed.), *Dimensions of forgiveness: Psychological research and theological perspectives* (pp. 9–28). Philadelphia: Templeton Foundation Press.

McCraty, R., Atkinson, M., Tiller, W., Rein, G., & Watkins, A. (1995). The effects of emotions on short term power spectrum analysis on heart rate variability. *American Journal of Cardiology, 76,* 1089–1093.

McCullough, M. E., & Worthington, E. L. (1994). Models of interpersonal forgiveness and their applications to counseling: Review and critique. *Counseling and Values, 39,* 2–14.

McCullough, M. E., Worthington, E. L., & Rachal, K. C. (1997). Interpersonal forgiving in close relationships. *Journal of Personality and Social Psychology, 73,* 321–336.

McEwen, B. S. (1998). Protective and damaging effects of stress mediators. *New England Journal of Medicine, 338,* 171–179.

McEwen, B. S., & Stellar, E. (1993). Stress and the individual: Mechanisms leading to disease. *Archives of Internal Medicine, 153,* 2093–2101.

Miller, T. Q., Smith, T. W., Turner, C. W., Guijarro, M. L., & Hallet, A. J. (1996). Meta-analytic review of research on hostility and physical health. *Psychological Bulletin, 119,* 322–348.

Oman, D., Thoresen, C. E., & McMahon, K. (1999). Volunteerism and mortality among the community-dwelling elderly [Special Issue: Spirituality and health]. *Journal of Health Psychology.*

Ornish, D., Brown, S. E., Scherwitz, L. W., & Billings, J. (1990). Can lifestyle changes reverse coronary heart disease? *Lancet, 336,* 129–133.

Pargament, K. I. (1997). *The psychology of religion and coping: Theory, research, and practice.* New York: Guilford Press.

Pennebaker, J. W., Kiecolt-Glaser, J. K., & Glaser, R. (1988). Disclosure of traumas and immune functioning: Health implications of psychotherapy. *Journal of Consulting and Clinical Psychology, 56,* 239–245.

Petrie, K. J., Booth, R. J., & Pennebaker, J. W. (1998). The immunological effects of thought suppression. *Journal of Personality and Social Psychology, 75,* 1264–1272.

Pickering, T. G., & Gerin, W. (1990). Cardiovascular reactivity in the laboratory and the role of behavioral factors in hypertension: A critical review. *Annals of Behavioral Medicine, 12,* 3–16.

Popper, K. R. (1965). *Conjectures and refutations.* New York: HarperCollins.

Price, V. A. (1988). Research and clinical issues in treating Type A behavior. In B. K. Houston & C. R. Snyder (Eds.), *Type A behavior pattern: Research, treatment, and intervention* (pp. 275–311). New York: Wiley.

Propst, L. R., Ostrom, R., Watkins, P., & Dean, T. (1992). Comparative efficacy of religious and non-religious cognitive-behavioral therapy for the treatment of clinical depression in religious individuals. *Journal of Consulting and Clinical Psychology, 60,* 94–103.

Raskin, R. N., & Hall, C. S. (1979). A narcissistic personality inventory. *Psychological Reports, 45,* 590.

Rhodewalt, F., & Morf, C. C. (1995). Self and interpersonal correlates of the Narcissistic Personality Inventory: A review and new findings. *Journal of Research in Personality, 29,* 1–23.

Richards, P. S., & Bergin, A. E. (1997). *A spiritual strategy for counseling and psychotherapy.* Washington, DC: American Psychological Association.

Richards, T. A., & Folkman, S. (1997). Spiritual aspects of lose at the time of a partner's death from AIDS. *Death Studies, 21,* 527–552.

Roberts, J. E., Gilboa, E., & Gotlib, I. H. (in press). Ruminative response style and vulnerability to episodes of dysphoria: Gender neuroticism, and episode duration. *Cognitive Therapy and Research.*

Rye, M. S., & Pargament, K. I. (1997, August). *Forgiveness and romantic relationships in college.* Paper presented at a meeting of the American Psychological Association, Chicago, IL.

Scheidt, S. (1996). A whirlwind tour of cardiology for the mental health professional. In R. Allan & S. Scheidt (Eds.), *Heart and mind: The practice of cardiac psychology* (pp. 15–124). Washington, DC: American Psychological Association.

Segerstrom, S. C., Taylor, S. E., Kemeny, M. E., & Fahey, J. L. (1998). Optimism is associated with mood, coping and immune change in response to stress. *Journal of Personality and Social Psychology, 74,* 1646–1655.

Shedler, J., Mayman, M., & Manis, M. (1993). The illusion of mental health. *American Psychologist, 48,* 1117–1131.

Smith, H. (1989). *The world's religions.* San Francisco: HarperCollins.

Smith, T. W. (1992). Hostility and health: Current status of a psychosomatic hypothesis. *Health Psychology, 11,* 139–150.

Spiegel, D., Bloom, J. R., Kraemer, H. C., & Gottlheil, E. (1989). Effect of psychosocial treatment on survival of metastatic breast cancer. *Lancet, 14,* 888–891.

Spielberger, C. D., Reheiser, E. C., & Sydeman, S. J. (1995). Measuring the experience, expression and central of anger. In H. Kassionone (Ed.), *Anger disorders: Definitions, diagnosis and treatment* (pp. 49–67). Washington, DC: Taylor & Francis.

Stone, A. A., Cox, D. S., Valdimarsdottir, H., & Jandorf, L. (1987). Evidence that secretory IgA antibody is associated with daily mood. *Journal of Personality and Social Psychology, 52,* 988–993.

Suppe, F. (1977). *The structure of scientific theories* (2nd ed.). Urbana: University of Illinois Press.

Tavris, C. (1989). *Anger: The misunderstood emotion.* New York: Simon & Schuster.

Taylor C. B., Fried, L., & Kenardy, J. (1990). The use of a real-time computer diary for data acquisition and processing. *Behaviour Research and Therapy, 28,* 93–97.

Tennen, H., & Affleck, G. (1990). Blaming others for threatening events. *Psychological Bulletin, 108,* 209–232.

Thoresen, C. E., & Hoffman Goldberg, J. (1998). Coronary heart disease: A psychosocial perspective on assessment and intervention. In S. Roth-Roemer, S. K. Robinson, & C. Carmin (Eds.), *The emerging role of counseling psychology in health care* (pp. 94–136). New York: Norton.

Thoresen, C. E., Luskin, F. M., & Harris, A. H. S. (1998). The science of forgiveness interventions: Reflections and suggestions. In E. L. Worthington (Ed.), *Dimensions of forgiveness: Psychological research and theological perspectives* (pp. 163–192). Philadelphia: Templeton Foundation Press.

Thoresen, C. E., & Powell, L. H. (1992). Type A patterns: New perspectives on theory, assessment, and interventions. *Journal of Consulting and Clinical Psychology, 60,* 595–604.

Walsh, R., & Vaughn, F. (1993). *Paths beyond ego: The transpersonal vision.* New York: Plenum Press.

Weil, A. (1997). *8 weeks to optimal health.* New York: Knopf.

Weiner, B., Graham, S., Peter, O., & Zmuidinas, M. (1991). Public confessions and forgiveness. *Journal of Personality, 59,* 281–312.

Whitehead, A. (1967). *Science and the modern world.* New York: Macmillan.

Williams, R., & Williams, V. (1993). *Anger kills: Seventeen strategies for controlling the hostility that can harm your health.* New York: Harper Perennial.

Worthington, E. L. (Ed.). (1998). *Dimensions of forgiveness: Psychological research and theological perspectives.* Philadelphia: Templeton Foundation Press.

℘ CHAPTER 13

Forgiveness in Pastoral Care and Counseling

John Patton

THE POINT OF VIEW EXPRESSED IN THIS CHAPTER

The understanding of forgiveness presented in this chapter is that forgive-ness or, more accurately, the quality of forgiving-ness, is an important characteristic of a life lived in right relationship with God and one's fellow human beings. It is better understood as a process of discovering how to live ones life in relationship than a program of action one should follow in order to achieve particular goals. This view of forgiveness is that of a Christian pastoral counselor and theologian, and in a book conceived and edited by psychologists, it seems important to suggest that a pastoral per-spective can influence how one might understand and interpret the data of human forgiveness.

Pastoral care is the effort of a religious tradition or faith group to of-fer healing, sustaining or guiding to those who acknowledge it as a source for help. Pastoral counseling is a more structured form of the religious tradition in which the person needing care has acknowledged it and openly sought it. It is different from other forms of counseling in that it is provided by those whom the religious tradition or faith group has autho-rized to offer care on its behalf.

Pastoral counseling is not primarily or necessarily "religious" in the sense of using or providing information about religious concepts. Neither is it simply counseling by one who is a religious person. Rather, it is a part of what a particular religious group understands as its ministry to persons, structured in relation to counseling or psychotherapeutic methods by one who is recognized by and accountable to that religious community.

A pastoral counselor—a practitioner of a particular kind of ministry to persons—thinks about or interprets what he or she does according to a pastoral theological method. The method begins with an issue or problem that has emerged from practice. It moves to theory in order to gain insight into the problem. Although it looks to theory to interpret practice, there is also the expectation that theory will be informed by practice. Particular problems in forgiveness, for example, challenge and sometimes change theories about forgiveness as well as being informed by them.

Forgiveness is necessarily a religious or theological term for a pastoral counselor because of his involvement in a religious tradition. Forgiveness has to do with the relationship between God and humankind, and with the relationship of human beings to each other. The pastoral counselor's experience of forgiveness in her practice must be interpreted in relation to the tradition of which she is a part, and to which she is accountable as a minister. What has been experienced in practice may modify or change the pastoral counselor's understanding and interpretation of the religious tradition, but what the tradition says cannot be ignored. It must be seriously engaged.

Because forgiveness also has to do with what human beings are, how they think, and what they do, it uses psychological as well as theological theory. Pastors and theologians, in their concern for persons, have always used some kind of psychological theory whether or not they were aware of it. The obligation of a pastoral counselor in using a theory from another discipline is to use it in a way that enriches and informs his or her own primary discipline, neither allowing the new data to dominate that discipline nor to reduce it to something it is not. A theologian, Theodore Jennings, has suggested that dialogue between disciplines such as theology and psychology "should be directed toward a common subject matter. The subject matter common to both is not the existence or nature of God but the nature and possible transformation of human existence" (Jennings, 1990).

Forgiveness is this type of subject matter. According to Jennings, a useful test of the seriousness and fruitfulness of a psychological–theological dialogue on forgiveness might be "whether the conceptuality and vocabulary of both sides is altered and enriched through the process. . . . The sign of a mature, responsible, and fruitful dialogue is that both sides come to require revision in the light of the discussion" (p. 864).

Although theology is commonly understood as a normative discipline, both theology and psychology make use of descriptive and normative views—statements of and assumptions about what human beings are and what they should be. In this chapter, written by a pastoral counselor and theologian, normative views may be more evident than in other chapters. Nevertheless, it is impossible to discuss a topic such as forgiveness without bringing into play norms and values about what is good. One simply should question the adequacy, reliability, and source of those norms.

Having described the perspective of the pastoral counselor, I turn now to the topic of forgiveness itself and how my concern with it developed. For another view of forgiveness by a pastoral counselor, see David Augsburger's *Helping People Forgive* (1995).

THE STRUGGLE WITH FORGIVENESS AS OBSERVED IN PASTORAL COUNSELING

In the 1970s and early 1980s, I did a great deal of pastoral counseling with couples, families, and individuals troubled with family relationships. I found that many of the persons with whom I worked made explicit use of forgiveness as an interpretive concept for their experience, but often they insisted that they could never forgive the one who had so deeply hurt them. They were unable to respond either to the threats they had heard about what might happen to them if they did not forgive, or to the affirmations of how forgiveness was "good for them." There were some who claimed to have forgiven the offender, but their forgiveness seemed so easily accomplished that I had difficulty in believing them. On occasion, I found myself thinking, "I believe in God's forgiveness, but I sometimes wonder if human forgiveness is really possible."

In the early stage of counseling with those concerned with forgiveness, what was even more prominent was the shame that these persons experienced. As a result of the injustices they had suffered, they did not feel that they were the same people they were before the injustice. Perhaps the people they were before the injury could have forgiven those who had hurt them, but now, they were estranged from their former identities and, thus, in no position to forgive.

What I observed later in the process of pastoral counseling was a gradual broadening of these persons' focus of concern. No longer was their agenda narrowly focused on the injury they had experienced and the one who had injured them. The frame of their life picture was enlarged, and we dealt with a number of different concerns in their lives. The injury was still there in the picture, but it was placed in relation to other things. Life was going on in spite of it.

As I reflected upon my clinical experience with these persons who were struggling with forgiveness in one way or another, two things were most evident: (1) the shame these persons experienced as a result of the injuries they had received; and (2) that forgiveness, or something like it, seemed to occur when they were able to see the people who had injured them as different people. I became convinced that forgiving was not primarily a behavior—something done or not done—but a process discovered retrospectively, after it had already begun.

As a result of these reflections and my subsequent research on shame and human forgiveness, the thesis for the book I wrote was stated in the following way:

> Human forgiveness is not doing something but discovering something—that I am more like those who have hurt me than different from them. I am able to forgive when I discover that I am in no position to forgive. Although the experience of God's forgiveness may involve confession of, and the sense of being forgiven for specific sins, at its heart it is the recognition of my reception into the community of sinners— those affirmed as God's children. (Patton, 1985, p. 16)

The first part of the thesis is based on an understanding of human forgiveness as part of a larger process of dealing with a shamed and estranged self and, as the self experiences healing, gradually being able to recognize the humanness of one's injurer as well as discovering one's own. The remainder of the thesis is essentially a theological affirmation. It claims that no one is "in position" to forgive another except in response to God's forgiveness of oneself. This is not the place to argue for that part of the thesis, but I must acknowledge that the theological conviction expressed certainly influences the way that I interpret both the human problem and the human possibility.

SHAME AND HUMAN FORGIVENESS

The shame experienced by persons I worked with in pastoral counseling resulted not only from the personal injury they had experienced, but also from the shame they had incorporated from what they understood their religious tradition to be saying to them. An example of this comes from a commentary on the New Testament Gospel of Matthew that is still used for personal religious devotion and study by members of the major Protestant denominations. In his discussion of the Lord's Prayer, the author states:

> Jesus says in the plainest possible language that if we forgive others, God will forgive us; but if we refuse to forgive others, God will refuse to forgive us. . . . If we say, "I will never forget what so-and-so did to me," and then go and take this petition on our lips, we are quite deliberately asking God not to forgive us. . . . No one is fit to pray the Lord's prayer so long as the unforgiving spirit holds sway within his heart. (Barclay, 1959, pp. 223–224)

Most of my counselees would not have been, in the judgment of this Biblical scholar, "fit to pray the Lord's prayer," but, in fact, they did pray it. They believed that forgiveness was important, but they were caught in the shame of what had happened to them, confirmed in it by what they understood their religious tradition was telling them they must do.

Emmie, whose story I presented in *Is Human Forgiveness Possible?*, was one of the persons with whom I became acquainted in her struggle to forgive in the midst of shame. She was the 50-year-old wife of a Presbyterian elder who had left her and moved in with another woman. When Elmer left, he never came back, so that much of the time prior to their divorce, she did not even know where he was. She, who had given close to 30 years of her life to marriage and children, was left without either. Her children had already grown up and moved away, and, in what seemed to her like another act of infidelity, they still wanted to have a relationship with their father in spite of what he had done.

Emmie, who was referred to me for pastoral counseling by her pastor, was left with her shame about what Elmer had done, and with what that might say about the kind of person she was. Much of what I experienced with her in the early part of our relationship was her anger at what had happened and her struggle to figure out how it could have happened. Such bad things should not happen to good people. She continued to worship in the church where she taught children in the Sunday School and tried to set a good example. Each Sunday, she joined the congregation in praying that fifth petition of the Lord's Prayer, "Forgive us our debts as we forgive our debtors," but was unable to think of forgiving as a possibility for herself.

As time went on, however, Emmie's life situation improved. She got a job, improved her relationships with her siblings and her children, and, as a part of her counseling with me, came to terms with her mother's death. She fell in love—not just with me this time, but with a married man whom she had met at her place of employment. One day in our regular twice-per-month interview, I said something like the following (Patton, 1985):

PASTOR: As I listen to you talking about your friend, I found myself wondering if you ever saw yourself as in the same position as Elmer [her husband].

EMMIE: (*Quickly*) No!

PASTOR: I see. It occurred to me that there might be some similarities.

EMMIE: Well, *I* don't see them.

Not long after that, Elmer, who had moved with his new wife to another city, lost his job and was unable to pay his alimony. Emmie was angry, financially pressed, but was able to write him a letter in which she expressed both her anger and her concern about his circumstances. In a matter-of-fact way, she described her financial needs and requested resumption of alimony payments as soon as he was reemployed. When she told me about this in our next interview, I commented:

PASTOR: Elmer sounds almost human!

EMMIE: What?

PASTOR: I never had heard you speak of him as an ordinary human being before, but listening to you then, that's all that he seemed to be. You sounded as if you were concerned about his predicament.

EMMIE: Well, he got himself into it.

PASTOR: I know. I was just noticing how you sounded. For the first time I can remember, he didn't just seem like the enemy, but just an ordinary human being.

(*Emmie remained silent.*)

Shortly after this, Emmie terminated her relationship with me, suggesting that it was getting in the way of the relationship with her now-divorced friend.

Throughout my experience with Emmie, I was aware of the question, "How is the petition in the familiar Lord's Prayer, 'Forgive us our debts as we forgive our debtors,' related to Emmie?" The hurt she felt because of the rejection by her husband resonated with an earlier feeling of rejection in never quite measuring up to her mother's expectations. Emmie's way of dealing with this, both with her mother and her husband, was to be good, or to do what was right. If she could not be sure she was loved, she could at least know that she was doing the right thing. She held on tightly to this view of herself, until she could feel love and affirmation as a person through her counseling and other developing relationships. Only when she felt affirmed in spite of the shame at being rejected did something like forgiveness—seeing her former husband not just as someone who had injured her but as an ordinary human being—become possible for her. I will return to Emmie's move toward forgiveness later in the chapter, but first it seems important to note some of the major defenses that are mobilized against shame.

IMPORTANT DEFENSES AGAINST SHAME

One of the major writers on shame, Gershen Kaufman (1989), has identified eight strategies used to defend against it: rage, contempt, striving for perfection, striving for power, internal withdrawal, humor, and denial. As a pastoral counselor, I found that three of these seemed most important: rage, righteousness, and power—more specifically, the power to forgive. Although these defenses are psychological phenomena, they are also phenomena that are interpreted ethically and theologically in the light of a person's religious tradition and practice. No doubt I have "seen" them so often in clinical experience because of my own involvement in and commitment to my religious tradition (Patton, 1985).

The defenses most evident in Emmie were rage and righteousness— her intense anger at Elmer and her claim to be the one in the right. I have used the term "righteousness," rather than simply "being right," to describe the latter defense because of its association with religion. Some of its strength seems to come from its appearing to be what our religion tells us to do. It is probably the defense that is most familiar to a pastor or marital therapist in beginning to work with a troubled marriage. Each spouse is insistent that he or she is right and the other is wrong. Those who question a significant other's care for them are quite likely to retreat into righteousness and deal with their shame by searching for the other's guilt. Much more could be said, but I move to another defense against shame and a counselee who used it.

Tom, another person whose story appeared in *Is Human Forgiveness Possible?* (Patton, 1985), was less angry in his defense against shame than was Emmie. Nevertheless, like many others I have known, he was very aware of his "power to forgive." A graduate student in psychology, Tom had originally consulted me about his relationship to women and his occasional sexual impotence, but he soon moved on to spend a great deal of time dealing with his relationship to his father. He wondered if he could ever forgive his father for divorcing his mother, when Tom was in his early teens, leaving Tom to be the "man of the house." Forgiving or not forgiving functions as a way to hold on to an old and familiar relationship through maintaining an incomplete transaction, a debit on what Boszormenyi-Nagy has called the "ledger of justice" (1987). As long as Tom withheld his forgiveness, his father still owed him something, and their relationship was maintained. If the forgiveness is offered, and the debit removed, relationship to the father may be lost.

In addition to the "advantage" that withholding forgiveness offered by preserving the past, it gave Tom something that his father did not appear to have—forgiveness understood, almost like a possession. It was a trump card that could be played at any time to show who was really in charge. Uncertain about his personal power because, among other things, of his inability to substitute for his mother's absent husband, Tom could always have his power to forgive available. Should he offer it, however, his advantage would be lost, and his strength in relation to his father would have to be evaluated on other grounds. Moreover, his father would no longer need him for forgiveness, and the relationship would be broken. There are clear advantages to Tom in not forgiving—advantages that may be thought of in terms of power to defend oneself against the shame of inadequacy and inferiority.

In both Emmie and Tom, there was intense anger at the way they had been injured, as well as righteousness and the power to forgive. In addition to defending against shame with righteousness and power, they used the defense of rage. Emmie's rage was more intense and held onto longer, but virtually every shamed person that I have encountered in counseling has experienced rage at the person who has injured them. Although this is too simple a distinction, I am distinguishing between rage and anger, rage being more intense and more personal. It is directed not to the injury, but to the injurer.

The most helpful interpretation of rage for me is found in Heinz Kohut's self psychology. I make this judgment because Kohut's self theory is not only an approach to a particular kind of pathology, but also a broadly based anthropological principle that makes significant affirmations about what is normatively human. The shame-prone individual, according to Kohut, does not recognize the person who has injured him as a center of independent initiative with whom he happens to be at cross-purposes. He is experienced only as an offending part of the shamed person's self. This phenomenon is what I believe I observed in Emmie and in many others who were caught up in the struggle to forgive.

According to Kohut, the transformation of this defensive rage does not take place by directly attacking it, but by relating empathically to the defending person. What the therapist does is to offer empathy, patient understanding, and a significant relationship through which additional emotional nourishment can be offered. The injury, and the rage caused by it, are not directly addressed but are dealt with in the context of an empathic response to the shamed and impoverished self (Kohut, 1972).

Empathy may involve warmth and kindness, but it is not primarily that. Rather, empathy is a disciplined, intuitive understanding that offers to the counselee a positive model of a caring human being, useful information to the counselee about himself, and an actual experience of what it means to be in relationship with a significant other. This is not Kohut's language for describing empathy, but it seems to me an accurate expression of his point of view. An empathic relationship provides useful experience in addressing life. It strengthens the person by eventually providing a more functional self, not by attempting to erase his or her problems (Kohut, 1984).

I have used Kohut's theory to interpret my experience with persons in pastoral counseling because his understanding of rage is a strong reminder that behavioral attempts to deal with anger are seldom adequate to confront life as it is or people as they are. Persons who have suffered self-injury do not "get over" their anger by either suppressing or expressing it. Their perception of reality is so influenced by what has happened to them that their rage cannot be dealt with apart from the way in which they are experiencing themselves. The person who has injured them is, as

Kohut puts it, "a flaw in a narcissistically perceived reality," so that discussing what should be done in relation to that person—forgiveness or anything else—is seldom worth the trouble (p. 644). The prior task is relationally binding their wounds without concern for what should be done to get life back in order again (Kohut, 1972).

Unfortunately, religion's response has too often been to try to fix things, expecting lasting results, for example, from simply announcing God's forgiveness. If we are forgiven, then we should be forgiving. This may be true—and in many ways I believe it is—but human beings have significant capacities for avoiding the truth. They simply are not what they ought to be, nor do they do what they should, in spite of impressive religious announcements and expectations. Undoubtedly, the announcement of forgiveness by the religious community is important, but the schedule upon which that announcement is apprehended by the forgiven one remains highly unpredictable.

FORGIVENESS AFTER VIOLENCE OR ABUSE

One of those who helpfully questioned my thesis about forgiveness was my daughter. As one who had been a rape victim, she made clear to me that seeing herself as "like" the stranger who had threatened her life and victimized her was not very realistic. It just made her more angry. Although because of the circumstances of my clinical practice and my own choice, I had been concerned in my book about forgiveness in the family, I had not dealt at all with the physical, psychological, and sexual abuse perpetrated by family members. Moreover, much of the literature on abuse makes it clear how the demands for forgiveness from those who have been victimized by family members can itself be abusive.

An illustration of this comes from Karen Olio, a psychotherapist writing in *Voices* (1992). Her article is a structured response to a statement in a children's book. The book, *I Can't Talk about It: A Child's Book about Sexual Abuse* (Sanford, 1986), insists that the abused child must forgive the father who abused her. Olio argues instead that such insistence on forgiveness "contributes to the re-victimization of survivors, who for so long were forced to conform to an external version of reality, by insisting the path to wholeness and freedom can only be found by adopting one particular way of thinking and feeling toward the abuser" (Olio, 1992, p. 73).

She challenges this "one-way" forgiveness by noting its presumption that the victim's judgment must be suspended. She argues to the contrary that, in fact, judgments offer a significant contribution to the healing process for survivors of sexual abuse. She comments that the "defense mechanisms, denial and dissociation, which are developed to cope with the emotionally overwhelming and physically over-stimulating abuse experiences, render survivors particularly susceptible to the suggestion that forgiveness is a necessary step toward resolution of the abuse trauma" (p. 74).

It is "no doubt crucial for resolution of the trauma that survivors be able to view the abuser as a human being, and that they not depersonalize him or her in the same manner that they themselves were depersonalized." But, she insists, compassion and forgiveness "are optional." Olio denies the argument of the recovery movement and 12-step programs that taking responsibility for forgiveness is an important part of an abused person's empowerment. Instead, she argues that survivors "who already must struggle with the feelings of self-blame caused by the abuse," should not have to take on the further blame of not being able to forgive (p.78).

In another treatment of human forgiveness after abuse, Sidney and Suzanne Simon argue that forgiveness is not forgetting and that victims of abuse should not forget. Their experiences and the pain caused by those experiences have a great deal to teach them about living. Forgiving is not excusing, or condoning, either. It is important that the victim not say that what was done to him or her was acceptable or "not so bad." Forgiveness is not absolving the abuser of all responsibility for what he has done. He is still responsible for what he did and must deal with it himself. Most important, forgiveness is not a clear-cut, one-time decision. A person cannot simply decide that today, he or she is going to forgive. If it happens, it happens as a result of confronting painful past experiences and healing old wounds.

The Simons argue that forgiveness is a discovery (Simon & Simon, 1990), as I did in *Is Human Forgiveness Possible?* It is the by-product of an ongoing healing process. Failure to forgive is not a failure of will. Instead, people are unable to forgive because wounds have not yet healed. Forgiveness is not something done (i.e., a behavior). It is something that happens as a sign of positive self-esteem, when the victim is no longer building his or her identity around something that happened in the past. The injury is not all of who one is, but is rather a part of life that has at least started to move out of the center of the frame (see also Fortune, 1988).

Another aspect of the problem with forgiveness as accentuated by assumptions and beliefs about forgiveness in religion comes from a situation presented by pastor Richard P. Lord (1991) in an article in *The Christian Century*. He was called upon to deal with the situation of a woman whose sons were killed and who herself was shot and left for dead by an unknown group of men who broke into her house. One of the men later wrote her from prison, saying that he had "found Christ," and asked her to forgive him. She asked her pastor, "Am I obligated as a Christian to forgive in this situation? Just what does the church mean by 'forgiveness'? He did not say, 'I'm sorry . . . just forgive me' " (p. 902).

In the pastor's answer to the question, he identifies two problems in forgiving: forgiveness as forgetting, and forgiveness as excusing. With respect to forgetting he comments, "When we forgive someone, it usually implies that we will try to act as though nothing has happened. Can we do this without showing massive disrespect for the victim of violence when those close to him or her are deeply concerned that their loved one not be forgotten?" With respect to excusing, he asks the question, if an abuser has a religious experience after the abuse has taken place, does this mean that "now we should act as though a crime wasn't committed?"

And, in reflecting on his proclamation in worship, "Your sins are forgiven," Pastor Lord imagines a battered wife thinking, "Who gave you the right to forgive the one who beats me?" As a consequence of this reflection, he argues that forgiveness cannot be "a commodity that can be handed out" by the church or anyone else, and he concludes that pastors and other well-intentioned Christians "have no right to insist that the victim establish a relationship with his or her victimizer to effect a reconciliation" (p. 902) .

Pastor Lord's answer to his parishioner was based on an understanding of repentance as involving three conditions: remorse, restitution, and regeneration. None of the three was evidenced in the prisoner who had "found Christ." Thus, the pastor concluded that to "offer forgiveness when these conditions are not met is not gracious. It is sacrilegious." His answer to the victim was "no." She did not have to forgive.

Almost more striking than the original article was the negative response it stirred up among *The Christian Century* readers. For example: "How can I be a Christian and refuse to forgive? . . . If you do not forgive others their trespasses, neither will your Father forgive you. I cannot call myself a Christian and refuse to forgive others or hope to have my sins forgiven" ("Readers' Response," 1991, p. 34).

Those who deal with forgiveness after abuse and violence remind us that expecting or demanding forgiveness from a person can itself be abusive. They also emphasize that forgiveness, if it takes place, is part of a broader healing process, not an isolated event.

THE STORY OF EMMIE RECONSIDERED

Another helpful challenger to my thesis about forgiveness is Professor Brad Binau of Trinity Lutheran Seminary in Ohio, who has reinterpreted my story of Emmie in *Is Human Forgiveness Possible?* using the understanding of shame in the Erikson developmental theory (Binau, 1997). Erikson related shame to the anal stage of development identified by Freud, and noted that in early childhood, muscles develop that allow the child both to hold on and to let go (E. Erikson, 1950). Erikson, however, was concerned with much more than this physical ability.

The holding on and letting go that Erikson identified have emotional as well as physical dimensions. Holding on can, on one hand, be a cruel restraint on oneself or, on the other hand, a part of the capacity "to have and to hold" another in relationship. Letting go sometimes means lashing out destructively, but it can also mean a more healing kind of release—letting things pass by, or letting them be. In this stage and ever after, according to Erikson, working with both sides of this issue becomes part of our lives. Through that kind of "working through," we develop the capacity to choose as a part of our autonomy.

Autonomy, which involves exercise of the will, does not simply overcome shame and doubt. Instead, it is developed in dialogue with them. Shame and doubt are not overcome. They become a part of the exercise of our will in making the choices that are appropriate for ourselves and for the communities of which we are a part. Erikson's wife, Joan, has noted that many people infer from the two-sided nature of the Eriksonian stages of development that optimal human development occurs when the good side overcomes the bad side.

> Regardless of a consistent effort to mention, even to applaud, the dystonic element present in conjunction with the syntonic basic strength at every stage of the life cycle, a certain positive thrust seems to prevail. Is it because we first called these strengths *virtues*, a word we used because it denoted vitality? Or is an American optimism apparent here? . . . The syntonic without the dystonic is meaningless. . . . None of the basic strengths is ever permanently achieved. . . . The properties of the dystonic elements not only as they show themselves each at their own critical stage of development, but throughout the life cycle, should be understood and respected. (J. Erikson, 1988, pp. 113–114)

In the light of this understanding of Erikson's theory, Binau (1997) sees something in Emmie's struggle to have a will of her own that I had not noted. I think he sees this also because of his Lutheran tradition, which in its theological context has affirmed the dystonic as well as the syntonic. With theologian Marjorie Suchocki's (1996) insight that forgiveness includes knowing as fully as possible the extent of the evil caused by the wrong that was done, Binau comments that this knowing may involve "holding on" to the grievance long enough to comprehend its magnitude so that we might gain adequate appreciation for the damage done. Moreover, "holding on" can also help the injured person discover that she is not alone in her suffering and that health is through pain, not around it. This, of course, is what should happen in a helping relationship with a shamed person, and what I think did happen with Emmie.

Then, noting that holding on too long allows the wrong done to repeat itself again and again, Binau moves to the other side of the polarity—

letting go. He relates Erikson's "letting go" to Suchocki's (1996) concept of "willing"—understood as "a reality-based flourishing that trusts God to deal with both sinner and self" (p. 97). This, in Emmie's case, is related to her moving on with life and at the same time having dealt enough with her shame to begin to see herself as a sinner, not just as someone who has been wronged. Her increased autonomy could now be expressed as letting go as well as holding on.

Letting go, as Binau interprets it theologically, does not mean letting go of reality. It means that "we let ourselves go into the arms of God—not to be carried away from our pain, but to be carried through it" (p. 35). Just as the resurrected Jesus bore the marks of the nail prints, so, Suchocki suggests, "the future made possible for us through forgiveness is not as if the sin never happened, but a future marked precisely in and through the scars of our experiences." Binau further suggests that I might have been better able to address the importance of forgiving more directly with Emmie if I had utilized Erikson's bipolar understanding of shame and the concepts of "holding on" and "letting go." And I think he is right.

FORGIVENESS AS A PART OF A LARGER PROCESS OF LIVING

Reflecting upon what has been discussed thus far in this chapter, my conviction that it is important to understand forgiveness as a part of something else should be evident. In my pastoral counseling, persons struggling with forgiveness seemed to discover something like forgiveness in themselves when they had moved on in their lives to deal with something other than "forgiving or not forgiving." The isolation they had felt in their shame at what had happened was at least partially overcome through the relationship they had experienced in their counseling and, usually, through a reconnection with a significant community in life outside their counseling.

Moreover, defenses against shame can be gradually abandoned, not by concentrating on forgiving or not forgiving the abuser, but when wounds to the self have been empathically bound up. As abuse and violence are overcome or at least partially overcome, a broader healing can take place. One overcomes shame and develops autonomy, including the capacity to will and to choose, by holding on and letting go in the context of significant relationship. For the child in the anal stage of psychosexual development, this takes place in relation to significant parental figures. For the shamed adult whose injury has caused the loss of autonomy, it takes place in relation to those who care in his or her adult world. The implication for forgiveness in each of these instances is that forgiveness is best understood as an important part of something larger. It may simply be going on with life "in spite of," or developing the good life of which forgiveness is a part.

Earlier, I noted the way that the Lord's prayer could be interpreted to add to the shame of having difficulty in forgiving. Although this chapter is not the place for any extensive interpretation of a religious text, a brief alternative interpretation might be in order. The phrase about "forgiving as we are forgiven" appears in the context of a prayer describing the believer's relationship to God, who is understood as a loving and forgiving parent. In relation to such a God, the believer is surprisingly empowered to be forgiving. Human forgiveness, understood in this theological way, is not primarily something to be done to improve our health or secure our salvation, but it is an illustration of a quality of life when it is lived in relation to God and one's fellow human beings. I make no claim that this is the only way to understand the teaching about forgiveness in the New Testament, but I am convinced that what I have said is not inconsistent with the main thrust of that teaching.

A life of faith in such a God is described theologically as a continual discovery and rediscovery of grace—the fact that we do not have to be, but we are. We do not have to forgive, but sometimes we discover the capacity to forgive in ourselves. Human beings worship God to celebrate that fact. Human forgiveness is not a condition of God's forgiveness but something enabled by God's response to human life.

Theologian L. Gregory Jones (1995) describes the life of which forgiveness is a part using the image of learning a craft. Just "as Aristotle emphasized the importance of learning a 'craft' for learning how to live, so there is a craft of forgiveness that Christians are called to learn from one another" (p. xii, 1995). The craft of forgiveness, according to Jones, involves the ongoing and ever-deepening process of learning to live in communion with God, with one another, and with the whole of creation.

As one who has been learning how to play music again after a recess of 35 years, I find Jones's image of learning a craft to be a powerful one. I play scales or exercises on my piano or saxophone so that the scales and chords become a part of me that I know how to embody in what I play— almost without thinking. When I practice learning my craft, I can feel where a note is to be played with my hand without a conscious decision about it. When I am able to practice my craft, I become less awkward, and music becomes a part of me. Someone said to me recently, "You must have been practicing. You're better than when I heard you last year." The craft becomes a part of who one is, not just what one does.

The religious life as the Christian tradition describes it is an ongoing communal activity of learning to live into the forgiveness that characterizes our relation to God. My way of saying this has been that it is a discovery in the process of living, in spite of the brokenness that I or another has created or has been responsible for. Although much of my concern over the years has been with human forgiveness, human and divine forgiveness cannot be separated theologically. I am committed to the view that we forgive as we are forgiven. God is a part of any forgiveness we give or receive. The way I ended my book on forgiveness was to suggest that what we do in responding to those who have been hurt by life and relationships is not to encourage or insist that they forgive, but to be with them in the pain of being themselves. It is an attempt to break the isolation of shame and rejection, so that they are freed from their need to view themselves as victims of life and can accept responsibility for their lives and the guilt that inevitably arises in human relationships. The task of the religious community and its ministers is not to supervise acts of forgiveness, but to provide relationships in which genuine humanity, including the possibility of forgiving one's transgressions, can be discovered.

REFERENCES

Augsburger, D. M. (1995). *Helping people forgive.* Louisville, KY: Westminster/John Knox.

Barclay W. (1959). *The Gospel of Matthew.* Philadelphia: Westminster Press.

Binau, B. (1997, October). *Wholeness and holiness: Forgiveness in light of shame and autonomy, and the dynamics of "holding on" and "letting go."* Unpublished lectures to the West Virginia Conference Pastors School of the United Methodist Church.

Boszormenyi-Nagy, I. (1987). *Foundations of contextual therapy: Collected papers of Ivan Boszormenyi-Nagy, M.D.* New York: Brunner/Mazel.

Erikson, E. H. (1950). *Childhood and society.* New York: Norton.

Erikson, J. M. (1988). *Wisdom and the senses.* New York: Norton.

Fortune, M. (1988). Forgiveness: The last step. In A. L. Horton & J. A. Williamson (Eds.), *Abuse and religion: When praying isn't enough* (pp. 215–220). Washington, DC: Heath.

Jennings, T. (1990). Pastoral theological methodology. In R. J. Hunter (Ed.), *Dictionary of pastoral care and counseling* (pp. 862–864). Nashville, TN: Abingdon Press.

Jones, L. G. (1995). *Embodying forgiveness: A theological analysis.* Grand Rapids, MI: Eerdmans.

Kaufman, G. (1989). *The psychology of shame: Theory and treatment of shame-based syndromes.* New York: Springer.

Kohut, H. (1972). Thoughts on narcissism and narcissistic rage. In P. H. Ornstein (Ed.), *The search for the self: Selected writings of Heinz Kohut* (Vol. 2, pp. 615–658). New York: International Universities Press.

Kohut, H. (1984). *The nature of psychoanalytic cure.* Chicago: University of Chicago Press.

Lord, R. P. (1991). Personal perspective. *The Christian Century, 108,* 902–903.

Olio, K. (1992). Recovery from sexual abuse: Is forgiveness mandatory? *Voices, 28,* 73–74.

Patton, J. (1985). *Is human forgiveness possible?: A pastoral care perspective.* Nashville, TN: Abingdon Press.

Readers' response. (1991, November 20–27). *The Christian Century, 108,* 34.

Sanford, D. E. (1986). *I can't talk about it: A child's book about sexual abuse.* Portland, OR: Multnomah.

Simon, S. B., & Simon, S. (1990). *Forgiveness: How to make peace with your past and get on with your life.* New York: Warner Books.

Suchocki, M. H. (1996). Reflections on forgiveness: A transformation. *Dialog, 35,* 95–100.

PART IV

Conclusion

The Frontier of Forgiveness

Seven Directions for Psychological Study and Practice

Kenneth I. Pargament, Michael E. McCullough, and Carl E. Thoresen

Forgiveness is an exciting new frontier for psychological research and practice. Before 1985, only a handful of empirical studies of forgiveness had been conducted (Worthington, 1998). Although scientific interest in this topic has increased sharply over the last 14 years, questions about forgiveness continue to outnumber answers. Thus, the frontier of forgiveness remains largely unexplored.

In this book we have assembled a set of chapters that advances the study of forgiveness. In this final chapter, we try to crystallize seven of the themes that run throughout these contributions (see Table 14.1). These themes, we believe, can provide guidance and direction to researchers and practitioners who would like to venture further into this new frontier.

FROM DISTANT TO CLOSE-UP: CONDUCTING PROXIMAL STUDIES OF FORGIVENESS

Advances in the study of many phenomena are marked by a progression from the general to the specific. For example, psychotherapy research initially focused on the general question of whether psychotherapy works.

TABLE 14.1. Seven Directions for the Psychological Study and Practice of Forgiveness

1. From distant to close-up: Conducting proximal studies of forgiveness
2. From one to many meanings: Exploring the variety of meanings of forgiveness
3. From isolation to integration: Weaving forgiveness into psychological theory
4. From single to multiple levels of analysis: Drawing on multiple perspectives of forgiveness
5. From the expected to the unexpected: Openness to the downside of forgiveness
6. From conceptualization to research: Expanding the empirical study of forgiveness
7. From intuition to information: Building an empirically informed approach to forgiveness in clinical practice

The form of the question itself suggested that psychotherapy is a uniform process that operates in the same way for different people. With further study, however, what looked to be a uniform process from a distance became sharply differentiated closer at hand (Kiesler, 1966). General questions were not sufficient to the task of understanding the psychotherapy process. "What kind of psychotherapy for what kind of problem works in what kind of way for what kind of person?" became the more refined and more answerable question that continues to drive research on psychotherapy today.

In the forgiveness arena, we are beginning to witness a similar shift from general questions about forgiveness, and its value in life to more specific questions. As we get closer to the process of forgiveness we see the limitations of our current conceptual and methodological tools. We are unlikely to find a simple neuropsychological basis for forgiveness, as Newberg, d'Aquili, Newburg, and deMarici note (Chapter 4, this volume). Single-item self-report measures of forgiveness, the standard in the field for 20 years, cannot capture the ways people experience and express forgiveness (McCullough, Rachal, & Hoyt, Chapter 4, this volume). Simplistic bromides (e.g., turn the other cheek, forgive and forget) can do little to help people struggling with the deeply disturbing feelings and profound questions raised by the encounter with mistreatment and injustice (Patton, Chapter 13, and Thoresen, Harris, & Luskin, Chapter 12, this volume). Uniform forgiveness interventions are not likely to be sensitive or responsive to the needs of different populations that approach forgiveness in disparate ways (Worthington, Sandage, & Berry, Chapter 11, this volume).

Forgiveness is more dimensional and more complex than we initially imagined. And the richness of the phenomena calls for more refined and more varied concepts, measures, methods, and programs. We are beginning to see progress in this direction. McCullough et al. (Chapter 4, this volume), for example, present an elegant method for answering an important question: "What goes into a score on a measure of forgiveness?" Generalizability theory, they assert, can help us determine the degree to which this score is a reflection of characteristics of the victim of the offense, the offender, or the offense itself. Thoresen, Harris, and Luskin (Chapter 12, this volume) detail a number of methods for studying forgiveness that take us beyond our reliance on self-report surveys collected at one point in time, such as structured interviews, narrative analyses, intensive study of individual cases, daily monitoring, and assessments of nonverbal communication. Malcolm and Greenberg (Chapter 9, volume) challenge forgiveness researchers to go beyond the question, "Do forgiveness interventions work?" to the question, "What about forgiveness interventions works?" Their method of task analysis illustrates the value of an intensive "close-up" investigation of the critical ingredients of forgiveness interventions; the method is both clinically rich and empirically valuable.

Future studies are likely to continue in the direction of more proximal investigations of forgiveness that involve more refined questions, concepts, methods, and programs. Does it follow that this field of study will become hopelessly complex? Not necessarily. In some instances, empirical studies may reveal that simpler models do a better job of capturing forgiveness phenomena than more complex ones. In this vein, Mullet and Girard (Chapter 6, this volume) found that a complex interactive model was not needed to account for the propensity to forgive. Instead, the likelihood of forgiving could be best explained by a simple additive combination of several factors, including whether the offender apologized to the victim, the degree of intent behind the offense, the severity of the offense, and whether the victim is still being affected by the consequences of the offense. Nevertheless, we suspect that researchers and practitioners interested in forgiveness will continue to be challenged by the richness and intricacies of this process. Ultimately, we believe, the study of forgiveness will require a level of knowledge, experience, and expertise commensurate to that needed to study other key psychological constructs, such as intelligence, morality, psychopathology, and prejudice.

FROM ONE TO MANY MEANINGS: EXPLORING THE VARIETY OF MEANINGS OF FORGIVENESS

What is forgiveness and what is not forgiveness? "In order to discern any 'thing,' " Zerubavel (1991) writes, "we must distinguish that which we attend from that which we ignore" (p. 1). Entities that are not clearly differentiated from their surroundings, he goes on to note, become almost invisible. There is no shortage of opinions about the meaning of forgiveness. There is, however, a lack of consensus. Although theorists and researchers generally agree about those things forgiveness is not (it is not to be confused with pardoning, condoning, excusing, forgetting, and denying) (Enright & Coyle, 1998), they do not agree about what forgiveness is. Currently, we can identify at least three points of disagreement about the meaning of forgiveness.

Intrapersonal or Interpersonal?

Theorists and researchers have, for the most part, defined forgiveness as an intrapersonal process, something that occurs within a person. That "something" involves a change in cognitions, behaviors, emotions, and/or motivations that can unfold even if the individual is no longer engaged in a relationship with the offender, even if the offender is no longer alive. Research based on this perspective has been largely "victim-centered," focusing on predictors of forgiveness, the process through which victims forgive, and the consequences of forgiveness for the victim.

In contrast, others conceptualize forgiveness as an interpersonal process (e.g., Exline & Baumeister, Chapter 7, and Gordon, Baucom, & Snyder, Chapter 10, this volume). For example, Exline and Baumeister note that transgressions often involve people who are well-acquainted with each other (e.g., family, friends, coworkers, romantic partners). It is critical, they believe, to understand forgiveness in the context of ongoing relationships. "How do people *behave* toward one another after incidents of transgression," they ask, "and what are the sources and consequences of their choices" (p. 210)? From this perspective, the relationship rather than the victim is the appropriate unit of analysis for studies of forgiveness. How offenders affect victims, how victims affect offenders, and how each partner contributes to the character of their relationship (i.e., forgiveness transactions, Worthington et al., Chapter 11, this volume) are all important objects of study from an interpersonal point of view.

Letting Go of the Negative or Embracing the Positive?

Several writers define forgiveness as a process involving a decrease in negative thoughts, feelings, and actions toward the offender (Gordon et al., Chapter 10, Temoshok & Chandra, Chapter 3, and Thoresen et al., Chapter 12, this volume). For example, Gordon et al. conclude from their review that forgiveness involves "(1) regaining a more balanced view of the offender and the event, (2) decreasing negative affect toward the offender, and (3) giving up the right to punish the offender further" (p. 360). They make a sharp distinction between "letting go of bitterness and anger" and reconciliation with the individual who committed the offense (p. 376), noting that one can forgive without reconciliation.

Others, however, maintain that forgiveness involves more than the release of the negative; expressions of positive feelings, thoughts, and behaviors to the offender are essential elements of forgiveness. North (1987), for example, writes that the forgiving individual can "view the wrongdoer with compassion, benevolence, and love while recognizing that he has willfully abandoned his right to them" (p. 502). Similarly, Enright and Coyle (1998) believe genuine forgiveness takes place when "one who has suffered an unjust injury chooses to abandon his or her right to resentment and retaliation, and instead offers mercy to the offender" (p. 140). The line between forgiveness and reconciliation can become less clear in these definitions. Worthington et al. (Chapter 11, this volume) explicitly incorporate reconciliation into their definition of forgiveness, with some caveats. "[Forgiveness is] a motivation to reduce avoidance of and retaliation (or revenge) against a person who has harmed or offended one, and to increase conciliation between the parties if conciliation is safe, prudent, or possible" (pp. 384–385). Those who define forgiveness in terms of expressions of positive thoughts, feelings, and actions toward the offender will likely measure forgiveness, teach forgiveness, and evaluate the efficacy of forgiveness interventions quite differently than those who define forgiveness as a "letting go" of the negative.

Ordinary or Extraordinary?

To what extent is forgiveness an extraordinary event, a less-than-commonplace process that involves a fundamental metamorphosis in living? Theorists have generally defined forgiveness as a profound life change. To put it another way, they describe a forgiveness with a capital "F." According to Pargament (1997), for example, forgiveness is a process of re-creation, a transformational method of coping, often religious in nature, that involves a basic shift in destinations and pathways in living. Through this process, the individual departs from a life centered around pain and injustice and begins to pursue a dream of peace. Toward this end, the person starts to think, feel, and act in very different ways about him- or herself, the offender, and the world more generally. Other writers also speak of forgiveness in terms of violations of basic beliefs, fundamental changes in assumptive worlds, large-scale changes in understandings and actions, motivational transformations, and part of a larger process of living (see Gordon et al., Chapter 10, Malcolm & Greenberg, Chapter 9, and Patton, Chapter 13, this volume; McCullough, Sandage, & Worthington, 1997).

It is important to note that theorists who define forgiveness with a capital "F" have often focused on victims who have experienced especially powerful violation, mistreatment, and injustice at the hands of others (e.g., incest, rape, Holocaust, marital infidelity). To respond to such massive assaults with forgiveness may, in fact, require a profound change in living. However, interpersonal hurts vary in magnitude. The disappointments and transgressions that take place between friends, family, romantic partners, and coworkers are certainly more commonplace and may elicit a form of forgiveness that is less rare and less profound. This is forgiveness with a lowercase "f," the kind that may be captured by developmental and sociopsychological studies of people who transgress, apologize, confess, repent, and forgive in the course of daily experience (see Exline & Baumeister, Chapter 7, and Mullet & Girard, Chapter 6, this volume).

What is the relationship between forgiveness with a capital "F" and lowercase "f"? The two may be qualitatively different phenomena. In recent years, researchers have suggested that there may be fundamental differences between the kind of depression captured by self-report instruments of depressive mood (e.g., Beck Depression Inventory) and the kind of depression captured by a clinical assessment and diagnosis of major depressive disorder (e.g., Coyne, 1994). Thus, it might be inappropriate and empirically unjustifiable to think of negative mood as an analog of major depression. Similarly, there may be important structural and functional distinctions between extraordinary and ordinary forms of forgiveness. Considering one to be an analog for the other might be, simply put, incorrect. On the other hand, the two types of forgiveness may be closely related to each other. In fact, they may lead into each other. The individual who has experienced the extraordinary form of "Forgiveness" may be more likely to respond to more commonplace insults and injuries with forgiveness in its ordinary form (Pargament, 1997). Conversely, experience and practice with ordinary forms of forgiveness in response to minor insults and injuries may set the stage for the profoundly re-creative expressions of "Forgiveness" in response to major life traumas.

Whether forgiveness with a capital "F" and lowercase "f" are the same is an empirical question that requires further study. Nevertheless, these differences in the meanings of forgiveness are not necessarily problematic in this early stage of study. They may, in fact, contribute to a more fully dimensional picture of forgiveness. To avoid confusion, however, researchers, theorists, and practitioners will need to be quite explicit about the definitions that guide their work and the phenomena of interest that fall within and outside of the boundaries of the forgiveness construct. Ultimately, however, a more complete understanding of forgiveness will require better integration of these various perspectives under one definitional umbrella.

Towards this end, we defined forgiveness in the introductory chapter of this book as "intraindividual, prosocial change toward a perceived transgressor that is situated within an interpersonal context" (McCullough, Pargament, & Thoresen, Chapter 1, this volume, p. 12). In light of the subsequent chapters, we (immodestly) believe that our definition held up well. It cuts to the core of the construct that attracts the attention and interest of a diverse group of researchers and practitioners, yet it retains the breadth and flexibility necessary to capture forgiveness in its varied forms. Our definition allows for the study of forgiveness as both an intraindividual and an interpersonal process, as a process of change that covers the full range of potential response to an offender (from letting go of the negative to expressions of the positive), and as a phenomenon that can be extraordinary for some and ordinary for others. Will other researchers find this definition useful? That remains to be seen. However, what we are interested in is definitional progress, so we welcome responses to our proposal.

FROM ISOLATION TO INTEGRATION: WEAVING FORGIVENESS INTO PSYCHOLOGICAL THEORY

The meaning of forgiveness and its implications for personal and social functioning can also be sharpened by integrating the construct into well-established theoretical and conceptual frameworks. The benefits of this theoretical integration are twofold. First, connecting forgiveness to other psychosocial phenomena that have already received theoretical attention and empirical validation may shed important new light on forgiveness, reducing the "fuzziness" of this construct (Gordon et al., Chapter 10, this volume). Second, forgiveness can, in turn, add richness and dimension to existing theories that have neglected this important process. These points have been illustrated by Robert Enright and his colleagues (e.g., Enright and the Human Development Study Group, 1991). Their integration of forgiveness within theories of moral and cognitive development has helped both to penetrate the process of forgiveness and to elaborate on the nature of morality. Elsewhere, we have suggested other potentially valuable theories and conceptual frameworks for the study of forgiveness, including social cognitive theory (Thoresen, Luskin, & Harris, 1998), theoretical work on altruism (McCullough, Rachal, Sandage, Worthington, Brown, & Hight, 1998; McCullough, Worthington, & Rachal, 1997), and coping theory (Pargament, 1997). Unfortunately, this kind of work has been an exception to the rule. Prominent theorists have either ignored or made only brief mention of forgiveness, and much of the research on this topic has been atheoretical (McCullough et al., Chapter 1, this volume). In the future, researchers will need to extend existing theories to incorporate the process of forgiveness.

   In this book, we have presented for the study of forgiveness a number of theoretical frameworks and perspectives drawn from virtually every major subdiscipline of psychology: developmental, social, health,

cognitive, cross-cultural, personality, pastoral, clinical, community, physiological, and evolutionary. We highlight just a few of these promising
frameworks.

The Forgiving Personality

Emmons (Chapter 8, this volume) makes some exciting links between forgiveness and an extensive literature on other personality traits, including
narcissism, empathy, and Type A behavior (see also Thoresen et al., Chapter 12, this volume). The sense of entitlement, grandiosity, self-admiration,
hypersensitivity to criticism, and lack of empathy that define the narcissistic personality likely inhibit forgiveness. Forgiveness itself, Emmons suggests, may be a higher order personality construct defined by a number of
special qualities: sensitivity to anger-mitigating circumstances, emotion-
management skills, empathy, humility, gratitude, and the desire to be in
harmonious relationships. The relationship of the forgiveness "trait" to
other traits, such as the five-factor model, or forgiveness "stories" to other
personality narratives (cf. McAdams, 1993), brings up important questions for personality research.

Confession and Forgiveness

Working from an interpersonal perspective, Exline and Baumeister
(Chapter 7, this volume) point to the close link between repentance on
the part of the offender and forgiveness by the victim. Empirical studies
indicate that a lack of repentance discourages forgiveness and repentant
acts promote it. Is the reverse true? Exline and Baumeister raise the critical and, as yet, unanswered, question: "Might expressions of forgiveness
also promote repentance" (p. 214)? Their interpersonal orientation also
brings with it several relevant theoretical and empirical literatures (e.g.,
guilt, confession, self-serving perceptions of events). For instance, recent
studies on the physical and psychological benefits of emotional self-disclosure have important implications for our understanding of repentance
and expressions of forgiveness.

Marriage and Forgiveness

Marriages are natural laboratories for studying the process of forgiveness
within the context of intense, ongoing relationships. Gordon et al. (Chapter 10, this volume) bring two theoretical frameworks to bear on the topic
of forgiveness within marriage. Drawing from cognitive-behavioral theory,
they describe betrayal within marriage as a violation of one critical part of
the victim's assumptive world, the "view that marriage is a place where
one can feel safe, secure, and put total trust in another person" (p. 350).

The violation can elicit a traumatic response that bears many similarities to posttraumatic stress disorder, including flashbacks triggered by cues that remind the individual of the betrayal. Drawing from insight-oriented theory, Gordon et al. describe how betrayal may grow out of a long-term history of violations of trust in the family. The individual who feels he or she has been betrayed in a prior relationship develops a destructive sense of entitlement, one that serves as a justification for the mistreatment of others. The victim's history of trust and betrayal in earlier relationships is also likely to impact on his or her ability to forgive within marriage. These theoretical perspectives have important implications for conceptualizing and treating marital transgressions, as Gordon et al. illustrate in their three-stage model of forgiveness in marriage.

Forgiveness over the Life Span

Developmental theories of cognition, morality, and personality often focus much of their attention on the early years of life, starting with infancy and ending in late adolescence. Forgiveness, however, is a process that seems to call for higher levels of personal and social maturity; to understand this process more fully requires a life-span developmental perspective. In support of this point, Mullet and Girard (Chapter 6, this volume) cite data that showed the elderly to be more likely to forgive others for transgressions than adolescents, young, and middle-aged adults. Furthermore, the willingness of the elderly to forgive was less dependent on circumstances than was the case for adolescents and younger adults. Thus, the frequency of forgiveness and quality of forgiveness itself may change at different points in the life cycle. Mullet and Girard's work underscores the significance of theory and research that captures the ways forgiveness evolves over the entire course of life.

Forgiveness and Spirituality

In his chapter on forgiveness in pastoral care and counseling, Patton (Chapter 13, this volume) makes a critical point: Forgiveness is best understood as "a part of a larger process of living" (p. 496). In fact, pastoral care for people who have suffered injuries at the hands of others involves a broadening of the individuals' concerns from a narrow focus on the injury and the offender to an enlarged "frame of their life picture." Forgiveness, Patton feels, is one element in the greater process of dealing with "a shamed and estranged self" and an ability "to recognize the humanness of one's injurer as well as discovering one's own" (p. 478). And, it is important to add, the kind of forgiveness Patton describes is not a secular process; it is profoundly spiritual, "an illustration of a quality of life when it is lived in relation to God and one's fellow human beings" (p. 497). Thus,

Patton reminds us that forgiveness should be viewed not in isolation, but as part of the entire tapestry of an individual's life.

In the chapters of this book, we see a number of exciting opportunities to weave forgiveness into the cloth of other theories and perspectives. In the process of integration, we may elucidate the character of forgiveness and enrich theories that have, until recently, overlooked this dimension of life.

FROM SINGLE TO MULTIPLE LEVELS OF ANALYSIS: DRAWING ON MULTIPLE PERSPECTIVES OF FORGIVENESS

As noted earlier, much of the study of forgiveness (like much of psychology as a field) has focused on the individual level of analysis (McCullough, Rachal, & Hoyt, Chapter 4, this volume). This body of work may leave the impression that forgiveness occurs within a self-contained individual operating in a social and cultural vacuum. Forgiveness, however, is a multilevel phenomenon, one that needs to be understood at biological, psychological, marital, familial, community, and cultural levels of analysis. Indeed, explanations that cross levels of analysis might be our best hope for rendering scientific facts about forgiveness "consilient" (see Wilson, 1998). It would be a mistake to assume that we can apply knowledge from one of these levels of analysis directly to another. Watzlawick (1988) describes the unfortunate consequences of this process, what he calls "errors of logical typing." For example, when the National Aeronautic and Space Agency needed to build a hangar to protect their larger space rockets from the weather, they simply magnified their old hangar design 10 times. They overlooked the fact that a hangar this size creates its own climate, complete with clouds, rain, and dangerous electricity (precisely the problem the larger hangar was designed to prevent)!

Similarly, we cannot assume that conceptualizations of forgiveness as a personality trait directly apply to the ways forgiveness unfolds in marital or familial relationship. Neither can we assume that our knowledge of forgiveness within marital and familiar relationships translates directly into the forgiveness that expresses itself in response to community or cultural conflicts. As McCullough et al. (Chapter 4, this volume) emphasize, researchers must be careful to select concepts, methods, and measures of forgiveness that are tailored to the appropriate level of specificity and analysis. Temoshok and Chandra (Chapter 3, this volume) note that there is a dearth of theory and research on the nature of forgiveness at the community and cultural levels. Unfortunately, however, there is no shortage of deep-seated social and political conflict, mistrust, and hatred that represent powerful naturalistic laboratories for the study of forgiveness.

Cross-level analyses represent another frontier for forgiveness research. Considerable work, for example, is needed to understand the social context and the way it shapes and is shaped by the experience of individual forgiveness. The social context may affect the very meaning of this construct. In the chapter by Rye et al. (Chapter 2, this volume), we learned that Hinduism, Buddhism, Judaism, Islam, and Christianity offer different definitions of forgiveness to their members. The social context may also support or discourage the expression of forgiveness. Patton (Chapter 13, this volume) notes that forgiveness develops in a social and spiritual community that supports and encourages it. Along similar lines, Thoresen et al. (Chapter 12, this volume) suggest that the participation of the spouse of the client in forgiveness interventions may facilitate the treatment process. On the other hand, some social contexts may erect special challenges to forgiveness. This appears to be the case in India, where many women are doubly victimized: first, by HIV infection through a spouse or partner and, second, by culturally supported stigma, discrimination, and isolation in response to their infection (see Temoshok & Chandra, Chapter 3, this volume). The prevailing "culture of narcissism" in Western society may represent our own particular social barrier to forgiveness (Emmons, Chapter 8, this volume).

Finally, it is important to consider the impact of forgiveness by an individual on the social context. Most studies have considered the effect of forgiveness on the individual's own mental health. Far less is known about the ways forgiveness affects the individual's social system. And yet the effects of forgiveness might conceivably ripple out toward others, including not only the offender but family, friends, coworkers, and the larger community. For example, the ex-wife who succeeds in forgiving her former husband may achieve greater peace of mind and emotional well-being not only for herself but for her children and next spouse as well. Conversely, in their study of Indian men and women infected with HIV, Temoshok and Chandra (Chapter 3, this volume) found that unforgiving attitudes were tied to persistence in risky sexual behaviors that increase the risk of further transmission. In their chapter, Newberg et al. (Chapter 5, this volume) suggest that forgiveness reduces bellicosity and elicits empathy for the person by his or her social network. They go even further, noting that by breaking the cycle of aggression and revenge, forgiveness may hold distinctive evolutionary advantages for humankind.

In summary, multilevel analyses are necessary to develop a more complete appreciation of forgiveness. Forgiveness should be understood as a phenomenon that is expressed at biological, psychological, marital, familial, community, and cultural levels (see Temoshok & Chandra, Chapter 3, this volume). Cross-level studies are also needed to understand how forgiveness at one level is shaped by forces from other levels, and how forgiveness at one level, in turn, impacts on other levels of human functioning. Toward these ends, forgiveness researchers should try to include a broader array of predictors and criteria in their studies. To reiterate an earlier theme, multiple measures are needed to assess the multilevel character of forgiveness and its correlates.

FROM THE EXPECTED TO THE UNEXPECTED
OPENNESS TO THE DOWNSIDE OF FORGIVENESS

Researchers and therapists have, for the most part, viewed forgiveness as a constructive, healthy process. A number of studies have indeed shown forgiveness to be associated with decreases in emotional distress and increases in personal well-being. However, research in this area is still developing and it is premature to conclude at this point that forgiveness is invariably helpful. Like most psychological processes, forgiveness may have a downside.

A few researchers have suggested that forgiveness in its more superficial or less-than-genuine forms has detrimental consequences. For instance, Trainer (1981) articulated different motivations for forgiveness and found that each had a distinctive set of correlates. A forgiveness that was used as a weapon of vengeance against others or to make the forgiver feel morally superior to others was associated with more negative emotions and attitudes; in contrast, a forgiveness offered because of its intrinsic value was tied to more positive emotions and attitudes. Similarly, Patton (Chapter 13, this volume) warns against the destructive effects of a social system that pressures people (who have already suffered a loss of control through their victimization) to forgive. It is important to note that Patton includes mental health professionals as well as pastors, family, friends, and God in this potentially coercive social system.

Exline and Baumeister (Chapter 7, this volume) propose some potential costs to more genuine forms of forgiveness. Perhaps forgiveness results in feelings of weakness and vulnerability on the part of the forgiver. Perhaps the forgiver is left with feelings of unfairness and injustice. Perhaps the forgiver loses the benefits of "victim status" in relationships with others. And perhaps forgiveness places the forgiver at greater risk of future harm. Katz, Street, and Arias (1997) conducted a study that hinted at this latter danger. Undergraduate women responded to a series of hypothetical episodes of relationship violence by their dating partners. Intentions to forgive the partner, they found, mediated the relationship between self-attributions and intentions to end the relationship. Specifically, students who were more likely to attribute the cause of the violence to themselves were also more likely to forgive their partner. Forgiving the partner, in turn, was associated with less likelihood of leaving the violent relationship. Of course, this study focused only on hypothetical scenarios. Yet it raises the disturbing possibility that forgiveness may increase the risk of remaining in potentially destructive relationships.

Unfortunately, there is very little research, experimental or naturalistic, on this and other potential costs to forgiveness. Further research is clearly needed. Studies of the impact of forgiveness on offenders are especially important and may help to answer some critical questions. Does forgiveness promote growth in the offender, constructive problem resolution and closer emotional connectedness between the forgiver and the offender? Or does it, in essence, "reward" the offender for his or her behavior, thereby perpetuating or exacerbating a destructive pattern of interrelationship?

Answers to questions such as these may not necessarily be simple. Forgiveness may be beneficial at certain times, in certain situations, for certain people, and irrelevant or even harmful in others. On this note, McCullough and Worthington (1994) caution against forgiveness when the perpetrator has not shown remorse, when the violation is too severe, or when the wounds from the offense are too fresh. Using a wider range of criterion measures, as Worthington et al. (Chapter 11, this volume) suggest, may reveal both costs and benefits of forgiveness. Perhaps forgiveness, in some situations, reduces psychological distress and increases the risk of future interpersonal violations. Conversely, forgiveness, at times, might reduce relational conflicts at the cost of psychological well-being.

Finally, researchers should be open to the potential benefits of the "flip-side" of forgiveness; namely, the experience of anger and pain. Several theorists, in fact, argue that without an appreciation for the nature of the offense and the pain it has caused, forgiveness can never be complete. As Patton (Chapter 13, this volume) puts it, the path to forgiveness and health is "through pain, not around it" (p. 495). Thoresen et al. (Chapter 12, this volume) add that it is important to distinguish constructive from destructive forms of anger expression. After all, some people are able to express their anger through constructive channels that rectify social injustices and provide meaning and purpose to their lives (Baures, 1996). The health risks of anger, Patton suggests, may lie not in the immediate physiological reactivity that accompanies the emotion, but rather in the failure to reach an emotional resolution in a reasonable period of time.

In summary, researchers and practitioners should maintain an openness to the unexpected, to the possibility that forgiveness may have some surprising consequences for the individual, the offender, and the larger social system. In particular, we should keep an eye open to the possibility of costs as well as benefits to forgiveness. As important and potentially valuable as forgiveness may be, it is not likely to be a panacea to the complex problems that arise out of interpersonal violations.

FROM CONCEPTUALIZATION TO RESEARCH: EXPANDING THE EMPIRICAL STUDY OF FORGIVENESS

There is no shortage of ideas or opinions about forgiveness, its value, and its effects. Empirical studies, however, have been in short supply. Fortunately, the picture may be beginning to change. There are signs of an expanding scientific study of forgiveness. The authors of the chapters in this volume have pointed to a number of important future research directions. We have highlighted several of these questions in this chapter, and summarized many of them in Table 14.2.

Some of the questions are very basic. For instance, as yet, we do not know how commonplace forgiveness is. Augsberger (1981) has said that forgiveness is one of the hardest things in the world to do. Some initial findings suggest that many people do, in fact, have difficulty forgiving. Recall that in Temoshok and Chandra's (Chapter 3, this volume) study of Indian men and women infected with HIV, 67% of their family members blamed them for their condition, and 45% reported that they would never be able to forgive them. As one father whose son died of AIDS at age 26 said: "He should not have been born into our family, and I can never forgive him for what he did to us. We did not perform any funeral rites for him, and we feel he should suffer the way he has made us all suffer" (pp. 70–71). On the other hand, a few other studies suggest that forgiveness may not be unusual. For instance, in a study of people from three Lebanese religious communities (Catholic, Maronites, and Orthodox), higher than expected levels of forgiveness were reported in response to vignettes describing the shooting of a child during the Lebanese Civil War (Azar, Mullet, & Vinsonneau, 1999). Many people extended the willingness to forgive to members of other religious communities on opposing sides of the civil war. In short, basic data are needed that describe the frequency of forgiveness across time, place, and person.

Some of the important questions for future research are exploratory. For example, a number of authors in this volume suggested that the construct of shame may be central to any understanding of forgiveness. They argue that a sense of personal unworthiness, dirtiness, sinfulness, and even responsibility lie at the heart of the response to interpersonal violations. For instance, Malcolm and Greenberg (Chapter, this volume) describe one client who is particularly moved by a role play of his mother in which the mother says: "And I don't want you to feel guilty. You didn't cause it. . . . This is not about you. It's about my life. It's about me being

TABLE 14.2. Critical Questions for Research on Forgiveness

- How commonplace is forgiveness?
- What roles does shame play in the forgiveness process?
- To what extent do members of different cultural, religious, and ethnic groups define forgiveness in different ways?
- What are the most powerful predictors of forgiveness?
- How do early childhood experiences affect the development of forgiveness?
- What is the relationship of forgiveness to physical health?
- Can people be trained to forgive through brief therapy?
- What impact does forgiveness have on the perpetrator and the likelihood of future offenses?
- What impact does forgiveness have on the individual's larger social network?
- How do various motivations for forgiveness affect the outcomes of forgiveness?
- What makes forgiveness interventions work?
- What impact does forgiveness have on the behavior of the forgiving person toward others?
- What is the empirical relationship between forgiveness and reconciliation?
- What is the relationship between forgiveness as a personality trait and other models of personality?
- What is the relationship between an individual's history in prior relationships and forgiveness within marriage?
- How does forgiveness evolve and change over the life span?
- What are the potential personal and social costs of forgiveness?
- What is the relationship between the values of forgiveness and social justice?
- When should forgiveness not be encouraged in a clinical context?
- How do we determine an individual's readiness to forgive?
- What personal, social, and culture variables promote and impede forgiveness?
- What factors are associated with forgiveness by larger social systems, such as nations, communities, and religious groups?
- To what extent and in what ways should forgiveness interventions be tailored to particular groups?

out of control. I take responsibility for what I did. . . . I was out of control" (p. 317). Overwhelmed by the sense of shame, people may respond with a range of defenses, from rage to arrogance to the search for perfection. The central problem here, Patton (Chapter 13, this volume) notes, is the failure to see the offender as an independent person; the offender instead becomes "an offending part of the shamed person's self" (p. 486). Through empathy and participation in a community, the individual can experience a healing of the self and a new capacity to see the offender as a separate human being struggling with his or her own problems in living.

Ultimately, forgiveness may grow out of this process of personal healing. These are, we believe, potent but untested ideas that are well worth exploring though empirical study.

Some future research questions have both theoretical and practical implications. One such intriguing question has to do with differences in the ways members of different cultural, ethnic, and religious groups may define forgiveness. As noted earlier, theorists and researchers have defined forgiveness in a variety of ways. The same point is likely to apply to those we study. Forgiveness may mean different things to members of different groups. For example, although the world's major religions place a value on forgiveness, they do not define forgiveness identically. Rye and his coauthors (Chapter 2, this volume) find a number of distinctions in the ways Hindu, Buddhist, Jewish, Christian, and Muslim scholars conceptualize forgiveness. Within Judaism, forgiveness is conceptualized as an interpersonal process, one that involves repentance on the part of the offender, followed by forgiveness on the part of the victim. Within Christianity, forgiveness is described as a more intrapersonal process, one less dependent on the attitudes and actions of the offender. While forgiveness is described as a "letting go" of the negative within Hinduism (Temoshok & Chandra, Chapter 3, this volume), Christianity describes forgiveness in terms of positive expressions of love, compassion, and mercy. Furthermore, the line between forgiveness and reconciliation appears to be more sharply drawn within Judaism and Islam than within Christianity, Buddhism, and Hinduism. To the student of comparative religion, these differences are interesting in and of themselves. From a psychological perspective though, the key question is whether the differences in the belief systems of these traditions translate into differences among their adherents. Do Christians, Jews, Buddhists, Hindus, and Muslims, in fact, define forgiveness differently? To what extent do members of these traditions incorporate and adhere to the teachings of their religions with respect to forgiveness?

It is important to understand the meanings of forgiveness to those we study and work with, including members of diverse religious, ethnic, and cultural groups. Lens model studies have been useful in learning about differences in the meanings of other complex constructs, such as religion and spirituality (e.g., Pargament, Sullivan, Balzer, Van Haitsma, & Raymark, 1995; Zinnbauer, 1997). They may also be helpful in learning about the meanings people attribute to forgiveness (e.g., Boon & Sulsky, 1997). On a more practical note, differences in meanings of forgiveness are also important to consider in efforts to promote forgiveness. Groups that define, experience, and express forgiveness in special ways may require different types of forgiveness interventions. In this vein, Worthington et al. (Chapter 11, this volume) solicit definitions of forgiveness in the early phases of their groups and use them as a starting point for intervention.

FROM INTUITION TO INFORMATION: BUILDING AN EMPIRICALLY INFORMED APPROACH TO FORGIVENESS IN CLINICAL PRACTICE

Opportunities abound for practitioners interested in addressing forgiveness in their clinical work. It is not difficult to generate a variety of potential targets for a forgiveness-oriented psychotherapy: to name a few, victims of crime, persons facing major illnesses and disability (e.g., HIV/AIDS), adult children of alcoholics, abused spouses, couples struggling with marital infidelity, combat veterans, divorced individuals, survivors of suicide, prison inmates, and people at the end of their lives. Psychotherapy with a forgiveness focus can also be targeted to individuals, couples, families, or groups. For example, Thoresen et al. (1998) cite the potential of structured, small-group, forgiveness-oriented therapy for a variety of populations.

Forgiveness-related interventions need not be limited to psychotherapy. Education for forgiveness has the potential to prevent or mitigate some of the long-term pain that follows a trauma. Forgiveness could become a topic of discussion, if not training, in primary, secondary, and higher education within secular as well as religious institutional settings. More focused educational programs could target groups that are especially likely to benefit from information about forgiveness, such as "bullies" and violent teens, couples entering marriage, workers in job training, couples preparing to become foster parents, and human service professionals. And forgiveness can be conceptualized as a sociopolitical intervention that may be applied to larger scale conflicts between tribes (e.g., Hutus and Tutsis in Rwanda), religious groups (e.g., Protestant and Roman Catholics in Ireland), racial groups (e.g., whites and blacks in South Africa), and nations (e.g., Bosnia, Serbia, and Albania).

In short, opportunities for forgiveness-related work are plentiful. Information to guide these efforts, however, is in shorter supply. Until recently, practitioners have had to work largely from intuition in their efforts to understand, evaluate, and intervene in this process in the context of clinical practice. Recently, several theorists have proposed promising theoretically based models to guide forgiveness interventions (e.g., Enright & Coyle, 1998; Gordon et al., Chapter 10, this volume; Worthington, 1998). An expanded scientific study of forgiveness, however, would advance the practice of forgiveness further by integrating models such as these with the knowledge gained by empirical evaluations.

Initial evaluations of forgiveness interventions have, in fact, yielded promising results (e.g., Freedman & Enright, 1995; Coyle & Enright, 1997; McCullough & Worthington, 1995; Thoresen et al., 1998). As several authors in this volume have pointed out, though, we need to take the next step in the scientific study of forgiveness and identify the "active ingredients" of these interventions (Malcolm & Greenberg, Chapter 9,

Thoresen et al., Chapter 12, and Worthington et al., Chapter 11, this volume). Can forgiveness occur without full appreciation of the enormity of the offense? How critical is empathy to forgiveness? Are issues of shame central to the resolution of long-standing resentments? Is insight into early relational and developmental impediments to forgiveness necessary for forgiveness to unfold? Is education in the forgiveness process itself necessary for forgiveness to occur? What types of motivational appeals (e.g., egoistic, altruistic, spiritual) are most effective in promoting forgiveness? What role does the individual's social context, including ethnicity, play in encouraging or discouraging forgiveness? And do forgiveness-oriented interventions produce effects equal to or exceeding those of bona fide treatments?

Answers to questions such as these will not come from a single study, but rather from a program of research of the kind described by Thoresen et al. (Chapter 12, this volume) and Worthington et al. (Chapter 11, this volume). Malcolm and Greenberg's (Chapter 9, this volume) task-analytic approach to therapy dealing with unfinished business seems particularly appropriate in this regard, for it offers a compelling method for identifying the most critical elements of forgiveness interventions.

We hope this program of research and others as well (e.g., Thoresen et al., 1998) will lead to an empirically informed approach to forgiveness in clinical practice, one that will be theoretically eclectic, relatively efficient, and maximally effective in promoting change. Of course, it is unlikely that any one approach will be applicable to all groups. When it comes to efforts to promote forgiveness, one size may not fit all. As Worthington et al. (Chapter 11, this volume) notes, forgiveness interventions may require "tailoring" to different groups with different needs and different norms.

Finally, it will be important to compare the effects of forgiveness-oriented interventions with those of well-established psychological treatments. In a recent meta-analysis by Wampold et al. (1997), the efficacy of bona fide psychological therapies was found to be roughly equivalent across a spectrum of psychological difficulties. Perhaps forgiveness interventions can demonstrate added value above and beyond current approaches to treatment. Would, for example, forgiveness interventions add to the effectiveness of established treatment programs for clinical depression or marital distress? At the very least, advocates for forgiveness treatments will have to show that such treatments are at least as helpful as existing psychological interventions.

We should not conclude this section before underscoring Patton's (Chapter 13, this volume) caveat. He warns against treating forgiveness as a "technique." To define forgiveness as a "skill" that can be "taught" to "clients or patients" by educators, therapists, health professionals, or pastors, without appreciation for its larger spiritual character, he cautions, may be, at best, ineffectual and, even worse, counterproductive. Forgiveness, he asserts, is more craft than science. In comments reminiscent of Viktor Frankl's (1984) seminal work on the search for meaning, Patton suggests that forgiveness is something that cannot be pursued directly but must be approached obliquely. It is part of an orientation to the world in which people see themselves as finite, limited beings, living in less-than-perfect relationships with other limited beings. In this sense, forgiveness is not a way to get healthy; it is a way of life.

How can researchers apply their scientific methods to this topic in ways that capture the richness and complexity of one of the most essentially human of all psychological processes? How can practitioners apply the knowledge gleaned from the scientific study of forgiveness in ways that reflect a respect for the essential humanity of those they try to touch? These are, perhaps, the greatest challenges of all for researchers and practitioners.

CONCLUSIONS

We would like to conclude with one final word of advice for individuals interested in studying forgiveness. Many people have deep-seated convictions about this topic. Very few people are neutral when it comes to forgiveness. This point applies as much to researchers and practitioners as it does to the people they study and serve. Those who enter this field of study would do well to assess their own attitudes and values toward this construct before they take it on. Forgiveness cannot be studied with dispassion and complete objectivity. It can, however, be studied fairly if we are willing to recognize our biases and our values, if we are willing to put them to test, and if we are willing to be surprised and learn from whatever the world has to teach us about this enigmatic yet utterly human process.

Our contributors have covered a lot of territory in this book. Nevertheless, as we noted earlier, the frontier of forgiveness remains largely unexplored. The frontier is also vast, spanning the physical, the psychological, the social, and the cultural world. The frontier is now drawing explorers from a variety of occupational "shores": social workers, psychologists, theologians, philosophers, clergy, physicians, nurses, and social scientists. This is an exceptionally challenging frontier, filled with thickets, swamps, pitfalls, and surprises. To negotiate this difficult terrain, the adventurer needs to come equipped with the full range of theoretical, methodological, and practical tools. And yet, despite the difficulties, the explorer who enters this frontier is likely to encounter some of the most striking vistas that can be found in the human landscape.

318CONCLUSION

REFERENCES

Augsberger, D. (1981). *Caring enough to forgive: Caring enough not to forgive.* Scottsdale, PA: Herald Press.

Azar, F., Mullet, E., & Vinsonneau, G. (1999). The propensity to forgive: Findings from Lebanon. *Journal of Peace Research, 36,* 169–181.

Baures, M. M. (1996). Letting go of bitterness and hate. *Journal of Humanistic Psychology, 36,* 75–90.

Boon, S. D., & Sulsky, L. M. (1997). Attributions of blame and forgiveness in romantic relationships: A policy-capturing study. *Journal of Social Behavior and Personality, 12,* 19–44.

Coyle, C. T., & Enright, R. D. (1997). Forgiveness interventions with post-abortion men. *Journal of Consulting and Clinical Psychology, 65,* 1042–1045.

Coyne, J. C. (1994). Self-reported distress: Analog or ersatz depression? *Psychological Bulletin, 116,* 29–45.

Enright, R. D., & Coyle, C. T. (1998). Researching the process model of forgiveness within psychological interventions. In E. L. Worthington, Jr. (Ed.), *Dimensions of forgiveness: Psychological research and theological perspectives* (pp. 139–161). Philadelphia: Templeton Foundation Press.

Enright, R. D., & the Human Development Study Group. (1991). The moral development of forgiveness. In W. Kurtines & J. Gewirtz (Eds.), *Handbook of moral behavior and development* (Vol. 1, pp. 123–152). Hillsdale, NJ: Erlbaum.

Frankl, V. (1984). *Man's search for meaning.* New York: Washington Square Press.

Freedman, S. R., & Enright, R. D. (1996). Forgiveness as an intervention goal with incest survivors. *Journal of Consulting and Clinical Psychology, 64,* 983–992.

Katz, J., Street, A., & Arias, I. (1997). Individual differences in self-appraisals and responses to dating violence scenarios. *Violence and Victims, 12,* 265–276.

Kiesler, C. (1966). Some myths of psychotherapy research and the search for a paradigm. *Psychological Bulletin, 65,* 110–130.

McAdams, D. (1993). *Stories we live by.* New York: Guilford Press.

McCullough, M. E., Rachal, K. C., Sandage, S. J., Worthington, E. L. Jr., Brown, S. W., & Hight, T. L. (1998). Interpersonal forgiving in close relationships: II. Theoretical elaboration and measurement. *Journal of Personality and Social Psychology, 75,* 1586–1603.

McCullough, M. E., Sandage, S. J., & Worthington, E. L., Jr. (1997). *To forgive is human: How to put your past in the past.* Downers Grove, IL: Intervarsity Press.

McCullough, M. E., & Worthington, E. L., Jr. (1994). Encouraging clients to forgive people who have hurt them: Review, critique, and research prospectus. *Journal of Psychology and Theology, 22,* 3–20.

McCullough, M. E., & Worthington, E. L., Jr. (1995). Promoting forgiveness: A comparison of two brief psychoeducational group interventions with a waiting-list control. *Counseling and Values, 40,* 55–68.

McCullough, M. E., Worthington, E. L., Jr., & Rachal, K. C. (1997). Interpersonal forgiving in close relationships. *Journal of Personality and Social Psychology, 73,* 321–336.

North, J. (1987). Wrongdoing and forgiveness. *Philosophy, 62,* 499–508.

Pargament, K. I. (1997). *The psychology of religion and coping: Theory, research, practice.* New York: Guilford Press.

Pargament, K. I., Sullivan, M. S., Balzer, W. E., Van Haitsma, K. S., & Raymark, P. H. (1995). The many meanings of religiousness: A policy capturing approach. *Journal of Personality, 63,* 953–983.

Thoresen, C. E., Luskin, F. M., & Harris, A. H. S. (1998). The science of forgiveness interventions: Reflections and suggestions. In E. L. Worthington, Jr. (Ed.), *Dimensions of forgiveness: Psychological research and theological perspectives* (pp. 163–192). Philadelphia: Templeton Foundation Press.

Trainer, M. F. (1981). *Forgiveness: Intrinsic, role-expected, expedient, in the context of divorce.* Unpublished doctoral dissertation, Boston University, Boston, MA.

Wampold, B. E., Mondin, G. W., Moody, M., Stich, F., Benson, K., & Hyun-nie, A. (1997). A meta-analysis of outcome studies comparing bona fide psychotherapies: Empirically, "all must have prizes." *Psychological Bulletin, 122,* 203–215.

Watzlawick, P. (1988). *Ultra-solutions or how to fail most successfully.* New York: Norton.

Wilson, E. O. (1998). *Consilience: The unity of knowledge.* New York: Vintage.

Worthington, E. L., Jr. (1998). Introduction. In E. L. Worthington, Jr. (Ed.), *Dimensions of forgiveness: Psychological research and theological perspectives* (pp. 1–8). Philadelphia: Templeton Foundation Press.

Worthington, E. L., Jr. (1998). The pyramid model of forgiveness. In E. L. Worthington, Jr. (Ed.), *Dimensions of forgiveness: Psychological research and theological perspectives* (pp. 107–137). Philadelphia: Templeton Foundation Press.

Zerubavel, E. (1991). *The fine line: Making distinctions in everyday life.* New York: Free Press.

Zinnbauer, B. J. (1997). *Capturing the meanings of religiousness and spirituality: One way down from a definitional tower of Babel.* Unpublished doctoral dissertation, Bowling Green State University, Bowling Green, Ohio.

Author Index

Subject Index